# BIOLOGICAL CONTROL OF PESTS, PATHOGENS AND WEEDS: DEVELOPMENTS AND PROSPECTS

# BIOLOGICAL CONTROL OF PESTS, PATHOGENS AND WEEDS: DEVELOPMENTS AND PROSPECTS

PROCEEDINGS OF
A ROYAL SOCIETY DISCUSSION MEETING
HELD ON 18 AND 19 FEBRUARY 1987

ORGANIZED AND EDITED BY
R. K. S. WOOD, F.R.S., AND M. J. WAY

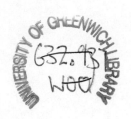

LONDON
THE ROYAL SOCIETY
1988

Printed in Great Britain for the Royal Society
by the
University Press, Cambridge

ISBN 0 85403 347 5

First published in *Philosophical Transactions of the Royal Society of London*,
series B, volume 318 (no. 1189), pages 109–376

**British Library Cataloguing in Publication Data**
Biological control of pests, pathogens and weeds;
  developments and prospects.
  1. Crops.  Pathogens.  Biological control.
  I. Wood, R. K. S. (Ronald Karslake Starr), *1919–*
  II. Way, M. J.   III. Royal Society.
  632

  ISBN 0-85403-347-5 ✓

Published by the Royal Society
6 Carlton House Terrace, London SW1Y 5AG

# PREFACE

Biological control is the use of an important natural process to decrease damage to useful plants caused by pests, mainly insects and nematodes, by pathogens such as fungi, bacteria, viruses and related agents, and by weeds. The term 'biological control' is sometimes used to include almost all methods other than the use of synthetic chemicals to protect plants, in particular control by breeding and selection of resistant plants. But more commonly biological control is regarded as being based on the use of organisms, and agents such as viruses, but not of the useful plant that is to be protected, or of the weed that is to be controlled (Waage & Greathead, this volume). As such, it was the subject of the meeting the proceedings of which are recorded in the pages that follow.

Plant breeding and selection is usually the most favoured method of control and will continue to be used on a large scale in many important crops. But often the level of control attained is inadequate, or can be obtained only at the expense of other more desirable plant characteristics such as yield or quality. In such circumstances the usual alternative has been to apply pesticide chemicals. The scale of such chemical control is indicated by the end-user value of crop protection chemicals of *ca.* U.S.\$12 $\times$ 10$^9$ in 1985 and a forecast of a continuing annual increase of 2–3% (Jutsum, this volume). These figures reflect the success and benefits of chemical control which, no doubt, will continue as the most used and economic method of controlling losses in many circumstances. Nevertheless, despite its success, there are serious problems from dependence on chemical control, particularly if the resistance of pests, pathogens and weeds to pesticides becomes still more prevalent and severe, and because of increasing pressures to decrease greatly the release of chemicals into the environment because of harm they are known or perceived to cause. Biological control is seen as an alternative as well as a method with which chemicals can be integrated, so decreasing the loading of the environment with undesirable chemicals. Its great virtue, like that of host-plant resistance, is that it makes use of the natural mechanisms by which damage to plants by pests and pathogens is kept at the low values usually found in natural populations. Because of its advantages biological control has continued to attract a reasonable share of research and there have been many and striking successes, particularly in the control of some insect pests (Waage & Greathead, this volume). Nevertheless, its overall impact so far on crop production has remained much less than that of the other two methods, partly because there has not been the will or sufficient incentive to develop commercial products or economic practices from promising research results. However, interest in biological control has increased greatly during the past few years, partly for reasons given above and also because developments based on striking advances in biotechnology and in recombinant DNA technology are likely to expand greatly the practicality of large-scale commercial developments. Such current interest made the case for a Discussion Meeting in 1987 and for its proceedings. Our aim was to review the achievements of biological control, to assess its potential for expansion and to provide bases for analyses of the interactions between organisms on which control depends.

We thank the lecturers for agreeing so readily to attend and for contributing so much to the meeting and to this volume; also those who participated in the discussions and the many others who attended. We are much indebted to Miss Christine Johnson for all she did in organizing the meeting, and to Mr Christopher Purdon for his part in publishing these proceedings.

R. K. S. WOOD

M. J. WAY

*December 1987*

# CONTENTS

*Phil. Trans. R. Soc. Lond.* B **318**, 111–128 (1988)

*Printed in Great Britain*

# Biological control: challenges and opportunities

BY J. K. WAAGE AND D. J. GREATHEAD

*C.A.B. International Institute of Biological Control, Silwood Park, Ascot, Berkshire SL5 7PY, U.K.*

Biological control, the use of living organisms as pest control agents, has enjoyed varying popularity over the past century, but today is well established as an important component of integrated pest management. We examine some current challenges to the use of biological control and particularly to classical biological control, the introduction of exotic natural enemies. These include conflicts of interest (1) with the conservation of native species and (2) between agricultural lobbies. On a scientific level, we examine two debates over the ecological and genetic basis of successful control. The challenge of Murdoch *et al.* (*Am. Nat.* **125**, 344–366 (1985)) to the notion of stability in pest populations under biological control, reveals that the stabilizing mechanisms may differ between pest taxa with different patterns of spatial dynamics. With respect to the hypothesis of Hokkanen & Pimentel (*Can. Ent.* **116**, 1109 (1984)) on the better chances of 'new associations' in biological control, we present an analysis that reaches different conclusions. Finally, we discuss future prospects for the different approaches to biological control, and suggest that long-term control methods, such as introduction and inoculation, will be used increasingly in the future.

## INTRODUCTION

The term biological control was first used by Smith (1919) to describe the introduction of exotic insect natural enemies for the permanent suppression of insect pests. It has since been applied, at times, to include virtually all pest control measures except the application of chemical pesticides: plant breeding for resistance to pests, autocidal controls, application of semiochemicals and cultural controls. We prefer to restrict the term to the use of living organisms (natural enemies) as pest control agents. These natural enemies include parasites, parasitoids, predators, antagonists, competitors and phytophages for weed control. The targets include weeds, plant-feeding invertebrates, plant pathogens and disease vectors.

Biological control was first applied, long before its definition, when man began keeping cats to protect stored grain from damage by rodents. All early efforts employed general predators: mongooses, owls, toads, ants and the like. During the 19th century, after microbes were discovered and insect life cycles began to be understood, some (usually unsuccessful) attempts were made by far-sighted scientists to use other kinds of organism (Ordish 1967). However, the spectacularly successful and well publicized introduction of the vedalia beetle, *Rodolia cardinalis*, into California from Australia in 1888 to control the cottony cushion scale, *Icerya purchasi*, is usually taken as the formal beginning of biological control as a recognized discipline (Doutt 1958).

The excitement that was generated stimulated interest in many parts of the world, and ladybirds and other predatory insects were soon being despatched haphazardly from continent to continent, usually to no avail (Lounsbury 1940). It was not long before an insect parasitoid was successfully introduced, in 1906, from the U.S.A. into Italy for control of the mulberry

8-2

scale, *Pseudaulacaspis pentagona*, (Berlese 1915). However, the poor success rate during this period led to the realization that a more scientific approach was needed, and it stimulated study of the taxonomy, ecology and, above all, population dynamics of insect natural enemies. The lead in systematic foreign exploration was taken by the United States Department of Agriculture which set up a laboratory in France for the study of the natural enemies of the gypsy moth, *Lymantria dispar*. The report on this work (Howard & Fiske 1911) began the study of insect population dynamics, which was taken up by W. R. Thompson, F.R.S., who in 1928 became superintendent of the Farnham House Laboratory, which became the C.A.B. International Institute of Biological Control (Thompson 1930).

Biological control thrived in the absence of effective alternatives, until World War II put an end to foreign exploration in Europe, followed by the advent of powerful synthetic organic insecticides. However, the limitations of these new chemicals soon became apparent as insects developed resistance. Later, the adverse effects of persistent organochlorine chemicals on the environment were exposed (Carson 1962) and the cost of pesticides rose sharply after the oil crisis of 1973. These and other factors resulted in a return to a more rational approach to pest control, exemplified by the integrated pest management concept, and led to the resurgence of interest in biological control. The fluctuating course of interest in biological control is well reflected in the pattern of scientific publications on the subject over the past 60 years (Commonwealth Institute of Biological Control (CIBC) 1981).

Today, biological control is seen to comprise several techniques. The 'introduction' of exotic agents for long-term depression and regulation of pest populations is often now called 'classical biological control'. 'Inoculation' is a similar strategy, involving the periodic establishment of agents in conditions where they cannot persist all the year round, hence each inoculation provides control over a number of pest generations. 'Augmentation' involves the supplemental release of indigenous natural enemies to increase control of a pest, often strategically timed for a vulnerable stage of pest population growth. Finally, 'inundation' involves the release of large numbers of agents to control a single pest generation, with no anticipation of effects on subsequent generations. It is this method that has been the focus of much recent development of insect and plant pathogens as biological pesticides.

Although the popularity of classical biological control has waxed and waned over its first hundred years, its cumulative achievements have been many. Table 1 presents some estimates of the number of introductions of insect agents and an approximate measure of the successful controls achieved, i.e. where the establishment of an agent has greatly reduced or eliminated the need for other control measures. Data for weeds come from the Silwood International Project on the Biological Control of Weeds (Moran 1985) and data for insects from the CIBC database.

TABLE 1. RECORDS OF ESTABLISHMENTS OF INSECTS FOR THE BIOLOGICAL CONTROL OF INSECT AND WEED PESTS TO DATE (SEE TEXT FOR EXPLANATION)

|  | insects | weeds |
|---|---|---|
| agent species | 563 | 126 |
| pest species | 292 | 70 |
| countries | 168 | 55 |
| establishments | 1063 | 367 |
| substantial successes | 421 | 113 |
| (percentage) | (40) | (31) |

Classical biological control using pathogens is relatively new, but can claim about four successes against insects and two against weed pests.

Dozens of species of insect predators and parasitoids are now reared worldwide for augmentation, inoculation and inundation, and in some instances these programmes have been shown to be economically competitive with alternative methods of control (Reichelderfer 1981; Hassan 1981). The most popular agents, the egg parasitoids *Trichogramma* spp., are currently used for control of moth pests over an estimated 15 million ha† of cropland worldwide (J. Voegele, personal communication). Pathogen control agents have been the most recently developed, with commercial products that incorporate nematodes, fungi, bacteria, viruses or Protozoa for the control of weeds, insects and plant diseases. Other pathogen preparations are being developed non-commercially as cottage industries in developing countries.

Increasingly, serious consideration is given to biological control in the development of new pest control programmes – a striking change from the past two decades. Despite the fact that public and private investment in research and development of chemical pesticides far exceeds that of biological methods, and is likely to continue to do so for the forseeable future (Jutsum, this symposium), biological control has won a firm place in pest management, from which it is not now likely to be dislodged.

General papers such as this often extol the virtues of biological control, detailing spectacular examples and drawing pointed (and often defensive) comparisons with chemical control methods. This is not our intention. Having established above what we feel is the strong position of biological control today, we will look at some of the current controversies that challenge it, particulary problems raised by conflicts of interest and public perception, and conflicts raised among ecologists about how biological control works and how it should be done. This is necessarily a sample of the many current developments in biological control, and it focuses on introduction or classical biological control, because of the permanent nature and scientific complexity of this method.

## BIOLOGICAL CONTROL AND PUBLIC OPINION

The disastrous use of generalist vertebrate control agents in the early days of biological control has left a frustratingly persistent public view that a natural enemy, once it has eliminated the pest, will become a pest itself. This notion has recently been joined by a growing aversion to things alien to the environment, which has perhaps accompanied the progress of genetic engineering research, and together these fears pose a new challenge in the development of biological control.

A typical example is to be found in the programme for the control of cassava mealybug, *Phenacoccus manihoti*, and mites, *Mononychellus tanajoa, sensu lato*, in Africa (Neuenschwander & Herren, this symposium), financially the largest biological control project in operation today, and perhaps ever. Early in this project the Organization of African Unity hesitated to sanction introductions into Africa of non-African insects, despite several very successful classical biological control programmes that had been done there (Greathead 1971). This is understandable given the havoc that non-African insects were causing on cassava at that time. Such seemingly simple misunderstandings can interfere with even very major projects, and show that scientists must not naïvely underestimate the privilege they enjoy in understanding

† 1 hectare = $10^4$ m².

[ 3 ]

114          J. K. WAAGE AND D. J. GREATHEAD

trophic associations, host specificity and other concepts that make it unlikely that invertebrate natural enemies will become pests in their own right.

The risk of control agents becoming pests is minimized in biological control by the selection and screening of host-specific agents against economically important species. This is now routine for weeds, where agents are usually tested for oviposition, feeding or development or both, against all important crop plants in the proposed region of introduction (Schroeder 1983). These tests are conservative in that they do not consider ecological or behavioural factors that may isolate an agent from a non-target plant (Dunn 1978). Experience to date shows that the methods currently in use are reliable, because there have been only two reported cases of insects consistently damaging useful plants among the 126 species successfully introduced: these involved species first introduced against *Lantana camara* in Hawaii in 1902 (Perkins & Swezey 1924), which pre-dated systematic screening tests, and indeed they were not screened at all. There is some concern that current screening methods may not be as satisfactory for pathogen agents. Some rusts, for instance, are known to exhibit host shifts in new environments (Alcorn 1976), possibly making a single screen a poor measure of potential host range.

Insect and pathogen control agents against insect pests are, by contrast, not extensively screened before introduction, because of the very few insects of direct benefit to man. No serious mistakes have been made, although introduced parasitoids have been implicated as a factor in the failure of an introduced weed control agent in Hawaii (Howarth 1983), Mauritius and South Africa (Greathead 1971).

Thus current procedures for ensuring the safety of classical biological control are directed at protecting agriculture. Recent public concern for the environment is rapidly changing this situation, causing increasing demands that agents for introduction pose no threat to the native fauna and flora of the country of introduction, and particularly to its endangered species. The risks involved are as yet poorly assessed, because it was not previously required that screening be done on native species. Shifts of weed control agents to native plants have been documented, although none has as yet involved a serious threat to a species (Turner 1985). The same is probably occurring for insect control agents (Howarth 1983).

Legislation that could require assessment of the impact of exotic biological control agents on native fauna and flora exists, or is under development, in countries like U.S.A., Australia and the U.K. In the U.K., the Wildlife and Countryside Act 1981 can be applied in this respect, and the current project on the biological control of bracken (Lawton, this symposium) may prove to be its first test case. In some countries, legislation has been linked with concern over genetic engineering: hence in the U.S.A. draft legislation exists for a Biological Control and Biotechnology Act which would treat biological control agents as imported germplasm subject to the same restrictions as recombinant DNA (Klassen & Dorschner 1985).

As biological control practitioners, we are confident that these new requirements would not seriously reduce the possibility of finding safe control agents for exotic pests. Further, we are keen to provide the public with the information they need to resolve any conflict between the agricultural and conservation consequences of an introduction. The problem is primarily one of cost, complicated by the availability of rare plant species for testing. Screening of control agents is expensive, and is already a large part of limited programme budgets. An analysis of programmes for the biological control of 28 weeds in Canada, for instance, has revealed that about 52% of pre-release costs involve host specificity screening (Harris 1979). To include

[ 4 ]

native flora in screening may make the cost of some programmes prohibitive to the public institutions that usually fund them. For instance, the European thistle, *Cirsium arvense*, an introduced weed of North American pastures, has about 130 native congeners there, some of which may be endangered species (Turner 1985): how many would have to be screened to satisfy concern for the native flora? Clearly, the risk is that many potentially safe and successful biological control programmes may never be done, committing farmers in many cases to the continued use of pesticides, the environmental hazards of which can often be predicted.

Risks to native flora and fauna do not pose the only conflicts of interest in the future development of biological control. More straightforward are conflicts of interest between agricultural lobbies, a striking example of which is the recent Australian court case in which private citizens succeeded in obtaining an injunction against the Australian Government's programme of introduction of insect control agents against the pasture weed *Echium plantagineum* (L.), commonly known as Patterson's curse (Cullen & Delfosse 1985). These citizens, beekeepers and graziers (who know it as Salvation Jane), felt that this plant was beneficial to their interests. The long-term consequence of this case was the Biological Control Bill 1984 which requires the government to advertise its intention to control specified target organisms biologically, and its intention to introduce specified agent organisms for this programme. Conflicts of interest can then be resolved during a public enquiry before programmes proceed too far.

An example of the potential scale and complexity of conflicts of interest in biological control is the recent development of tree legumes as sources of fodder, wood and fuel for small farmers in developing countries. Species of tree in genera such as *Leucaena, Albizia, Acacia, Mimosa* and *Prosopis* are being actively developed as new crops throughout the tropical world (Nitrogen Fixing Tree Association 1985). At the same time, their desirable attributes of rapid growth, high seed production and an ability to colonize and stabilize poor soils make them invasive weeds, and species in all these genera are targets for proposed biological control programmes. This conflict is complicated by the recent appearance in Asia of a neotropical legume-feeding psyllid, *Heteropsylla cubana*, which defoliates the major cultivated tree legume, *Leucaena leucocephala*, (Mitchell & Waterhouse 1986). At CIBC, we have been asked to explore the possibility of classical biological control for this insect pest by using agents from Central America. However, for those who consider *L. leucocephala* a weed, now under increasingly effective (if fortuitous) biological control by *H. cubana*, such a programme would be a disaster! A final twist to this story is that another species of *Heteropsylla* is being considered as a control agent for the neotropical *Mimosa invisa*, a weed of plantations in Asia. Introduction of control agents for the *Heteropsylla* on *L. leucocephala* might interfere with the success of the programme against *M. invisa* (Waterhouse & Norris 1986).

How we quantify, let alone resolve, complex conflicts of interest such as these is a new and exciting challenge to agricultural economists. An equivalent challenge for basic research is to understand the genetic and ecological basis of host specificity in insects and pathogens, so helping to evaluate better the limits to host range and the risk of host shifts in biological control agents.

## WHAT MAKES BIOLOGICAL CONTROL WORK?

A practitioner of biological control might answer this question with 'money, time, luck and a little bit of scientific insight'. The logistic constraints on mounting successful biological control, particularly on an international scale, are formidable and (as discussed above) likely to become more so. But in this forum, we would like to concentrate on scientific constraints, namely those that limit our understanding of how biological control works and hence of what makes a good biological control agent.

The greatest challenge to understanding biological control must certainly be associated with programmes involving introduction and inoculation, where change in pest populations depends not only on the mortality imposed by natural enemies in a generation, but that imposed over time by the progeny of established natural enemy populations. By contrast, understanding how inundative biological control works over a single generation is relatively simple: for pathogens it can involve dose–response studies similar to those used for chemicals (Huber & Hughes 1984), whereas for mass-released nematodes, predators and parasitoids, where searching behaviour and hence host distribution must be considered, the functional response model (Holling 1959) offers a good conceptual framework. Surprisingly, this model has been little used in practical inundation studies (Knipling & McGuire 1968; Ridgway *et al.* 1979; Zhou Li-Tzu 1988) but recent improvements for field quantification (see, for example, Hopper & King 1986) hold promise for its wider use.

For inoculation and introduction, satisfactory predictive modelling of long-term population dynamics has been possible only over short time periods in simple systems such as glasshouses. Retrospective modelling of classical biological control has been possible when data are sufficient (Hassell 1980) and current detailed studies on cassava green mites in Africa may provide the basis for the first prospective modelling of classical biological control, if satisfactory agents can be found (A. P. Gutierrez, personal communication).

Apart from these few instances, understanding of biological control has rested on ecological theory, the predictions of which are often compared with the broad patterns of success and failure of previous programmes (see, for example, DeBach 1964). Although this is a rather unsatisfactory approach, it has been much improved recently by the compilation of large data sets on past programmes, which permit quantitative analyses of factors related to success.

For programmes against insect pests a number of databases have been assembled (Clausen 1978; Luck 1982; Laing & Hamai 1976; Greathead 1986), and studies have concentrated on the relation between success and the taxonomic group to which the natural enemy and pest belong, the stability of the pest's habitat and the continuity of its populations (Ehler & Miller 1978; Hall & Ehler 1979; Hall *et al.* 1980; Noyes 1985; Hokkanen 1985; Greathead 1986). For the biological control of weeds, there now exists a database of introductions involving insect, vertebrate and disease agents (Julien 1982), which has provided information on the relation between success and the taxonomic group of both agent and pest (Julien *et al.* 1984).

The lack of precise and detailed quantitative information on most biological control programmes severely limits these analyses, as does the difficulty in establishing a consistent measure of success (Greathead 1986). To the extent that they are of value, the way forward must certainly be the elaboration of these databases with biological and ecological information on agents and pests, to explore how life history and population parameters are correlated with known outcomes. This has recently been done for weed control agents by scientists from CIBC, Imperial College and elsewhere, who have incorporated available information on the ecological niche, behaviour, population growth, release patterns and impact of each agent used into existing databases (Moran 1985). Preliminary analyses reveal intuitively satisfying results such as a positive correlation between success and intrinsic growth rate of the agent (Crawley 1986, 1987), and indicate their value in improving ecologically based scoring systems already used for selecting agents (Harris 1973; Goeden 1983; but see Schroeder & Goeden 1986). In another study using the same original database (Julien 1982), Burdon & Marshall (1981) have shown that success is greater against asexually reproducing than against sexually reproducing weeds.

Another popular approach to understanding biological control has been the exploration of theoretical models. Most of these have focused on the use of arthropod natural enemies (Hassell 1978), particularly parasitoids, which are relatively easy to model. More recently, models for the use of pathogens have been explored (Anderson 1982; May & Hassell, this symposium). The kinds of models used, and their structure, are discussed in more detail by May & Hassell (this symposium).

As a general comment, we feel that the past five years have seen a dramatic and valuable shift in the emphasis of these models, from one directed at the desirable properties of control agents, for which their general form was perhaps not best adapted, to one of exploring broad interactions between different kinds of agents and between biological control agents and other pest management practices. This includes studies of interactions between generalist and specialist natural enemies (Hassell & May 1986), natural enemies acting at different stages of the pest life cycle (Wang & Gutierrez 1980; May et al. 1981), parasitoids and insecticides (Barclay 1982; Waage et al. 1985), and pathogens and arthropod agents (Carpenter 1981), some of which are discussed by May & Hassell (this symposium). The broad, and often simple, conclusions that emerge from these studies will, we feel, be of much greater value in planning future biological controls, particularly in integrated pest management (IPM) systems, than further elaboration of models that explore the minutiae of dynamical interactions between agents and pests.

In the current profusion of database analyses and theoretical models, little has emerged to challenge the conventional ecological wisdom used in biological control, with two striking exceptions. The first deals with the role, even the existence, of population stabilizing processes in biological control (Murdoch et al. 1985), and the second with the role of genetic variation in successful biological control (Hokkanen & Pimentel 1984). We will now consider both challenges, which if real, might greatly alter our views of what makes biological control work.

*Stability in successful biological control*

According to theory, successful biological control is associated with two population processes: the depression of pest population size and the maintenance of pest populations at a new lower level: depression and stability (Waage & Hassell 1982; May & Hassell, this symposium). It has long been accepted that stability in biological control is conferred by some kind of refuge generated in space or time that protects the pest population from being driven to extinction by the control agent, which itself would otherwise die out.

In an important paper, Beddington et al. (1978) used analytical parasitoid–host models to compare the ability of different biological properties of parasitoids and hosts to create these refuges and thereby stabilize pest populations at the high levels of depression observed in biological control. Comparing sigmoid functional responses, relative parasitoid–host generation times, mutual interference between parasitoids and non-random distribution of attacks by parasitoids on hosts, only the last mechanism was able to regulate pest populations several

[ 7 ]

orders of magnitude below the equilibrium generated by density-dependent food limitation acting on the host in the absence of the parasitoid.

Although other possible stabilizing factors were not examined (e.g. temporal synchrony (Griffiths 1969)) or have since emerged (e.g. variation in susceptibility between hosts (Hassell & Anderson 1984); density-dependent parasitoid sex ratios (Hassell *et al.* 1983)), the bold conclusion of Beddington *et al.* (1978) has left non-random search the single most popular explanation of stability in successful biological control. In addition, it has engendered a veritable explosion of studies on spatial density dependence in parasitoid–host systems (see, for example, Morrison & Strong 1980, 1981; Morrison *et al.* 1980; Hassell 1980; Heads & Lawton 1983; Weis 1983; Waage 1983; Murdoch *et al.* 1984).

Initially, the concept of non-random search was associated with aggregation by natural enemies on high density 'patches' of hosts, perhaps because concurrent studies on optimal foraging by predators and parasitoids predicated that aggregation would be adaptive and widespread (Charnov 1976; Cook & Hubbard 1977). As a result, aggregative behaviour was identified as a desirable attribute for a control agent.

The discovery that parasitism between patches is frequently not positively density dependent, led Murdoch *et al.* (1984, 1985) and others to challenge the contention that non-random search is an important stabilizing mechanism in parasitoid–host interactions, and therefore that aggregative ability is an important attribute in a control agent.

However, more recent studies have reaffirmed that spatial patterns of parasitism need not be positively density dependent to be stabilizing (Hassell 1984; Chesson & Murdoch 1986): stability is conferred simply by the concentration of attacks in some patches and not others. In addition aggregation is not always adaptive (Lessells 1985; Iwasa *et al.* 1981), but depends upon parasitoid behaviour and host distribution. Thus studies of the spatial distribution of mortality cannot, unless detailed, tell us much about the ability of parasitoids to depress or stabilize host populations.

A more basic challenge to the designation of stability-conferring attributes for selecting natural enemies is the argument of Murdoch *et al.* (1985) that successful biological control agents do not stabilize host populations at all. Rather, they suggest that the persistence of pest populations after successful biological control is a consequence of stochastic processes involving the creation of host patches by colonization and their extinction after discovery by the agent. In essence, they argue that spatial refuges are products of spatio-temporal patchiness, not of the non-random search of natural enemies. It might be argued that these are two ways of looking at the same process. None the less, it has led the authors to suggest that the most efficient natural enemies are not those showing patterns of search or activity that leave some hosts safe in refuges, but those that are efficient at finding and killing pests at any density and time. This, in turn, indicates a very different set of natural enemies as desirable candidates for selection.

Murdoch and his colleagues feel that their claim is supported by the frequent local extinction of pest populations in biological control which they argue would not arise simply from non-random search. Their most firm evidence comes from scale insect populations (Murdoch *et al.* 1984; but see Huffaker *et al.* 1986). However, extinction of host patches is characteristic of other biological control systems, including whiteflies (van Lenteren 1986) and mites (Sabelis & van de Meer 1986; Nachman 1987).

What is common to Homoptera and mites is that patches constitute populations of pests reproducing over several generations, on which natural enemies can exhibit not only a functional but a numerical response. Simulation studies have demonstrated the existence of stabilizing mechanisms in patchy mite-like predator–prey systems (Hastings 1977; Sabelis & Diekmann, unpublished data) which are not associated with non-random search between patches: indeed Huffaker's (1958) classical orange and mite system may be an example. This situation contrasts with that where spatial heterogeneity has been claimed as a stabilizing factor (e.g. Hassell 1980). Here, patches represent a transient life stage, say, eggs or caterpillars on plants, which do not reproduce or persist for more than a generation and where natural enemies are limited to a functional response only.

Perhaps Murdoch *et al.* (1985) have not refuted the importance of non-random search to stability of biological control interactions, but have found a mechanism of stability characteristic of certain kinds of natural enemy – pest interactions. If true, this would force us to rethink the argument of Beddington *et al.* (1978) for a stabilizing mechanism common to all biological control systems. It is interesting that, of the six examples given by Beddington *et al.* (1978), the four associated with the greatest depression involve Homoptera, and the other two involve 'life stage patch' interactions of parasitoids with Lepidoptera and Hymenoptera.

TABLE 2. HYPOTHETICAL CONTINUUM OF PEST TYPES, THE NATURE OF THEIR PATCHY DISTRIBUTION, AND THE SPATIALLY MEDIATED STABILIZING MECHANISMS THAT MAY OPERATE IN THEIR BIOLOGICAL CONTROL

| | | |
|---|---|---|
| patch duration: | many generations (colony) | single generation (life stage) |
| stabilizing mechanism: | asynchronous patch dynamics | non-random search |
| examples: | mites, Homoptera | Lepidoptera, Hymenoptera |

We believe that there may be a range of spatially mediated stabilizing mechanisms (table 2) associated with different degrees of patch permanence ranging from transient, 'life stage patches' where non-random search may be an important factor, to 'colonial patches' where other mechanisms may act, with or without non-random search. If this is true, it would suggest that desirable attributes for natural enemies may vary between pest systems, with obvious implications for selection of control agents.

### Genetics and the 'new association' theory

Although it is usual in classical biological control to seek agents from the target pest in its area of probable origin, highly successful control has been obtained from the introduction of natural enemies that are not naturally associated with the target pest, either because they do not come from the native area of the pest, or because they come from a related pest species. Pimentel (1963) used this evidence to suggest that coevolution between pest and control agent leads to increased resistance of the pest and decreased effectiveness of the agent, making it desirable to seek control agents that do not have a close evolutionary history with the pest.

This argument has been criticized (see, for example, Huffaker *et al.* 1971), but has re-emerged recently in an analysis of a large biological control database by Hokkanen & Pimentel (1984), incorporating releases of pathogens, insects, molluscs and vertebrates for the control of

[ 9 ]

insect and weed pests. They conclude that 'there is about a 75% greater chance for success if the parasite and its host are newly associated instead of an old association'. If this pattern is real, then current methods for selecting agents may need reappraisal.

Besides problems associated with the comparison of programmes as diverse as birds against insects and pathogens against plants, and the inclusion of only successful programmes in the analysis, more specific criticisms of the accuracy of both the database and analysis of Hokkanen & Pimentel (1984) have been levelled at its treatment of programmes for insect (Greathead 1986) and weed (Harris 1986; Goeden & Kok 1986) control. We feel a more refined and accurate analysis is necessary, and have therefore prepared one that uses a CIBC database and (1) considers only insect control agents for insect pests, and (2) expands the analysis to include all establishments, not just successes. (This is still conservative as it excludes failures to establish, which may be biased against new associations because of genetic or climatic incompatability, see, for example Crawley (1986) for biological weed control.) Like Hokkanen & Pimentel (1984) we identify new associations as those in which the agent came from a different geographical region to the host (and possibly from a different host), and we try to reduce the bias caused by the repetition of projects, particularly successful ones: in our case we select agent records from the first project ever mounted against a particular pest and ignore subsequent ones.

TABLE 3. SUCCESS RATINGS OF INSECT AGENTS IN FIRST PROGRAMMES AGAINST INSECT PESTS: A TEST OF THE 'NEW ASSOCIATION' THEORY (SEE TEXT FOR EXPLANATION)

| associations | complete (C) | substantial (S) | partial (P) | none (N) |
|---|---|---|---|---|
| new | 20 | 29 | 13 | 83 |
| old | 37 | 81 | 12 | 166 |

overall: $p < 0.09$.    $C+S$ against $P+N$: $p < 0.82$.    $C+S+P$ against $N$: $p < 0.82$.

Our results are shown in table 3. The distribution of agents attributed with complete, substantial, partial or no success does not differ significantly between new and old associations (goodness of fit test, $\chi^2 = 6.4$, $p$ less than 0.09). It is, perhaps, more realistic to pool some of these arbitrary ratings of success to give a more robust comparison, in which case we find even less difference ($\chi^2 = 0.05$, $p$ less than 0.82). This analysis, like its predecessor, has certain flaws: for instance, several species contributing to a completely successful programme are often given a 'complete' rating, even if the relative contribution of each species is unknown. More detailed analyses are necessary to avoid these errors. In balance, we do not feel that the evidence for the superiority of new associations justifies its being given precedence as a selection criterion for biological control agents. However, the underlying concept that natural enemies become less effective with time, needs more scrutiny, particularly as it could jeopardize the future of past biological control successes!

The notion that the effectiveness of biological control agents will generally decrease as a result of coevolution with their hosts is not supported by current theory (May & Anderson 1983). This phenomenon can arise where high virulence reduces transmission by insect vectors by killing hosts too rapidly, as has been suggested for the biological control of rabbits by myxoma virus, but seems unlikely to occur with pathogens attacking insect pests, where the hosts' life cycles are short and vectors are probably not so important. Biological control has made use of the fact that exotic strains of some widely distributed pathogens are more likely to promote epizootics than local strains (Milner *et al.* 1982; Milner & Mahon 1985). However, it is not clear that this variability indicates local evolution of reduced virulence, and direct evidence for this is limited (Briese 1986).

For insect parasitoids, long-term laboratory interactions with hosts have led to a decrease in parasitoid reproductive rate (see Boulétreau (1986) for a review), and hence have been used to support Pimentel's (1963) theory. However, this does not always lead to the increase in host population levels inferred in the 'new association' argument. Further, there is no clear evidence from the field that parasitoid effectiveness has decreased during the course of classical biological control (Boulétreau 1986). Even the textbook example of the evolution of resistance to a parasitoid – *Mesoleius tenthredinus* introduced into Canada for control of the sawfly *Pristiphora erichsonii* (Muldrew 1953; Ives & Muldrew 1984) – is likely to be the result of the introduction of a competitively superior resistant host population, and not of selection acting on the original parasitoid population (Ives & Muldrew 1984).

Although there is little evidence that parasitoids become less effective after prolonged exposure to hosts, there is some evidence from biological control that they get more effective (van den Bosch 1964; Messenger & van den Bosch 1971). Indeed, in classical biological control a long 'lag period' is sometimes found between the establishment of a control agent and the point at which its populations rise rapidly to control the pest (Doutt & DeBach 1964); could this indicate a period of natural selection for improved effectiveness?

Although as yet we have very little understanding of what causes spatial and temporal genetic variation in the effectiveness of control agents, the hypothesis of Hokkanen & Pimentel (1984) appears to explain some of the observed patterns.

### FUTURE TRENDS IN BIOLOGICAL CONTROL

Although classical biological control continues to fascinate ecologists, practical attention has focused recently on inundative methods, and particularly the potential for commercial biopesticides. Much venture capital is being put into the development of microbials, and as this happens a veil of secrecy is rapidly falling over research in this new and exciting field. However, the small firms that develop and market such products are often short-lived, as are their products: indeed, the United Kingdom's leading microbial pesticide firm has recently closed after only two years. A number of these firms are 'bought out' by large agrochemical and biotechnological companies. Although it might be argued that this is the logical path towards the expansion of microbial methods, it should be remembered that microbial products, once in the portfolio of an agrochemical firm, must compete with pesticides with larger markets and more conventional production problems. For this and other reasons, we do not see a substantial shift in industry to microbial products in the near future; enthusiasm must be maintained, but development will be slow.

What then of classical biological control and inoculative methods? Much of the future 'market' here will be created by the continuing ability of pests to escape quarantine restrictions. To give an idea of the scale of this invasion, van Lenteren *et al.* (1988) estimate that over 70 species of exotic pest have invaded The Netherlands since 1900, whereas in the U.S.A., between 1920 and 1980, at least 837 exotic insect species became established, about 10% of them becoming serious pests (Hoy 1985). Such immigration is a continuing process: for instance, CIBC is currently investigating biological control for an Asian mealybug,

*Rastrococcus invadens*, which appeared in 1982 as a pest in West Africa, a Central American psyllid, *Heteropsylla cubana*, which in 1984 began a whirlwind spread throughout the Pacific and Asia on the tree legume *Leucaena leucocephala*, and an Asian scale insect, *Aonidiella orientalis*, which appeared in 1986 as a threat to cultivated neem, *Azadirachta indica* (Meliaceae), in Central Africa.

Apart from this virtually guaranteed 'market', our increasing knowledge of how biological control works may make it profitable to re-attempt past failures (Hoy 1985), and to exploit genetic variability to find, or even produce, better or new agents for old pests. Introduction of exotic agents against native pests, still a relatively little-explored area (Carl 1982), may provide yet more opportunites as our knowledge develops. Finally, a trend is emerging away from inundative methods towards inoculative methods employing the same species. Thus recent studies in China have shown that single, carefully timed releases of the egg parasitoid *Trichogramma* early in a growing season can give as good control of moth pests on maize and sugar cane as the more conventional weekly or biweekly mass-releases later in the season (Shen Xiao-Cheng 1988; Guo Ming-Fang 1988).

To what extent will this increase in opportunities for biological control be met by an increase in demand? Biological control is generally appreciated today as an important component of IPM, and demand for it is likely to spread as IPM programmes develop worldwide. It should be remembered as well that, in economic terms, perhaps the greatest contribution of biological control to agriculture comes not through programmes of introduction, inoculation and inundation, but from the contribution of indigenous natural enemies to pest suppression in sprayed crop systems. This 'natural control' is increasingly appreciated in pest management, and has stimulated the development of selective pesticides, methods to reduce pesticide application and manipulation of cropping practices to encourage natural enemies. A paper of at least this length would be required to discuss properly this aspect of biological control; it can only be said here that the demand for improved natural control, and the need to understand how it works, are increasing rapidly (see van Emden, this symposium; Pickett, this symposium).

Thus the demand for biological control is likely to develop at least as fast as the adoption of IPM practices. In reality, we think it will develop much faster, as a result of another, less measured process, namely the rapid growth in public concern about pesticides and their effects on health and the environment. The past few years have seen many developments. In industrialized countries, these include increasing demand for organically grown produce, new laws requiring that pesticides for registration be screened for negative effects on natural enemies, and even state and federal taxes on broad spectrum compounds to fund research on non-chemical methods of control. In developing countries, where a high percentage of pesticides used are subsidized by aid organizations, a growing awareness of pesticide misuse and environmental pollution may lead to a decline in subsidies for broad-spectrum compounds, thereby leaving a gap in pest management that can be filled only by more rational management practices, and increased reliance on cultural and biological methods of control.

Whether the demand for biological control will grow at the careful pace of implementation of IPM practices, or at the rather more hurried pace of an environmental movement, the scientific skills that we need to understand and use it to implement and diversify, will be much called upon in years to come.

REFERENCES

Alcorn, J. L.  1976  Host range of *Puccinia xanthi*. *Trans. Br. mycol. Soc.* **66**, 365–367.

Anderson, R. M.  1982  Theoretical basis for the use of pathogens as biological control agents of pest species. *Parasitology* **84**, 3–33.

Barclay, H. J.  1982  Models for pest control using predator release, habitat management and pesticide release in combination. *J. appl. Ecol.* **19**, 337–348.

Beddington, J. R., Free, C. A. & Lawton, J. H.  1978  Dynamic complexity in predator–prey models framed in difference equations. *Nature, Lond,* **255**, 58–60.

Berlese, A.  1915  La destruzione della *Diaspis pentagona* a mazzo della *Prospaltella berlesei*. *Redia* **10**, 151–228.

Boulétreau, M.  1986  The genetic and coevolutionary interactions between parasitoids and their hosts. In *Insect parasitoids* (ed. J. Waage & D. Greathead), pp. 169–200. London: Academic Press.

Briese, D. T.  1986  Host resistance to microbial control agents. In *Biological plant and health protection* (ed. J. M. Franz). (*Fortschr. Zool.* **32**, 233–256.) Stuttgart: Gustav Fischer Verlag.

Burdon, J. J. & Marshall, D. R.  1981  Biological control and the reproductive mode of weeds. *J. appl. Ecol.* **18**, 649–658.

Carl, K. P.  1982  Biological control of native pests by introduced natural enemies. *Biocontrol News Inf.* **3**, 191–200.

Carpenter, S. R.  1981  Effect of control measures on pest populations subject to regulation by parasites and pathogens. *J. theor. Biol.* **92**, 1891–1894.

Carson, R.  1962  *Silent spring.* London: Hamish Hamilton.

Charnov, E. L.  1976  Optimal foraging; the marginal value theorem. *Theor. Popul. Biol.* **9**, 129–136.

Chesson, P. L. & Murdoch, W. W.  1986  Relationships among host–parasitoid models. *Am. Nat.* **127**, 696–715.

CIBC 1981  Is anyone there? *Biocontrol News Inf.* **2**, 273.

Clausen, C. P. (ed.)  1978  Introduced parasites and predators of arthropod pests and weeds: a world review. *Agric. Handb. Agric. Res. Serv. U.S.* no. 480. (551 pages.)

Cook, R. M. & Hubbard, S. F.  1977  Adaptive searching strategies in insect parasites. *J. anim. Ecol.* **46**, 115–125.

Crawley, M. J.  1986  The population biology of invaders. *Phil. Trans. R. Soc. Lond.* B **314**, 711–731.

Crawley, M. J.  1987  What makes a community invasible? In *Colonisation, succession and stability* (ed. A. J. Gray, M. J. Crawley & P. J. Edwards). Oxford: Blackwell Scientific Publications. (In the press.)

Cullen, J. M. & Delfosse, E. S.  1985  *Echium platagineum*: catalyst for conflict and change in Australia. In *Proceedings of the VI International Symposium on Biological Control of Weeds, Vancouver, Canada, 1984* (ed. E. S. Delfosse), pp. 249–292. Ottawa: Agriculture Canada.

DeBach, P. (ed.)  1964  *Biological control of insect pests and weeds.* London: Chapman & Hall.

Doutt, R. L.  1958  Vice, virtue and the vedalia. *Bull. ent. Soc. Am.* **4**, 119–123.

Doutt, R. L. & DeBach, P.  1964  Some biological control concepts and questions. In *Biological control of insect pests and weeds* (ed. P. DeBach), pp. 118–142. London: Chapman & Hall.

Dunn, P. H.  1978  Shortcomings in the classic tests of candidate insects for the biocontrol of weeds. *In Proceedings of the VI International Symposium on Biological Control of Weeds* (ed. E. S. Delfosse), pp. 51–56. Ottawa: Agriculture Canada.

Ehler, L. E. & Miller, J. C.  1978  Biological control in temporary agroecosystems. *Entomophaga* **23**, 207–212.

Goeden, R. D.  1983  Critique and revision of Harris' scoring system for selection of insect agents in biological control of weeds. *Prot. Ecol.* **5**, 287–301.

Goeden, R. D. & Kok, L. T.  1986  Comments on a proposed 'new' approach for selecting agents for the biological control of weeds. *Can. Ent.* **118**, 51–58.

Greathead, D. J.  1971  A review of biological control in the Ethiopian Region. *Tech. Commun. Commonw. Inst. biol. Control* no. 5. (162 pages.)

Greathead, D. J.  1986  Parasitoids in classical biological control. In *Insect parasitoids* (ed. J. Waage & D. Greathead), pp. 289–318. London: Academic Press.

Griffiths, K. L.  1969  Development and diapause in *Pleolophus basizonus* (Hymenoptera: Ichneumonidae). *Can. Ent.* **101**, 907–914.

Guo Ming-Fang 1988  New method of *Trichogramma* utilization. In *Second international symposium on Trichogramma*. (ed. J. Voegele, S. Hassan, J. C. van Lenteren & J. K. Waage). Paris: Institut National de Recherches Agronomique. (In the press.)

Hall, R. W., Ehler, L. E. & Bisabri-Ershadi, B.  1980  Rate of success in classical biological control of arthropods. *Bull. ent. Soc. Am.,* **26**, 111–114.

Hall, R. W. & Ehler, L. E.  1979  Rate of establishment of natural enemies in classical biological control. *Bull. ent. Soc. Am.* **25**, 280–282.

Harris, P.  1973  The selection of effective agents for the biological control of weeds. *Can. Ent.* **105**, 1495–1503.

Harris, P.  1979  Cost of biological control of weeds by insects in Canada. *Weed Sci.* **27**, 242–250.

Harris, P.  1986  Biological control of weeds. In *Biological plant and health protection* (ed. J. M. Franz). (*Fortschr. Zool.* **32**, 233–256). Stuttgart: Gustav Fischer Verlag.

Hassan, S. A. 1981 Mass production and utilisation of *Trichogramma*. 2. Four years successful biological control of the European corn borer. *Meded. Fac. Landbwet. Rijksuniv. Gent* **46**, 417–428.

Hassell, M. P. 1978 *The dynamics of arthropod predator–prey systems*. Princeton, New Jersey: Princeton University Press.

Hassell, M. P. 1980 Foraging strategies, population models and biological control: a case study. *J. Anim. Ecol.* **49**, 603–628.

Hassell, M. P. 1984 Parasitism in patchy environments: inverse density dependence can be stabilising. *I.M.A.J. math. appl. med. Biol.* **1**, 123–133.

Hassell, M. P. & Anderson, R. M. 1984 Host susceptibility as a component in host-parasitoid systems. *J. Anim. Ecol.* **53**, 611–621.

Hassell, M. P. & May, R. M. 1986 Generalist and specialist natural enemies in insect predator–prey interactions. *J. Anim. Ecol.* **55**, 923–940.

Hassell, M. P., Waage, J. K. & May, R. M. 1983 Variable parasitoid sex ratios and their effect on host–parasitoid dynamics. *J. Anim. Ecol.* **52**, 889–904.

Heads, P. A. & Lawton, J. H. 1983 Studies on the natural enemy complex of the holly leafminer: the effects of scale on the detection of aggregative responses and the implications for biological control. *Oikos* **40**, 267–276.

Hokkanen, H. M. T. 1985 Success in classical biological control. *CRC crit. Rev. Pl. Sci.* **3**, 35–72.

Hokkanen, M. & Pimentel, D. 1984 New approach for selecting biological control agents. *Can. Ent.* **116**, 1109–1121.

Holling, C. S. 1959 Some characteristics of simple types of predation and parasitism. *Can. Ent.* **91**, 385–398.

Hopper, K. R. & King. E. G. 1986 Linear functional response of *Microplitis croceipes* (Hymenoptera: Braconidae) to variation in *Heliothis* ssp. (Lepidoptera: Noctuidae) density in the field. *Envir. Ent.* **15**, 476–480.

Howard, L. O. & Fiske, W. F. 1911 The importation into the United States of the parasites of the gipsy moth and the browntail moth. *Bull. Bur. Ent. U.S. Dep. Agric.* no. 91, 1–344.

Howarth, F. G. 1983 Classical biocontrol: panacea or Pandora's box. *Proc. Hawaii. ent. Soc.* **24**, 239–244.

Hoy, M. A. 1985 Improving establishment of arthropod natural enemies. In *Biological control in agriculture IPM systems* (ed. M. A. Hoy & D. C. Herzog), pp. 151–166. London: Academic Press.

Huber, J. & Hughes, P. R. 1984 Quantitative bioassay in insect pathology. *Bull. ent. Soc. Am.* **30**, 31–34.

Huffaker, C. B. 1958 Experimental studies on predation: dispersion factors and predator–prey oscillations. *Hilgardia* **27**, 343–383.

Huffaker, C. B., Kennett, C. E. & Tassan, R. L. 1986 Comparisons of parasitism and densities of *Parlatoria oleae* (1952–1982) in relation to ecological theory. *Am. Nat.* **128**, 379–393.

Huffaker, C. B., Messenger, P. S. & DeBach, P. 1971 The natural enemy component in natural control and the theory of biological control. In *Biological Control* (ed. C. B. Huffaker), pp. 16–67. New York: Plenum.

Ives, W. G. H. & Muldrew, J. A. 1984 *Pristiphora erichsonii* (Hartig), larch sawfly, (Hymenoptera: Tenthredinidae). In *Biological control programmes against insects and weeds in Canada 1969–1980*. (ed. J. S. Kelleher & M. A. Hulme), pp. 369–380. Farnham Royal, England: Commonwealth Agricultural Bureaux.

Iwasa, Y., Higashi, M. & Yamamura, N. 1981 Prey distribution as a factor determining the choice of optimal foraging strategy. *Am. Nat* **117**, 710–723.

Julien, M. H. (ed.) 1982 *Biological control of weeds*. Farnham Royal, England: Commonwealth Agricultural Bureaux.

Julien, M. H., Kerr, J. D. & Chan, R. R. 1984 Biological control of weeds: an evaluation. *Prot. Ecol.* **7**, 3–25.

Klassen, W. & Dorschner, K. 1985 Biological control research in the United States. In *Development and operation of an international biological control network*. CAB International Institute of Biological Control. (Unpublished report.)

Knipling, E. F. & McGuire, J. U. Jr. 1968 Population models to appraise the limitations and potentialities of *Trichogramma* in managing host insect populations. *Tech. Bull. U.S. Dep. Agric.* no. 1387. (44 pages.)

Laing, J. E. & Hamai, J. 1976 Biological control of insect pests and weeds by imported parasites, predators, and pathogens. In *Theory and practice of biological control* (ed. C. B. Huffaker & P. S. Messenger), pp. 685–723. New York: Academic Press.

Lessels, C. M. 1985 Parasitoid foraging: should parasitism be density dependent? *J. Anim. Ecol.* **54**, 27–41.

Lounsbury, C. P. 1940 The pioneer period of economic entomology in South Africa. *J. ent. Soc. sth. Afr.* **3**, 9–29.

Luck, R. F. 1982 Parasitic insects introduced as biological control agents for arthropod pests. In *CRC Handbook of pest management in agriculture*, vol. II (ed. D. Pimentel), pp. 125–284. Boca Raton, Florida: CRC Press.

May, R. M. & Anderson, R. M. 1983 Epidemiology and genetics in the coevolution of parasites and hosts. *Proc. R. Soc. Lond.* B **219**, 281–313.

May, R. M., Hassell, M. P., Anderson, R. M. & Tonkyn, D. W. 1981 Density dependence in host–parasitoid models. *J. Anim. ecol.* **50**, 855–865.

Messenger, P. S. & van den Bosch, R. 1971 The adaptability of introduced biological control agents. In *Biological control* (ed. C. F. Huffaker), pp. 68–92. New York: Plenum Press.

[ 14 ]

Milner, R. J. & Mahon, R. J. 1985 Strain variation in *Zoophthora radicans*, a pathogen on a variety of insect hosts in Australia. *J. Aust. ent. Soc.* **24**, 195–198.

Milner, R. J., Soper, R. S. & Lutton, G. G. 1982 Field release of an Israeli strain of the fungus *Zoophthora radicans* (Brefeld) Batks for biological control of *Therioaphis trifolii* (Monell) f. *maculata*. *J. Aust. ent. Soc.* **21**, 113–118.

Mitchell, W. C. & Waterhouse, D. F. 1986 Spread of the *Leucaena psyllids*: their natural history, distribution, predators and resistant leucaenas. *Leucaena Res. Reps* **7**, 6–8.

Moran, V. C. 1985 The Silwood International Project on the biological control of weeds. In *Proceedings of the VI International Symposium on Biological Control of Weeds, Vancouver, Canada, 1984* (ed. E. S. Delfosse), pp. 65–68. Ottawa: Agriculture Canada.

Morrison, G. & Strong, D. R. 1980 Spatial variations in host density and the intensity of parasitism: empirical examples. *Envir. Ent.* **9**, 149–152.

Morrison, G. & Strong, D. R. 1981 Spatial variations in egg density and the intensity of parasitism in a neotropical chrysomelid (*Cephaloleia consanguinea*). *Ecol. Ent.* **6**, 55–61.

Morrison, G., Auerback, M., McCoy, E. D. 1980 Spatial differences in *Heliothis zea* egg density and intensity of parasitism by *Trichogramma* spp an experimental analysis. *Envir. Ent.* **9**, 79–85.

Muldrew, J. A. 1953 Population studies on some small forest mammals in eastern Canada. *J. Mammal.* **36**, 21–35.

Murdoch, W. W., Chesson, J. & Chesson, P. L. 1985 Biological control in theory and practice. *Am. Nat.* **125**, 344–366.

Murdoch, W. W., Reeve, J. D., Huffaker, C. B. & Kennett, C. E. 1984 Biological control of olive scale and its relevance to ecological theory. *Am. Nat.* **123**, 371–392.

Nachman, G. 1987 Systems analysis of acarine predator–prey interactions II. The role of spatial processes in system stability. *J. Anim. Ecol.* **56**, 267–281.

Nitrogen Fixing Tree Association 1985 *Annual report*. Waimanalo, Hawaii, U.S.A.

Noyes, J. S. 1985 Chalcidoids and biological control. *Chalcid Forum* **5**, 5–13.

Ordish, G. 1967 *Biological methods in crop pest control*. London: Constable.

Perkins, R. C. L. & Swezey, O. H. 1924 The introduction into Hawaii of insects that attack lantana. *Bull. Exp. Stn Hawaii Sug. Plrs Ass.* (Ent. Ser.) no. 16. (83 pages.)

Pimentel, D. 1963 Introducing parasites and predators to control native pests. *Can. Ent.* **95**, 785–792.

Reichelderfer, K. H. 1981 Economic feasibility of biological control of crop pests. In *Biological control in crop production* (ed. G. C. Papavisas), pp. 403–417. London: Granada.

Ridgway, R. L., Ables, J. R., Goodpasture, C. E. & Hartstack, A. W. 1979 *Trichogramma* and its utilisation for crop protection in the United States. Invitational Paper, *USSR–USA conference on use of beneficial organisms in control of crop pests, Washington, D.C.* August 1979.

Sabelis, M. W. & van der Meer, J. 1986 Local dynamics of the interaction between predatory mites and two-spotted spider mites. In *Dynamics of physiologically structured populations* (ed. J. Metz & O. Diekmann). Lecture notes in biomathematics, pp. 322–344. Springer: Berlin.

Schroeder, D. 1983 Biological control of weeds. In *Recent advances in weed research* (ed. W. W. Fletcher), pp. 41–78. Farnham Royal, England: Commonwealth Agricultural Bureaux.

Schroeder, D. & Goeden, R. D. 1986 The search for arthropod natural enemies of introduced weeds for biological control in theory and practice. *Biocontrol News Inf.* **7**, 147–155.

Shen Xiao-Cheng 1988 The inoculative release of *Trichogramma dendrolimi* for controlling corn borer and rice leafroller. In *Second international symposium on Trichogramma* (ed. J. Voegele, S. Hassan, J. C. van Lenteren & J. K. Waage). Paris: Institut National de Recherches Agronomique. (In the press.)

Smith, H. S. 1919 On some phases of insect control by the biological method. *J. econ. Ent.* **12**, 288–292.

Thompson, W. R. 1930 *Biological control of insect and plant pests*. London: HMSO.

Turner, C. E. 1985 Conflicting interests and biological control in weeds. In *Proceedings of the VI International Symposium on Biological Control of Weeds, Vancouver, Canada, 1984* (ed. E. S. Delfosse), pp. 203–225. Ottawa: Agriculture Canada.

van den Bosch, R. 1964 Encapsulation of the eggs of *Bathyplectes curculionis* (Thomson) (Hymenoptera: Ichneumonidae) in larvae of *Hypera brunneipennis* (Boheman) and *Hypera postica* (Gyllenhal) (Coleoptera: Curculionidae). *J. Invert. Path.* **6**, 343–367.

van Lenteren, J. C. 1986 Parasitoids in the greenhouse: successes with seasonal inoculative release systems. In *Insect parasitoids* (ed. J. Waage & D. Greathead), pp. 341–374. London: Academic Press.

van Lenteren, J. C., Woets, J., Grijpma, P., Ulenberg, S. A. & Minkenberg, O. P. J. M. 1988 Invasion of pest and beneficial insects into the Netherlands. *Proc. K. ned. Akad. Wed. C.* (In the press.)

Waage, J. K. 1983 Aggregation in field parasitoid populations: foraging time allocation by a population of *Diadegma* (Hymenoptera, Ichneumonidae). *Ecol. Ent.* **8**, 447–453.

Waage, J. K. & Hassell, M. P. 1982 Parasitoids as biological control agents – a fundamental approach. *Parasitology* **84**, 241–268.

Waage, J. K., Hassell, M. P. & Godfray, H. C. J. 1985 The dynamics of pest-parasitoid-insecticide interactions. *J. appl. Ecol.* **22**, 825–838.

Wang, Y. H. & Gutierrez, A. P. 1980 An assessment of the use of stability analyses in population ecology. *J. Anim. Ecol* **49**, 435–452.

Waterhouse, D. F. & Norris, K. R. 1986 *Biological control: Pacific prospects.* Australian Centre for International Agricultural Research Report. Melbourne, Australia: Inkata Press.

Weis, A. E. 1983 Patterns of parasitism by *Torymus capite* on hosts distributed in small patches. *J. Anim. Ecol.* **52**, 867–877.

Zhou Li-Tzu 1988 Study on parasitizing efficiency of *Trichogramma confusum* Viggiani in controlling *Heliothis armigera* Hübner and its modelling. In *Second international symposium on Trichogramma* (ed. J. Voegele, S. Hassan, J. C. van Lenteren & J. K. Waage). Paris: Institut National de Recherches Agronomique. (In the press.)

## Discussion

R. Brown (*ICI Plant Protection Division, Bracknell, U.K.*). What are Dr Waage's criteria for screening indigenous organisms against novel biocontrol agents and what level of confidence do you put in this process?

Are these criteria applied equally to both rich and poor countries, even if a poor country with an important and soluble pest problem could not afford the screening costs?

J. K. Waage. So far, routine screening is largely done for weed control agents and this is usually more concerned with crop plants than the native flora. However, especially in North America screening of endangered native species is having to be included. Screening of insect biological control agents is now being demanded by some countries, usually only against bees and species of concern to conservationists, e.g. birdwing butterflies in Papua New Guinea. We can never be absolutely sure, but we are confident that the methods used against weed and insect control agents are reliable: when they have been followed there have been no unforeseen consequences.

The same criteria are applied to potential introductions into all countries. If a country cannot afford screening then we help it find a donor to support this work.

R. R. M. Paterson (*C.A.B. International Mycological Institute, Kew, U.K.*). What are the procedures for screening weed control agents to be introduced so as to be sure that non-target plants will not be attacked?

D. J. Greathead. Nowadays, weed control agents are screened according to a centrifugal phylogenetic scheme (as Dr Hasan explains further in his paper) whereby the agent is tested first against different populations of the target weed, then species in the same genus, genera in the same tribe, and so on. Other plants are also checked, including important crops planted in the area where control is planned. Attention is also paid to any plants with similar secondary chemicals, host plants of species related to the candidate agent, and any other plants specified by the authorities who will have to decide on whether to introduce the agent. These protocols have so far avoided any unforeseen attacks on non-target plants be we can never be absolutely sure this will not happen. It is a matter of taking a calculated risk.

P. T. Haskell (*Department of Zoology, University College, Cardiff, U.K.*). Because it is impossible to give an absolute guarantee that a biocontrol agent after release will not cause any harm to non-target organisms, it is surely essential that some form of risk assessment procedure relating to release be worked out and agreed internationally? To begin with, this could be based on the 'centrifugal' procedure outlined by Dr Greathead, with extra safeguards appropriate for materials such as genetically engineered organisms. Such an international procedure could be formulated in the first place by organizations such as the CAB International Institute of Biological Control, the International Organization for Biological Control of Noxious Animals and Plants, the Food and Agricultural Organization of the United Nations and the World Health Organization.

D. J. GREATHEAD. The suggestion that there should be internationally accepted rules for screening is a good one. In fact, scientists concerned with weed control agents have taken action and the protocol I have outlined (in reply to R. R. M. Paterson) was debated and refined at successive International Symposia on Biological Control of Weeds, which take place every four years. No protocols have been worked out for insect control agents. Generally, it has been sufficient to show that they do not attack beneficial species. However, assurances that non-target native species will not be attacked are beginning to be demanded. It will, therefore, soon be necessary to adapt and apply the protocols for weed control agents to insect control agents.

It will be more difficult to obtain a consensus for an internationally accepted procedure from regulatory authorities who have differing agricultural priorities and concerns for the environment. This would require harmonizing of legislation (which has begun in Europe) and that would not be easy.

R. J. COOK (*United States Department of Agriculture Agricultural Research Service, Washington State University, Pullman, U.S.A.*). Are there any examples of a biocontrol agent, or any other potentially beneficial organism, having had a negative effect on the environment following its deliberate release into the environment? Please give examples from what you call the prescientific and postscientific areas of biological control, i.e. before and since 1888.

J. K. WAAGE. There are very few examples considering the large number of introductions that have been made, and most of these relate to the introduction of general predators, chiefly vertebrates such as mongooses, owls and the cane toad. Many of these introductions were made during the prescientific period but, unfortunately, some were made later when those concerned should have realized the dangers.

These aside, carefully selected, reasonably host specific invertebrate agents have led to few unanticipated side effects. In Hawaii and Mauritius there have been negative effects where parasitoids used to control crop pests have interfered with taxonomically similar insects introduced for weed control.

The most serious and widely publicized negative effect relates to the introduction of predatory snails (*Gonaxis* spp.) onto Pacific islands for control of the Giant African Snail (*Achatina fulica*). These non-specific predators have been blamed for the disappearance of endemic snails that were being studied by evolutionary biologists, particularly in Hawaii and Western Samoa.

K. KRISHNAIAH (*Directorate of Rice Research, Rajendranagar, Hyderabad, India*). Please indicate a few successes of biological control through conservation, and some methods practised in achieving these successes.

D. J. Greathead. Management of oil-palm estates to avoid outbreaks of defoliating caterpillars is widely practised, especially in Malaysia. Practices include growing ground cover to protect pupating parasitoids and to provide food for the adults. Measures to reduce road dust blowing into the plantations also help. Any incipient outbreaks can then usually be stopped by spraying virus that occurs naturally.

Recent work in southeast Asia by a team from the Food and Agriculture Organization of the United Nations has demonstrated that rice pests can be prevented from causing serious damage by encouraging predators, especially spiders, by such means as avoiding weeding the bunds around fields and piling up trash on them as refuges between crops.

In the U.S.A. there are several well known examples, for instance strip harvesting of alfalfa to allow natural enemy populations to move into uncut stips and maintain a high density.

*Phil. Trans. R. Soc. Lond.* B **318**, 129–169 (1988)

*Printed in Great Britain*

# Population dynamics and biological control

By R. M. May[1], F.R.S., and M. P. Hassell[2], F.R.S.

[1] *Department of Biology, Princeton University, Princeton, New Jersey 08544, U.S.A.*
[2] *Department of Pure and Applied Biology, Imperial College at Silwood Park, Ascot, Berkshire SL5 7PY, U.K.*

Using simple models for host–parasitoid and host–pathogen interactions, we present a basic framework for examining the outcome of releasing natural enemies against a target pest population in a classical biological control programme. In particular, we examine the conditions for the initial invasion and establishment of a natural enemy species, for the maximum depression of the host population, and for the persistence of the populations in a stable interaction. In these conditions there are close parallels between parasitoids and pathogens.

The practice of augmenting an existing natural enemy population by regular mass releases has been widely practised, especially with parasitoids. The conditions for eradication of the pest are very similar in host–parasitoid and host–pathogen models, namely that releases must be greater than the equilibrium production of natural enemies in the absence of releases. Any additional density dependence acting on the host population after the stage attacked by parasitoids can influence the effectiveness of augmentative releases. This is particularly the case with over-compensating density dependence when additional releases can actually lead to an increase in the host population.

A theoretical basis for biological control cannot be properly developed simply by considering the dynamics of releasing single natural enemy species. Biological control often involves the interplay among different types of natural enemies affecting the same host population. As a step in the direction of producing more complex, multispecies models, we examine the dynamics of three situations: (1) where the host is attacked by two parasitoid species; (2) by a generalist predator and a specialist parasitoid; or (3) by a parasitoid and a pathogen. The dynamics of these three-species systems can be complex, and with properties not easily foreseen from the separate pairwise interactions. These results caution us against formulating biological control strategies purely in terms of two-species systems.

For the main part we examine host–parasitoid interactions with discrete, synchronized generations. These would appear to be less suitable to tropical insects where continuous generations and life cycles of the host and parasitoid of different length are to be expected. We show, however, that cycles (with a period of one host generation) can be obtained from an age-structured simulation model, and that these are promoted by the parasitoids having a life cycle half as long as that of the host. Some implications for biological control are discussed.

Finally, we turn briefly to the dynamics of host–parasitoid and host–pathogen interactions where pesticides are also applied, and we discuss the evolution of pesticide resistance within the context of these models.

## Introduction

The broad objective of biological control is to reduce the average abundance of a pest by using one or more populations of natural enemies, and in so doing to reduce the chance of future outbreaks. These are issues that go to the very heart of population dynamics, involving the determinants of population abundance (measured by long-term average levels), the role of natural enemies in promoting the persistence of their hosts or prey, and the 'invasion' of new, natural, enemy species into established guilds. Biological control should thus be viewed as an application of the principles of population ecology; only in this way can it escape from its current state of *ad hoc* practices based mainly on poorly documented past experiences.

This does not mean, however, that such a basic ecological approach to biological control will lead to confident pronouncements on the outcome of particular programmes. Understanding the dynamics of populations in the field requires lengthy and intensive study, on time scales that are usually incompatible with the urgency imposed by heavy pest-inflicted losses. Predictions in population biology are, moreover, almost invariably probabilistic rather than deterministic. We should, therefore, look to population ecology to provide insights on general strategic problems (such as the relative merits of generalist versus specialist natural enemies, or of single versus multiple introductions), rather than detailed predictions on the use of particular natural enemies.

In this paper we shall consider for the main part the use of parasitoids and predators in biological control, although we shall also in several places draw parallels with the use of pathogens. It is encouraging that several principles apply irrespective of the type of natural enemy. We begin by considering basic components of the interactions between hosts and parasitoids, and between hosts and pathogens. This leads to a simple framework for discussing the dynamical properties of such interactions. We then extend the discussion to situations with more than one natural enemy species, with complex host and parasitoid life cycles, or with natural enemies regularly augmented by further releases or supplemented by the use of insecticides.

## BASIC FRAMEWORKS FOR THE DYNAMICS OF HOST–ENEMY INTERACTIONS

### (a) Hosts and parasitoids

More than 10% of all metazoan species are insect parasitoids, a term first applied by Reuter (1913) to describe insects that develop as larvae on the tissues of other arthropods, which they ultimately kill. Many previous studies have focused on the importance of particular attributes of parasitoids to biological control (see, for example, Hassell & May 1973; Beddington *et al.* 1978; Waage & Hassell 1982), drawing conclusions from simple models for the interaction of the population of a host and its coupled parasitoid:

$$N_{t+1} = Fg(fN_t) \, N_t f(N_t, P_t), \tag{1a}$$

and
$$P_{t+1} = cN_t\{1 - f(N_t, P_t)\}. \tag{1b}$$

Here, $N$ and $P$ are the host and parasitoid populations, respectively, within successive generations, $t$ and $t+1$; $Fg(fN_t)$ is the per capita net rate of increase of the host population (which is density dependent when the function $g$ is less than 1); $c$ is the average number of adult female parasitoids emerging from each parasitized host ($c$ therefore includes the average number of eggs laid per host parasitized, the survival of these progeny, and their sex ratio); and the function $f$ defines the fraction of hosts that are not parasitized. A feature of such interactions with discrete generations is the different dynamics that can occur depending upon the sequence of mortalities and reproduction in the host's life cycle (Wang & Gutierrez 1980; May *et al.* 1981; Hassell & May 1986). Equation (1) is for the case of parasitism acting first, followed by the density dependence defined by $g$ (see May *et al.* (1981) for a discussion of alternatives). In

[ 20 ]

effect, therefore, the model represents an age-structured host population with pre- and post-parasitism stages. The implications of this are discussed in a number of the contexts below.

Throughout this paper we shall use a particular form for the function $f$ in equation (1), namely the zero term of a distribution of parasitoid attacks on hosts that is assumed to be negative binomial (May 1978) (see figure 3):

$$f(N_t, P_t) = \left[1 + \left\{\frac{aP_t}{k(1 + aT_\mathrm{h}N_t)}\right\}\right]^{-k}. \tag{2}$$

Here, $a$ is the *per capita* searching efficiency of the parasitoids, $T_\mathrm{h}$ is their handling time (Holling 1959$a, b$) and $k$ is the parameter from the negative binomial determining the degree of contagion in the distribution of attacks. Contagion increases as $k \to 0$, whereas in the opposite limit, $k \to \infty$, the Poisson distribution is recovered to give the Nicholson–Bailey expression for independently random parasitoid attacks (Nicholson 1933; Nicholson & Bailey 1935). The use of (2), with the clumping parameter $k$ constant, enables us to explore the dynamical effects of parasitoid searching behaviour that is non-random or aggregated, without being engulfed in a proliferation of parameters characterizing the details of such behaviour; that is, (2) is no more than one among several ways in which some of the essentials of non-random search by parasitoids may be introduced in a simple way (Hassell & May 1973, 1974; Hassell 1978; May 1978; Perry & Taylor 1986). In reality, the outcome of a parasitoid's searching behaviour cannot usually be characterized so simply (Hassell & May 1974; Chesson & Murdoch 1986; Kareiva & Odell 1987; Perry & Taylor 1986). For example, the clumping parameter $k$ may depend explicitly on the overall host density, as shown in figure 1$a$. In this case the decrease in clumping as host density rises reflects the more even distribution of parasitism from patch to patch as the host population gets more abundant (Hassell 1980). Such changes in $k$ with host population size have only a minor effect on the dynamical properties of the interaction (see below).

In the simplest form of the model, defined by (1) and (2), we ignore density dependence

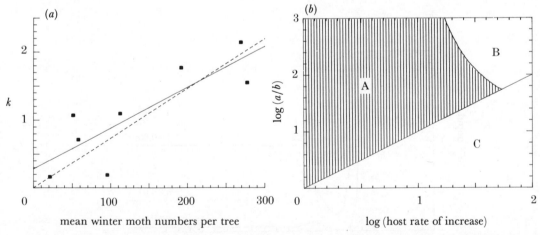

FIGURE 1. (a) The relation between the degree of clumping of parasitoid larvae per winter moth host (expressed by the parameter $k$ from the negative binomial distribution), and the mean winter moth numbers per tree. Solid line $Y = 0.28 + 0.006X$; $b_{yx}$ (slope) $\pm 0.004$. Broken line: regression constrained through the origin, $Y = 0.007X$. (b) Local stability boundaries for the model in equations (1) and (2), in terms of the parameter combination $a/b$ (where $a$ is the parasitoid searching efficiency and $b$ is the slope (equal to 0.006) of the regression in (a)). The model is stable in region A and shows expanding oscillation in regions B and C. (With $k$ constant, the model is locally stable in both regions A and B, which corresponds to the condition $k < 1$.) (After Hassell (1980).)

and handling time $(g(fN_t) = 1$ and $T_h = 0)$, whereupon the population dynamics are easily understood. The equilibrium populations are given by $N^* = P^*/(1-1/F)$ and $P^* = (k/a)\,[F^{1/k} - 1]$, and the system is stable, with disturbances damping back to the equilibrium state, for all $k$ less than 1. In short, increasing the contagion in the distribution of parasitoid attacks promotes stability. Interestingly, values of $k$ have been estimated for several species of insect parasitoid (see, for example, papers by Broadhead & Cheke 1975; Hassell 1980; Elliott 1982, 1983; Perry & Taylor 1986), and in almost all cases the mean value is less than unity. Making $k$ a function of host density, as in figure 1$a$, does not affect this conclusion; it merely makes the condition for stability a little more restrictive, as shown in figure 1$b$.

More generally, if we take account of other density-dependent factors (apart from parasitoids) influencing host abundance, the parasitoid population may not be able to maintain itself. Specifically, suppose that the host population in the absence of parasitoids fluctuates about some long-term average density or 'carrying capacity', $K$ (given from (1) by $Fg(K) = 1$). The parasitoids will be unable to invade and persist in this system (that is $P_t$ will not increase from low levels) if $K$ is below a threshold value $K_T$, given (for $T_h = 0$) by

$$K_T = 1/ac. \tag{3}$$

Note that, as expected, this threshold host density decreases (so that parasitoid persistence is easier) as parasitoid searching efficiency, $a$, increases.

Comparable models framed as differential equations, and thus appropriate to situations with completely overlapping generations, have also been developed (see, for example, Leslie & Gower 1960; Pielou 1969; Murdoch & Oaten 1975). We shall, however, restrict ourselves here to interactions in which generations are effectively discrete and non-overlapping. Not only are these common in temperate regions (e.g. univoltine insect pests attacking fruit and timber trees), but also they can arise in much less seasonal, uniform conditions, as a direct consequence of the host–parasitoid interaction itself (Auslander *et al.* 1974; and see below).

Classical biological control involves the introduction of a natural enemy against a pest

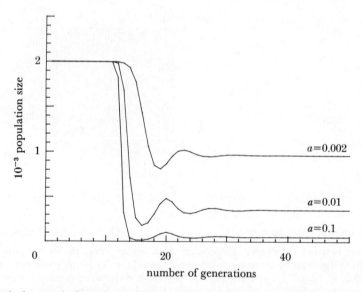

FIGURE 2. Numerical example from the model in equations (1) and (2), showing a host population reduced from its carrying capacity by the introduction of parasitoids in generation 10. The three lines show the different outcomes with parasitoids of different searching efficiencies as shown. Other parameters: $F = 3$, $k = 0.5$.

population fluctuating around its carrying capacity. Whether the parasitoid can establish itself and, if so, whether the host population is unstable or persists closely around a new lower level (as in the examples in figure 2) will depend upon several components of the interaction, such as the nature of the function $f$, whether the host rate of increase is density dependent, and whether $c$ is a function of parasitoid density (e.g. due to density dependence in parasitoid sex ratios (Hassell *et al.* 1983)). The degree of 'depression' of the host population below its carrying capacity was defined by Beddington *et al.* (1975) as the ratio, $q$, of host average abundances before and after the introduction of parasitoids (i.e. $q = K/N^*$, where $K$ is the carrying capacity in the absence of the parasitoid; see figure 2). The magnitude of $q$, and therefore the success of the parasitoid as a biological control agent, depends upon the balance between:

(1) the host's net rate of increase ($Fg(fN_t)$ in (1)), and

(2) the various factors affecting overall parasitoid performance, such as the *per capita* searching efficiency ($a$) and maximum attack rate of adult females, the spatial distribution of parasitism in relation to that of the host, and the sex ratio and survival of parasitoid progeny.

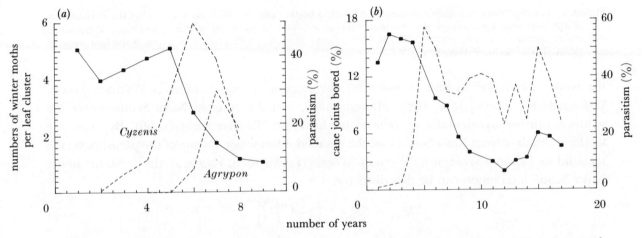

FIGURE 3. The biological control of two insect pests after the introduction of parasitoids. (*a*) The winter moth (*O. brumata*) in Nova Scotia by the tachinid *C. albicans*, and the ichneumonid *Agrypon falveolatum* (after Embree 1966). (*b*) Sugar cane stem borers (*Diatraea* spp.) by the tachinid *Lyxophaga diatraeae*, and the braconid *Apanteles falvipes* (after Anon 1980). Broken lines indicate percent parasitism (From Waage & Hassell (1982).)

Cases of successful biological control have never been monitored sufficiently before, during and after the release of natural enemies to enable convincing pictures to be drawn in the manner of figure 2. Figure 3*a,b* shows two of the best examples. In the case of the winter moth in Nova Scotia, although not properly quantified, it is known that the populations have persisted at very low levels since accurate sampling ceased (see below). A much clearer example of what natural enemies can do is given in figure 4, showing a resource-limited host population in the laboratory declining after the introduction of parasitoids, and then persisting in a relatively stable host–parasitoid interaction.

In one case, at least, the parameters in (1) and (2) have been estimated for a successful biological control programme; that of the winter moth (*Operophtera brumata*) in Nova Scotia, which was successfully controlled in hardwood forests after the establishment of the two parasitoids from Europe (figure 3*a*). The information comes from two independent studies on

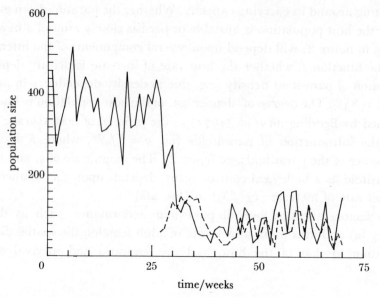

FIGURE 4. The depression in population size of the bruchid beetle *Callosobruchus chinensis* (——) after the introduction of the pteromalid parasitoid *Anisopteromalus calandrae* (----) in week 26 of the interaction. Populations maintained in the laboratory at 30 °C and 70 % relative humidity, with black-eyed beans as the host resource (V. A. Taylor & M. P. Hassell, unpublished results).

the winter moth and its natural enemies: one from a natural habitat in Wytham Wood, Oxford, U.K., (Varley *et al.* 1973; Hassell 1980), and the other in Nova Scotia where the winter moth was accidentally introduced in the 1930s (Embree 1965, 1966). By using the winter moth data from Nova Scotia and the detailed information on one of the parasitoids (the tachinid fly *Cyzenis albicans*) from Wytham Wood (Hassell 1968, 1969 *a*, *b*), the dynamics of the Nova Scotia interaction can be described by

$$N_{t+1} = FN_t s_e s_p \left\{ 1 + \left( \frac{aP_t}{k} \right) \right\}^{-k}, \qquad (4a)$$

and

$$P_{t+1} = 0.65 N_t \left[ 1 - \left\{ 1 + \left( \frac{aP_t}{k} \right) \right\}^{-k} \right]. \qquad (4b)$$

Here, $F = 89$; $s_e$ (equal to 0.02) is the mean fractional survival of winter moth between the estimated egg and prepupal stages; and $s_p$ (equal to 0.65) is the mean survival of winter moth pupae in the soil, probably due mainly to generalist predators (the same affects the *C. albicans* pupae, as shown in (4*b*)). Finally, $a$ (0.14 m$^2$ per generation) is the searching efficiency of *C. albicans* and $k$ ($0.28 + 0.006 N_t$) is the degree of clumping of parasitism within hosts, both determined at Wytham Wood (Hassell 1980); note the explicit dependence of the clumping parameter $k$ upon host density (see figure 1*a* above).

The predictions of this model are shown in figure 5. The small equilibrium populations are the result of the balance between (*a*) the low net rate of increase of the winter moth once it is discounted by the mortalities other than parasitism (i.e. $Fs_e s_p = 1.16$) and (*b*) the high overall *per capita* efficiency of the parasitoids (a combination of a high value of $a$ (equal to 0.18) and the relatively high survival of parasitoid progeny (0.65)). The persistence of the populations at these low levels is entirely due to the clumped distributions of parasitoid progeny among the total host population resulting from the small values of $k$ in (4). Without these clumping effects

[ 24 ]

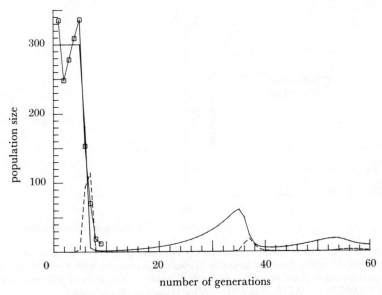

FIGURE 5. Biological control of the winter moth in Nova Scotia. Solid and broken lines give the host and parasitoid populations per square metre of canopy area, respectively, predicted from the model in equation (4). Parameter values: $F = 89$, $s_e = 0.02$, $s_p = 0.65$, $a = 0.14$ m² and $k = 0.28 + 0.006 Nt$. Solid points give the observed winter moth larval populations (data from Embree 1966). (For further details see Hassell (1980).)

(i.e. assuming random parasitism), there is no regulatory mechanism and the model is unstable.

The values of $k$ in figure 1a were obtained by fitting the negative binomial distribution to frequency distributions of *C. albicans* larvae within the salivary glands of dissected winter moth larvae collected at Wytham Wood (figure 6a). Behaviourally, these patterns arise from the tendency of adult *C. albicans* to oviposit preferentially in areas of high leaf damage, thus causing higher probabilities of parasitism in areas with higher winter moth density, as shown in figure 6b (Hassell 1968). Examples of such spatial density dependence are matched in the literature by as many others that are inversely density dependent, and by those that show no relation at all. They may all be explained, however, in the same terms of different allocations of foraging time between patches and differing constraints on the maximum attack rate within a patch (Hassell 1982a; Lessells 1985). Interestingly, both the direct *and* inverse patterns can contribute markedly to population regulation, with the details of the host distribution determining which is the more important in any particular case (Hassell 1984).

Such variation in the fate of host individuals in different patches is only one of several different ways in which within-generation heterogeneity can arise. Alternatively, some hosts may be protected from parasitism within some form of explicit physical refuge (Maynard Smith 1974; Hassell 1978), or there may be some degree of temporal asynchrony between parasitoids and hosts (a refuge in time; Griffiths (1969); Hassell (1969a)), or hosts may vary in some phenotypic character(s) that make(s) some individuals more able to resist parasitism than others (Hassell & Anderson 1984). All these mechanisms, however, share the property of rendering some individuals more susceptible to parasitism than others, giving different probabilities of parasitism for different host individuals or groups of individuals. This in turn creates a partial refuge for the host population, which promotes the stability of the interaction (Bailey *et al.* 1961; Hassell & May 1973).

[ 25 ]

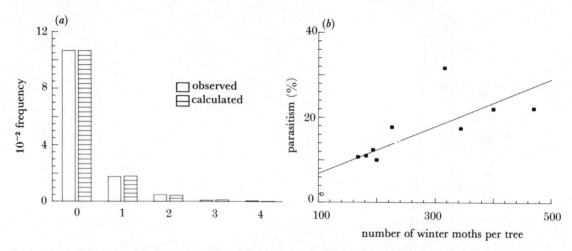

FIGURE 6. (a) The observed frequencies of winter moth larvae containing different numbers of C. albicans larvae, compared with the expected values from the negative binomial distribution with $k = 0.55$. (b) The same data as in (a), but now partitioned to show the different levels of parasitism on trees of different local winter moth density ($Y = 1.250 + 0.055X$; $r = 0.772$, $P < 0.01$). (After Hassell & May (1985).)

We have, therefore, a picture in which specialist, synchronized parasitoids can make effective biological control agents provided that their overall *per capita* efficiency (in relation to the discounted host's net rate of increase) is high enough to cause a marked depression of the host equilibrium. In general, however, this 'overall efficiency' is not simply the usual instantaneous measure, $a$, of equations (2) and ($4a, b$). Also included should be any constraints on parasitoid performance, such as a low maximum attack rate, male-biased sex ratios, mortalities of parasitoid progeny, and distributions of parasitism that are not well correlated with the distribution of hosts (i.e. course-grained). Including these factors gives more complex measures of parasitoid efficiency, such as

$$A = \frac{1}{n}\sum_{n=1}^{n}\left\{\frac{1}{P_iT_i}\ln\left(\frac{N_i}{N_i - P_e}\right)\right\}. \tag{5}$$

Here, $n$ represents the number of patches, $P_iT_i$, the number of adult parasitoids and the average time they spend searching for $N_i$ hosts, and $P_e$ the number of adult parasitoids emerging, all within patch $i$ (Hassell 1982b). Along with such high parasitoid efficiency, successful biological control also requires some regulatory mechanism(s) that minimize(s) the chance of future outbreaks. Obvious density-dependent processes, such as resource limitation on host density or mutual interference between parasitoids, are unlikely candidates when populations are sparse. The various mechanisms generating heterogeneity in the distribution of parasitoid attacks are, however, as marked, or more so, when populations are sparse, and so provide a plausible and potentially powerful means of regulating interactions associated with biological control (Beddington et al. 1978).

This conclusion stems from models in which there is complete redistribution of host and parasitoid individuals within the habitat in each generation. All patches are thus recolonized afresh each generation, and this is clearly appropriate for many, more mobile species. At the other extreme, however, there are interactions in which hosts and parasitoids can interact within a patch over several generations, with only a certain amount of mixing and recolonization of patches in each generation. Scale insects and their natural enemies, or predator–prey interactions involving mites, provide good examples. In such cases, local

[ 26 ]

extinction of hosts and parasitoids within patches can easily occur (Murdoch *et al.* 1985; Chesson 1981), and the persistence of the system as a whole is dominated by the degree of asynchrony between the state of the different patches rather than by the spatial distribution of parasitism *per se* (Sabelis & Laane 1986; Sabelis & van der Meer 1986). There is thus a continuum from cases of more or less complete mixing of the subpopulations each generation (e.g. winter moth) where heterogeneity in the distribution of parasitism is likely to be very important for regulation, to cases in which large fractions of the host and parasitoid populations do not move from their patches and where persistence is largely governed by the temporal refuge effect of host patches being colonized at different times by the natural enemies (J. K. Waage, M. Sabelis & M. P. Hassell, unpublished results; see Waage (this symposium) for further details). The ideal attributes of a successful biological control agent in the latter case have yet to be explored, but clearly they will include the ability of the natural enemies to locate host patches and, once there, to exploit the host sub-population rapidly by the natural enemies' combined functional and numerical responses.

### (b) Hosts and pathogens

Viruses, bacteria, Protozoa and fungi can kill insects, and such pathogens have been deliberately used in efforts to control particular insect pests. The use of the bacterium *Bacillus thuringiensis* against the gypsy moth, *Lymantria dispar*, in North America is probably the best-known example. A variety of other case studies are reviewed by Tinsley & Entwhistle (1974), Tinsley (1979) and Falcon (1982). Unlike the work involving parasitoids, such empirical efforts to use pathogens as agents of biological control have, until recently, not been accompanied by analysis of the underlying dynamics of insect host–pathogen systems. Such a theoretical framework has recently been explored by Anderson & May (1981), who indicate applications to specific interactions between some insect pests and viral or microspordian protozoan pathogens. What follows is a brief summary of this work, which is still in its formative stages.

Consider first a host population with discrete, non-overlapping generations, whose average density is regulated by a lethal pathogen that spreads in epidemic fashion through each generation before reproduction. The dynamics of this population is again described by equation (1 a) (where $g = 1$ in the absence of other density-dependent effects):

$$N_{t+1} = FN_t f(N_t). \tag{6}$$

The difference between this and (1 a) is that $f(N_t)$ now represents the fraction escaping infection (rather than escaping parasitoid attack). This fraction escaping infection as an epidemic spreads through a population of density $N_t$ is given implicitly by the Kermack–McKendrick expression, $f = \exp\{-(1-f)\,N_t/N_T\}$ (Kermack & McKendrick 1927); here $N_T$ is the threshold host density (which depends on the virulence and transmissibility of the pathogen). For $N$ less than $N_T$, the epidemic cannot spread ($f = 1$), whereas the infected fraction, $f$, falls to ever smaller values as $N$ increases above $N_T$. This simple, natural and purely deterministic model exhibits completely chaotic behaviour: the system has no stable equilibrium point, nor any stable cycles, but rather fluctuates (tending to alternate between relatively high and relatively low population densities) in such a way that the deterministic dynamics are effectively indistinguishable from the sample function of some random process (for a more detailed discussion, see May (1985)).

Equation (6), with its bizarre dynamics, is the analogue (for regulation by a pathogen) of the familiar Nicholson–Bailey equation (for regulation by a parasitoid). Had (6) been studied sooner, chaotic dynamics may have forced themselves upon our attention earlier, and the history of several subjects might be different. As it is, the dynamical properties of (6) have been appreciated too recently for them yet to have motivated any systematic study of field or laboratory populations. Most of the insect host–pathogen systems that have received attention differ from the model of (6) in that transmission is via free-living infective stages of the pathogen (rather than by direct contact between susceptible and infected hosts, as in the Kermack–McKendrick assumption), and/or host generations to some extent overlap (so that differential, rather than difference, equations are appropriate). Largely for these reasons, studies of insect host–pathogen dynamics have mainly used differential equations, representing the approximation that populations of hosts and pathogens change in a continuous way.

In the simplest such model, the host population is assumed to have a *per capita* birth rate $a$ and a *per capita* death rate $b$ from all causes other than the pathogen, both of which rates are density independent. The total population $N(t)$ is partitioned into uninfected and infected hosts, with population densities $X(t)$ and $Y(t)$, respectively; $N = X + Y$. Although invertebrate species are usually able to mount cellular or humoral responses to infection, current evidence suggests they are not able to develop acquired immunity to agents of infectious disease (Anderson & May 1981). Thus the basic model is lacking the class of recovered-and-immune hosts found in conventional epidemiological models for vertebrates. The basic model further assumes that infections are transmitted directly from infected to uninfected hosts, so that the net rate at which new infections appears is $\beta XY$, where $\beta$ is a transmission parameter. This description of the infection process accords with some data (Anderson & May 1981). Infected hosts either recover (at a rate $\gamma$, so that the characteristic recovery time is $1/\gamma$), or are killed by the disease (at a rate $\alpha$).

When all this is put together, the dynamics of the model population are given by

$$dX/dt = a(X + Y) - bX - \beta XY + \gamma Y, \tag{7a}$$

and

$$dY/dt = \beta XY - (\alpha + b + \gamma) Y. \tag{7b}$$

New susceptibles appear by birth (from either infected or uninfected individuals) or by recovery from the infected state; infectious individuals appear at the rate $\beta XY$, and remain infectious for an average time of $1/(\alpha + b + \gamma)$ before they die of the disease or of other causes, or recover. The overall population density obeys

$$dN/dt = rN - \alpha Y. \tag{7c}$$

Here we have defined $r$ equal to $a - b$ as the *per capita* rate of population growth in the absence of the pathogen.

In the absence of infection ($Y$ equal to 0, $N$ equal to $X$), this model population will grow exponentially at the rate $r$. If a small number of infectious individuals are introduced into such a disease-free population (corresponding to $X$ approximately equal to $N$, $Y$ much less then $N$), the infection will spread and establish itself provided the right-hand side of (7b) is positive; this will be the case if $N > N_T$, where the threshold host density $N_T$ is defined as

$$N_T \equiv (\alpha + b + \gamma)/\beta. \tag{8}$$

[ 28 ]

Given the exponential growth of this host population in the absence of the disease, the threshold will always be attained eventually, and thus the infection can always establish itself sooner or later. More generally, if other density-dependent factors regulate the host population around some average value $K$ in the absence of disease, then the pathogen can invade only if $N_T < K$; this result is directly analogous to the earlier threshold results for parasitoid establishment.

Once established, the virus, bacterium, or other infectious agent can, in the absence of any other density-dependent effects, regulate the host population density, provided it is sufficiently pathogenic:

$$a > r. \tag{9}$$

If this regulatory criterion is met, then in the simplest model the host population is regulated to a constant equilibrium value, $N^*$, given by $N^* = [\alpha/(\alpha-r)] N_T$, with $N_T$ given by (8). The fraction of this equilibrium host population that is infected at any one time is simply $Y^*/N^* = r/\alpha$; perhaps surprisingly, the more virulent the infection (the larger $\alpha$), the smaller the equilibrium fraction infected. On the other hand if (9) is not satisfied, the host population continues to grow exponentially at a diminished *per capita* rate, $r' = r - \alpha$, until other kinds of regulatory effect can no longer be ignored.

Table 1 lists some estimates of *per capita* mortality rates induced by pathogens, $\alpha$, and from other natural causes, $b$, for a miscellany of invertebrate hosts and viral, bacterial, protozoan, and fungal infections. Table 1 lacks corresponding estimates of the *per capita* birth rates, $a$, and consequently lacks comparisons between $\alpha$ and $r$; there are, unfortunately, very few field studies that give estimates of all three parameters. Thus it is hard to say how often $\alpha$ exceeds $r$ in the field. The data compiled in table 1 do no more than indicate that many disease agents of invertebrates are highly pathogenic, with the most pronounced pathogenicity tending to arise among viral and bacterial agents. For a more full discussion, both of the theory and the data, see Anderson & May (1981).

Notice that, just as self-maintaining parasitoids cannot in general eradicate their hosts, so too pathogens will not in general be capable of eradicating the target pest species; once the host population is driven to sufficiently low densities, it will be below threshold for maintenance of the pathogen. Exceptions can arise by some of the complications discussed below; eradication could, for instance, be made possible by extreme cases of vertical transmission. Given that a self-sustaining pathogen is unable to eradicate the pest, the aim is usually to reduce the host population significantly below its disease-free average level, $K$ (around which the pristine population may have exhibited a greater or lesser degree of density-independent fluctuation). The question thus arises, what is the degree of pathogenicity, $\alpha$, producing maximum depression of the pest population?

First thoughts might suggest that the greater the pathogenicity, the better. Certainly, if $\alpha \to 0$ the pathogen has no effect on host population growth. But, at the other extreme, too large a value for $\alpha$ leads to too large a value of $N_T$ (essentially because the disease kills hosts so fast that a very large host population is needed to perpetuate the infection), and thence to the regulated population having high density. As emphasized by Anderson & May (1981), the optimum self-sustaining control, in the sense of lowest equilibrium levels of pest population density, will usually be attained from an infectious disease agent with intermediate pathogenicity. For the simple model of equation (7), we can see this explicitly from the expression $N^* = \alpha(\alpha + b + \gamma)/\{(\alpha - r)\beta\}$, which is minimized for the intermediate value

TABLE 1. NATURAL AND PATHOGEN-INDUCED MORTALITY RATES FOR INSECT HOSTS OF SOME VIRAL, BACTERIAL, PROTOZOAN AND FUNGAL INFECTIONS

(From Anderson & May (1981), where references are given. Ewald (1987) has in some cases given independent assessments of these mortality rates, by using a somewhat different estimation procedure; his estimates are within factor-of-two agreement.)

| pathogen | host | natural mortality rate, $b$ (per week) | pathogen-induced mortality rate, $\alpha$ (per week) | ratio $\alpha/b$ (one figure accuracy) |
|---|---|---|---|---|
| **Viruses** | | | | |
| sack brood virus | Apis mellifera | 0.170 | 1.200 | 7 |
| nuclear polyhedrosis virus | Cadra cautella | 0.061 | 0.540 | 9 |
| nuclear polyhedrosis virus | Hyphantria cunea | 0.003 | 0.800 | 300 |
| A.B.P. virus | Apis mellifera | 0.250 | 1.900 | 8 |
| nuclear polyhedrosis virus | Porthetria dispar | 0.060 | 0.630 | 10 |
| nuclear polyhedrosis virus | Malacosoma americanum | 0.070 | 0.370 | 5 |
| **Bacteria** | | | | |
| Bacillus thuringiensis | Simulium vittatum | 0.035 | 2.400 | 70 |
| B. thuringiensis | Choristoneura fumiferana | 0.001 | 4.000 | 4 000 |
| Aeromonas punctata | Anopheles annulipes | 0.360 | 2.900 | 8 |
| Erwinia spp. | Colladonus montanus | 0.031 | 0.170 | 5 |
| **Protozoa** | | | | |
| Nosema stegomyiae | Anopheles albimanus | 0.230 | 0.410 | 2 |
| Pleistrophora schubergi | Hyphantria cunea | 0.003 | 0.036 | 10 |
| Herpetomonas muscarum | Hippelates pusio | 0.170 | 0.430 | 3 |
| Tetrahymena pyriformis | Culex tarsalis | 0.260 | 0.660 | 3 |
| **Fungi** | | | | |
| Beauveria tenella | Aedes siemensis | 0.026 | 0.500 | 20 |
| B. tenella | Culex tarsalis | 0.110 | 0.840 | 8 |
| B. bassiana | Musca domestica | 0.270 | 0.740 | 3 |
| B. bassiana | Hylemya antiqua | 0.300 | 0.550 | 2 |
| B. bassiana | Phormia regina | 0.240 | 0.560 | 2 |
| Metarrhizium anisopliae | Musca domestica | 0.270 | 0.380 | 1 |
| M. anisopliae | Hylemya antiquia | 0.300 | 0.480 | 2 |
| M. anisopliae | Phormia regina | 0.240 | 0.420 | 2 |
| Aspergillus flavus | Culex peus | 0.020 | 0.170 | 9 |
| A. flavus | C. tarsalis | 0.061 | 0.220 | 4 |
| Fusarium oxysporum | C. pipiens | 0.027 | 0.620 | 20 |

$\alpha = r + \{r(a+\gamma)\}^{\frac{1}{2}}$ (and which becomes infinite for $\alpha \to \infty$ or $\alpha \to r$). This is an important point, because many control programmes assume that the most virulent pathogens are necessarily the best. This may to some extent be true for inundative release programmes, but it is not true for programmes that aim at a degree of self-perpetuation of the pathogen.

The basic model of (7) omits many biological features that can complicate host–pathogen systems. Briefly, pathogens may reduce the reproductive output of infected hosts (making it more likely that the pathogen will regulate the host population), may be transmitted 'vertically' from parent to unborn offspring (which decreases $N_T$, making it easier to maintain the infection in relatively low density populations of hosts), and may undergo an incubation or latent period within the host, during which time the host is infected but not yet infectious (this process tends to increase $N_T$, and also makes it less likely the infection will regulate the host population). The pathogenicity of the infection may, moreover, depend on the nutritional state of the host, which in turn is likely to depend on the host population density; under these circumstances, the host population may have two alternative stable states, and pass from one

TABLE 2. SUMMARY OF THE WAY IN WHICH SOME REALISTIC COMPLICATIONS CAN AFFECT THE ABILITY OF A PATHOGEN TO REGULATE ITS HOST POPULATION, AND TO PERSIST WITHIN A POPULATION OF HOSTS THAT EITHER IS OF LOW DENSITY OR FLUCTUATES WIDELY IN ABUNDANCE

| complicating factor | effect on regulatory capacity of pathogen (relative to basic model defined by equation (7)) | effect on threshold host density to maintain pathogen (relative to basic model) |
| --- | --- | --- |
| diminution in reproductive capacity of infected hosts | regulation is easier; regulated host population density is lower | no effect on threshold criterion |
| vertical transmission | no effect on regulatory condition; regulated host population density is lower | threshold host density lower (can be arbitrarily small) |
| latent period of infection | regulation is harder; regulated host population density is higher | threshold host density is higher |
| pathogenicity is stress related | can always regulate if pathogenicity is sufficiently strongly enhanced by stress | pathogen can persist provided transmission efficiency is high enough |
| other density-dependent constraints on host population growth | disease-related depression of host population density maximized for an intermediate degree of pathogenicity | pathogen cannot persist if threshold host density is too high (if $N_T > K$) |
| free-living infective stages of pathogen | regulatory criterion as for basic model; regulated state may be a stable point or cyclic oscillations | easier to maintain pathogen, especially if infective stages are long-lived |

to the other discontinuously. The effects of these complications are summarized in table 2, and discussed in detail elsewhere (Anderson & May 1981).

A major complication arises when the free-living transmission stages of the pathogen are long-lived, as happens for many pathogens of insects. Such free-living infective stages include the spores of many bacteria, protozoans and fungi, and the capsules, polyhedra or free particles of viruses (Tinsley 1979). In particular, baculoviruses of univoltine insects of temperate forests (principally of lepidopteran, hymenopteran and dipteran species) tend to have long-lived infective stages, partly because the soil environment of temperate forests affords relative protection from the ultraviolet components of sunlight (Jacques 1977). In the event of such complications, we define the population of free-living infective stages of the pathogen to be $W(t)$ at time $t$; in $(7b)$ the transmission term is now proportional to the rate of encounters between susceptible hosts and infective stages of the parasite, $vWX$:

$$\mathrm{d}Y/\mathrm{d}t = vWX - (\alpha + b + \gamma) Y. \tag{10}$$

Equation $(7c)$ for $N(t)$ remains unchanged. Infective stages are produced at a rate $\lambda$ from infected hosts, and are lost by death (at a rate $\mu$) or by absorption in hosts (at a rate $vN$), which gives

$$\mathrm{d}W/\mathrm{d}t = \lambda Y - (\mu + vN) W. \tag{11}$$

The three equations $(7c)$, $(10)$ and $(11)$ give a complete description of the dynamical behaviour of the variables $N(t)$, $Y(t)$ and $W(t)$. Provided infected hosts produce transmission stages of the parasite at a sufficiently fast rate (specifically, $\lambda > \alpha(\alpha + b + \gamma)/(\alpha - r)$), the pathogen will again regulate its host population so long as $\alpha > r$. However, the regulated state may be a stable point, or it may be a stable cycle. The cyclic solutions tend to arise for infections of high pathogenicity that produce large numbers of long-lived infective stages. In effect, the 'seedbank' of long-lived transmission stages can induce oscillations by the time lags it introduces into the system; the longer the life of transmission stages in relation to the characteristic regulatory time-scale (set largely by $1/\alpha$), the greater the propensity to oscillation.

Many microsporidian protozoan and baculovirus infections of insects appear to possess the combination of a relatively large $\alpha$ and a small $\mu$ that produces cyclic changes in host

TABLE 3. CYCLIC VARIATIONS IN THE ABUNDANCE OF FOREST INSECT SPECIES (FROM ANDERSON AND MAY (1981), WHERE REFERENCES ARE GIVEN)

| host insect species | locality | period of cycles in population abundance (years) | pathogen |
|---|---|---|---|
| *Orgyia pseudotsugata* (Douglas-fir tussock moth) | North America | 7–10 | nuclear polyhedrosis virus |
| *Acleris variana* (black-headed budworm) | eastern Canada | 10–15 | nuclear polyhedrosis virus |
| *Bupalus piniarius* (pine looper) | Europe | 5–8 | nuclear polyhedrosis virus |
| *Zeiraphera diniana* (larch bud moth) | Europe | 9–10 | granulosis virus |
| *Diprion hercyniae* (spruce sawfly) | North America | 8 | nuclear polyhedrosis virus |
| *Malacosoma disstria* (tent caterpillar) | North America | 8–12 | nuclear polyhedrosis virus |

abundance. For the forest insect pests listed (with associated pathogens) in table 3, insertion of reasonable estimates of $\alpha$, $\mu$, and $r$ in $(7c)$, $(10)$ and $(11)$ suggests cycles with periods in the general range 3–30 years, in approximate accord with the observed periods of 5–12 years for these pests. Only for the larch budmoth, *Zeiraphera diniana*, and an associated granulosis virus could Anderson & May (1980) find sufficient data to estimate all parameters in the relevant model. In this one instance they did find an encouraging fit between the observed and theoretically estimated periods of the oscillations in host density, and in the cyclic patterns of prevalence of infection (although the agreement between the observed and theoretically estimated amplitudes of the cycles in host density were less encouraging, with the observed amplitude being an order of magnitude larger than the theoretical estimate). McNamee *et al.* (1981) have refined the analysis, but there remains much scope for further research, particularly in field studies of forest insects and their pathogens.

## AUGMENTATIVE RELEASES

### (a) *Release of parasitoids*

The regular, inundative release of mass-reared parasitoids, most often *Trichogramma* spp. that attack the egg stage of a wide range of insect species, has been practised since early in this century as an alternative to classical biological control, particularly against lepidopterous pests (DeBach & Hagen 1970; Ables & Ridgeway 1981). The efficacy of such programmes is limited by a number of factors (Stinner 1977), which are now listed.

(1) Mass rearing can often decrease the fecundity, longevity and searching efficiency of parasitoids (Stinner *et al.* 1974).

(2) Released parasitoids may rapidly disperse away from the crop in question. Possible remedies for this are to 'pretreat' parasitoids with host kairomones to stimulate search after release (Gross *et al.* 1975), or to apply the kairomones directly to the crop to act as arrestants for the released parasitoids (Lewis *et al.* 1975; Waage & Hassell 1982).

(3) The released individuals may act as a kind of biological insecticide in the sense that none of the parasitoid progeny survive or remain in the area to parasitize future pest generations. This differs in spirit somewhat from programmes that aim to augment an established population of natural enemies of the same or different species.

(4) Lepidopterous pests generally suffer high mortality among early larval stages. This has led to controversy and conflicting reports on the potential impact of released egg-parasitoids in relation to other later occurring mortalities (see, for example, Myers 1929; Box 1932; Pickles 1936; Metcalfe & Breniere 1969). In addition, in the case of graminaceous stalk borers, this early larval mortality is likely to be density dependent owing to competition for the limited space within a stem, as shown by the example in figure 7 for the sorghum stalk borer, *Chilo partellus*, (van Hamburg & Hassell 1984). This raises additional problems for parasitoid release, as discussed in relation to the models below.

A theoretical treatment for several models of periodic mass release of parasitoids has been given by Barclay *et al.* (1985). Before this the only theoretical discussion of such inundative releases is that of Knipling & McGuire (1968) (see also Knipling 1972), who used simple numerical examples of the release of Nicholson–Bailey parasitoids to investigate how levels of parasitism were affected by the density at which parasitoids were released and by their searching efficiency. The examples considered by Barclay *et al.* (1985) are all for discrete

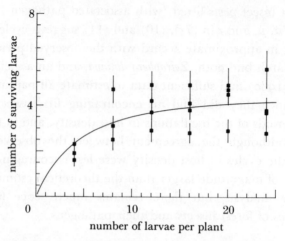

FIGURE 7. The density dependent relationship between the number of surviving larvae ($S$) of the sorghum stalk borer (*Chilo partellus*) and the first instar larvae per plant in a glasshouse experiment. Means ($\pm$ standard errors (s.e.)) of 15 replicates are shown, and the data are described by the model, $S = N(1+dN)^{-b}$, fitted by nonlinear least squares ($d = 0.15\pm0.09$, $b = 1.16\pm0.41$ (s.e.)). (After van Hamburg & Hassell (1984).)

host–parasitoid interactions, as in equation (1). In what follows, we revisit some of their results, and also discuss the impact of augmentative releases where the pest is already attacked by a different parasitoid species (see also Appendix 1). The analogous studies of criteria for eradicating pests by pathogen release are presented elsewhere (Anderson & May 1981), and are only briefly summarized here.

Consider a simple extension of the model in (1):

$$N_{t+1} = FN_t g(fN_t) f(P_t) \tag{12a}$$

and

$$P_{t+1} = cN_t\{1 - f(P_t)\} + R. \tag{12b}$$

Here, $R$ represents the population of the released parasitoids in each generation, and the function $f$ is given by (2). If we neglect for the moment the host density dependence in (12a) (i.e. put $g = 1$), our conclusions from this model are straightforward (the results are derived in Appendix 1).

(1) There is a linear decline in the host equilibrium level as $R$ increases, leading to eradication when $R > P^*$ (where $P^*$ is the pristine equilibrium density of parasitoid adults, before any programme of releases); see figure 8a.

(2) Parasitoid releases insufficient to eradicate the host promote stability, to the point where even a Nicholson–Bailey interaction (random search) can be stabilized if the releases are large enough; see figure 8b.

Equations (12a,b) are for the particular case of parasitism acting first in the host's life cycle, followed by an additional density-dependent mortality acting at a later host stage, as in the sorghum stalk borer example above. The degree of depression in the host population, caused by the releases of parasitoids, now depends critically on whether the host density dependence is under-, exactly or over-compensating (figure 9). Releases will always complement under-compensating density dependence ($b < 1$) and lead to lower equilibria than if either acted alone (figure 10a). However, as the density dependence becomes more severe, there is a growing risk that any parasitoid releases will be valueless (i.e. the density dependence compensates for the additional parasitism) or, worse still, may actually lead to higher pest

[ 34 ]

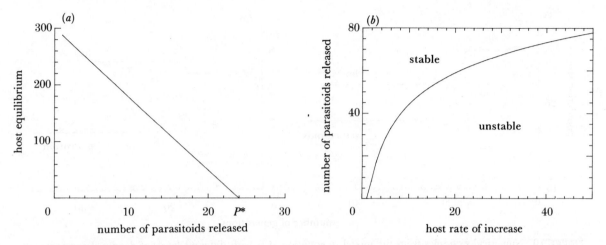

FIGURE 8. Equilibrium and stability properties of the model in equation (12). (a) The decline in host equilibrium levels ($N^*$) as $R$, the number of parasitoids released, increases. Eradication occurs when $R > P^*$, where $P^* = (k/a)\,(F^{\frac{1}{k}-1})$, $N^* = (P^* - R)/(1 - 1/F)$ and $a = 0.05$, $k = 0.5$ and $F = 5$. (b) Stable and unstable regions in relation to the number of parasitoids released, $R$, and the host rate of increase, $F$, with parameters as in (a) except $k \to \infty$ (i.e. random parasitism).

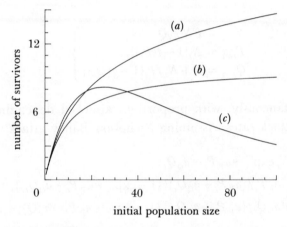

FIGURE 9. Examples of (a) under-compensating, (b) compensating and (c) over-compensating density dependence from the model $S = N(1 + dN)^{-b}$ (see also figure 7). Parameter values: (a) $d = 0.1$, $b = 0.8$, (b) $d = 0.1$, $b = 1$; (c) $d = 0.01$, $b = 5$.

populations if the density dependence is over-compensating ($b$ greater than 1), as shown by the example in figure 10b. It may well be that some of the conflicting results after releases of *Trichogramma* against stem borers, such as *Diatrea saccharalis* (see, for example, Box 1932; Tucker 1934 a,b; Metcalfe & van Whervin 1967) result from differences in the degree of larval density dependence in different situations and areas.

Often, augmentative releases are used where the pest is already attacked by parasitoids of a different species. Once again, the order of parasitism by the different species is important to the outcome (May & Hassell 1981). With species P already present and Q released augmentatively, the possibilities are:

(a) Q acts first:

$$\left.\begin{aligned}
N_{t+1} &= FN_t g(Q_t) f(P_t), \\
Q_{t+1} &= R + N_t\{1 - g(Q_t)\}, \\
P_{t+1} &= N_t g(Q_t)\,\{1 - f(P_t)\}.
\end{aligned}\right\} \qquad (13)$$

and

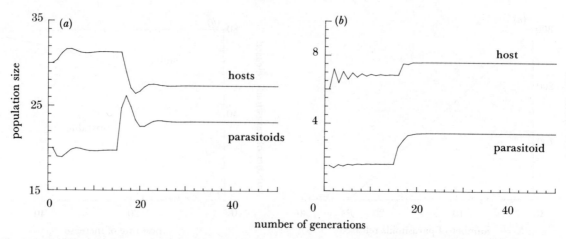

FIGURE 10. Numerical examples from the model in equation (12) with different levels of density dependence, $g$, defined by the expression used in figures 7 and 8. Parasitoid releases commence in generation 20. (a) The resulting depression in the host equilibrium when the density dependence is under-compensating ($d = 0.1$, $b = 0.8$, $F = 5$, $a = 0.1$, $k = 0.8$, $R = 5$). (b) The increase in host population level with over-compensating density dependence ($d = 0.05$, $b = 10$, $F = 10$, $a = 0.3$, $k = 0.8$).

(b)  P acts first:

$$
\left.
\begin{aligned}
N_{t+1} &= FN_t g(Q_t) f(P_t), \\
P_{t+1} &= N_t\{1-f(P_t)\}, \\
Q_{t+1} &= R + N_t f P_t \{1 - g(Q_t)\}.
\end{aligned}
\right\} \tag{14}
$$

and

(c)  P and Q act simultaneously, with proportions attacked depending on their relative abundance and relative attack rates. Assuming Nicholson–Bailey attack rates,

$$
\left.
\begin{aligned}
N_{t+1} &= FN_t \exp\left(-a_{\mathrm{P}} P_t - a_{\mathrm{Q}} Q_t\right), \\
P_{t+1} &= N_t\{a_{\mathrm{P}} P_t/(a_{\mathrm{P}} P_t + a_{\mathrm{Q}} Q_t)\}\{1 - \exp\left(-a_{\mathrm{P}} P_t - a_{\mathrm{Q}} Q_t\right)\}, \\
Q_{t+1} &= Nt\{a_{\mathrm{Q}} Q_t/(a_{\mathrm{P}} P_t + a_{\mathrm{Q}} Q_t)\}\{1 - \exp\left(-a_{\mathrm{P}} P_t - a_{\mathrm{Q}} Q\right)\} + R.
\end{aligned}
\right\} \tag{15}
$$

and

In all three cases, augmentative releases reduce host abundance leading to eradication when $g(R) > 1/F$ (figure 11). The picture is complicated, however, by the effect of releases on the coexistence of the two parasitoid species. For cases (a) and (c) above, which are most appropriate for the release of egg-parasitoids, releases of Q will always promote to some degree the instability of the established species P. Indeed, if there are no regulatory processes in the interaction other than the releases themselves (i.e. both P and Q are Nicholson–Bailey parasitoids) species P will always become extinct unless acting before Q in the host's life cycle (case b), in which case P and Q can coexist if $aN^* = (\ln F - R)/(1 - 1/F) > 1$.

The success of the augmentative release of egg-parasitoids clearly depends on a number of factors, including the efficiency of the parasitoids, the survival of parasitoid progeny for the next generation, any dispersal from the target area, the presence of other parasitoid species and any density-dependent processes affecting the host population. The mix of these will undoubtedly vary in importance in different systems, and will need to be carefully evaluated for each case to avoid costly and time-consuming investments where the likelihood of success is small.

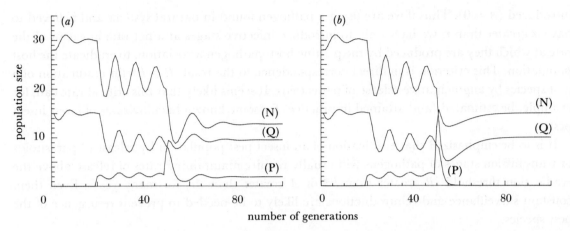

FIGURE 11. Numerical examples from the model in equation (14) showing the introduction and establishment of a second parasitoid species, Q, in generation 20. Augmentative releases of Q begin in generation 50, leading to a further reduction in the host population with (a) both P and Q coexisting ($R = 5$) or (b) Q replacing P ($R = 10$). Other parameters: $a_P = a_Q = 0.1$, $k_P = k_Q = 0.5$, $F = 2$, $g = 1$ (i.e. no additional host density dependence).

### (b) Release of pathogens

For the reasons outlined above, eradication of a pest species by a pathogen will usually require continual introduction of transmission stages. We summarize here the results of Anderson & May (1981) for the critical rate, above which such transmission stages must be introduced, to achieve extinction of the pest.

We established above that for the pathogen to be capable of regulating or eradicating the target-insect pest population we require $\alpha$ to be greater than $r$ (or some appropriately modified version of this relation if the infection decreases reproductive capacity, if pathogenicity is stress-related, or if other complications enter; table 2). If this criterion is obeyed, then the host population will be extinguished if free-living transmission stages of the pathogen are introduced at a rate $A$ in excess of a critical rate $Ac$ given by

$$Ac = \mu r(\alpha + b + \gamma) / \{v(\alpha - r)\}. \tag{16}$$

Here the parameters $\alpha$, $b$, $\gamma$, and $r$ have their usual meanings; $\mu$ is the death rate of free-living infective stages (whence their life expectancy is $1/v$); and $v$ is the rate at which infective stages successfully infect hosts (that is, $v$ is the transmission coefficient of free-living infective stages). Eradication efforts of this kind are more likely to be successful if they require relatively low rates of introduction of the pathogen. Thus, the criterion $A > Ac$, with $Ac$ defined by (16), is more likely to be met for infectious agents that are highly pathogenic ($\alpha$ large), have long-lived transmission stages ($\mu$ small), and have high transmission efficiency ($v$ large). In accord with common sense, both (16) and the overriding constraint $\alpha > r$ state that pest species with high population growth rates (large $r$) are relatively difficult to control.

With the exception of $v$, all the parameters in (16) can be measured, although there are very few host–pathogen systems for which all such measurements have been made. Direct assessment of the transmission parameter $v$ is, however, exceedingly difficult. It is therefore helpful to note that the critical introduction rate, $Ac$, can alternatively be expressed as $Ac = \lambda Y_0^*$. Here $Y_0^*$ is the equilibrium population of infected hosts, and $\lambda Y_0^*$ is the equilibrium net rate of production of infective stages by infected hosts, in a natural system when no pathogens are being artificially introduced ($A = 0$). Thus if we are using a pathogen found in natural systems and believed to have $\alpha$ greater than $r$, we have only to introduce infective stages at a net rate in excess of the rate at which they are produced by the pristine host–pathogen association, to eradicate the host population. This criterion is in direct correspondence to the result $R > P^*$ for eradication of a pest species by augmentative release of parasitoids. It seems likely that this critical rate can, for example, be estimated (and attained in practice) for some known baculoviruses of forest insect pests.

It is to be emphasized that eradication of an insect pest population by release of parasitoids or transmission stages of pathogens will usually require maintaining rates of release above the eradication threshold ($R$ greater than $P^*$ or $A$ greater than $Ac$) for many years. Even then, constant surveillance and reintroductions are likely to be needed to prevent resurgence of the pest species.

## MULTISPECIES INTERACTIONS

Many of the successes in biological control have involved the release of single parasitoid species (DeBach 1974; Messenger 1976), and of all predator–prey systems in the field, such examples come closest to the theoretician's delight of a closed two-species interaction. It is not possible, however, to develop a theoretical basis for biological control exclusively within such a simple framework. Many biological control programmes have led to the establishment of more than one parasitoid species (Clausen 1978), in others indigenous natural enemies have also played a part (Griffiths et al. 1984), and in yet others there has been the interplay between natural enemies and pathogens (Magasi & Syme 1984). Such interactions require the development of more complex, multispecies models involving mixes of parasitoids, predators and pathogens. These can show if the dynamics of simple multispecies systems are just the expected blend of the separate pairwise interactions, or if they have unexpected properties of their own. In biological control, the study of such systems may shed light both on how easily an introduced parasitoid can invade a community in which natural enemies of different types are already present and on how effective the introduced species (if it is indeed established) could be in lowering host populations and promoting persisting control.

### (a) Multiparasitoid introductions

A longstanding debate in biological control has centred on whether preliminary screening should be aimed at identifying the single most efficient parasitoid before release, or whether several species of parasitoids should be introduced for greatest effect. Some have suggested that interspecific interference between introduced parasitoid species may actually result in less depression of host abundance than achieved by introducing a single species (Turnbull & Chant 1961; Watt 1965; Kakehashi et al. 1984); others have suggested that multiple introductions will often provide a greater degree of host depression, or at least are a good way of identifying the best species without any attendant risks of diminished control (see, for example, van den Bosch & Messenger 1973; Huffaker et al. 1971; May & Hassell 1981; Waage & Hassell 1982).

The dynamics of multiparasitoid introductions can be conveniently considered within the framework of (13) and (14) (but without the augmentative releases; i.e. $R = 0$), and either with or without a density-dependent host rate of increase (May & Hassell 1981). In this case, it is assumed that species P is already established before the introduction of species Q, which either acts on the surviving hosts left by P or, if attacking the same host stage, is intrinsically inferior as a larval competitor whenever multiparasitism occurs. Three principle predictions emerge.

(1) As expected, the two species of parasitoids are most likely to coexist if each contributes to the stability of the interaction (e.g. if $k$ has a small value in (2)).

(2) Coexistence is also more likely if species Q has the higher searching efficiency (figure 12 $a$). If the efficiency is not high enough, Q will simply fail to become established (figure 12 $b$); if too efficient, however, Q will cause the replacement of P (figure 12 $c$). An apparent example

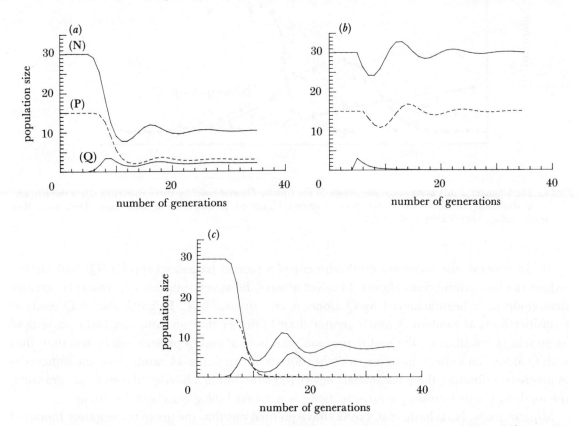

FIGURE 12. The effect of multiple parasitoid introductions from the model in equations (13) or (14), but with $g = 1$ and $R = 0$. Three possible outcomes are shown, after the introduction in generation 5 of a second parasitoid species, Q, where a stable host–parasitoid equilibrium already exists ($N^* = 30$, $P^* = 15$). ($a$) P and Q coexist; $a_P = 0.25$, $a_Q = 0.35$, $k_P = k_Q = 0.25$, $F = 2$. ($b$) Q fails to become established; $a_P = 0.1$, $a_Q = 0.05$, $k_P = k_Q = 0.5$, $F = 2$. ($c$) Q replaces P; $a_P = 0.1$, $a_Q = 0.4$, $k_P = k_Q = 0.5$, $F = 2$. (After Hassell (1978).)

of such 'competitive replacement' comes from the successive introductions of *Opius* parasitoids to control the fruitfly *Dacus dorsalis* in Hawaii (figure 13). If both species P and Q attack the same host stage rather than act in sequence, these criteria imply that coexistence is favoured if the intrinsically inferior species (Q) is also extrinsically superior to P in having the greater searching efficiency. A good natural example of this situation comes from the study of Zwolfer (1979) concerning the coexistence of two species of eurytomid parasitoids, *Eurytoma serratulae* and *E. robusta*, attacking a common host species, the knapweed gall fly, *Urophora cardui*, on creeping thistle. *E. serratulae* is the extrinsically superior species, being the more efficient searcher and having a preference for larger thistleheads containing more hosts. On the other hand, *E. robusta* is intrinsically superior in that its larvae will often kill those of *E. serratulae* if both occur within the same host individual. A model of the system predicts coexistence of both species due to just this balance between adult and larval competitive abilities.

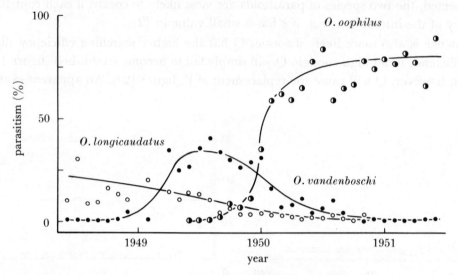

FIGURE 13. Changes in the percentage parasitism of the fruitfly *Dacus dorsalis* by three species of *Opius* parasitoids. Note that each successive parasitoid species causes a higher maximum level of parasitism. (Data from Bess *et al.* (1961), after Varley *et al.* (1973).)

(3) In general, the successful establishment of a second parasitoid species (Q) will further reduce the host equilibrium (figure 14). Not always, however, will this depression be greater than could have been achieved by Q alone, in the absence of P. In particular, if Q tends to parasitize hosts at random (*k* much greater than 1) rather than showing marked clumping of its attacks (*k* less than 1), the host depression with both P and Q present will be less than that with Q alone. This effect, however, is slight (dotted line in figure 14) and, given the difficulties in precisely estimating these parameters before introduction in a biological control programme, the analysis points to multiple introductions as a sound biological control strategy.

More recently, Kakehashi *et al.* (1984) have pointed out that the use of the negative binomial for the distribution of parasitism in these models represents a special case of each species causing quite independent contagious distributions of parasitism within the total host population. They then consider the other extreme where both parasitoid species respond in exactly the same way to host cues such as odour, density, etc., making a negative polynomial model with a common index of contagion, *k*, more appropriate. This difference has little effect on the stability of the models, but does change the equilibrium properties. In particular, it bears on the multiple introduction controversy argument because a single introduction of the superior searcher is now clearly the better strategy for maximizing the depression in host abundance. In the real world such complete covariance in the distributions of parasitism is probably less likely than more or less independent distributions (Hassell & Waage 1984), but in any event this is a cautionary example where general, strategic predictions can be affected by changes in the detailed model assumptions.

[ 40 ]

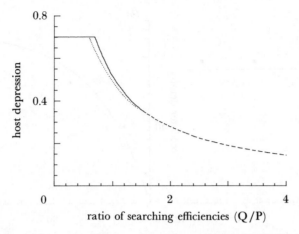

FIGURE 14. The depression in the host equilibrium, relative to the parasitoid-free carrying capacity, from the model in equation (13) with $R = 0$ and $g = \exp(-dNt)$. At very low searching efficiences of Q relative to that of P, Q cannot invade and there is a stable interaction with only the host and P present $(NP)$. As the searching efficiency of Q increases, Q invades and the host equilibrium is further reduced $(NPQ)$. Finally, at higher searching efficiencies, Q replaces P to give even lower host populations $(NQ)$ (which for the main part, however, are locally unstable). Dotted lines show the additional depression if only the host and Q were present. Parameter values; $d/(a_{\mathrm{p}} \ln F = 0.4$, $F = 2$, $k_{\mathrm{P}} = 0.25$, $k_{\mathrm{Q}} = 3$. (After May & Hassell (1981).)

### (b) Generalists and specialists

Introductions in biological control will often be made where the pest is already significantly affected by one or more generalist natural enemies, be they polyphagous parasitoids or generalist predators such as carabids, staphylinids or small mammals. Strategies for introduction should thus be based on a fundamental understanding of

(1) the general conditions necessary for a specialist to 'invade' an existing host–generalist interaction, and

(2) once established, how the specialist interacts with the generalist to affect the dynamics of the host population, and how this is altered if it acts before or after the generalist in the host's life cycle.

We commence by assuming that the generalists have a type II functional response based on a negative binomial distribution of encounters with the hosts (cf. equation (2)), and a simple numerical response given by

$$Gt = h\{1 - \exp(-N_t/b)\}. \tag{17}$$

Here, $h$ is the saturation number of predators and $b$ determines the typical prey density at which this maximum is approached (Southwood & Comins 1976) (figure 15). Such a numerical response might arise from reproduction on a much shorter time scale than that of the hosts or, more likely, from a behavioural response involving 'switching' from feeding elsewhere (Royama 1970) or on other prey species (Murdoch 1969). Combining these functional and numerical responses gives a density-dependent mortality over at least a range of host densities (figure 16), defined by the model

$$N_{t+1} = FN_t g(N_t), \tag{18}$$

where

$$g = [1 + a'G_t/\{k'(1 + a'T_{\mathrm{h}}'N_t)\}]^{-k'}. \tag{19}$$

[ 41 ]

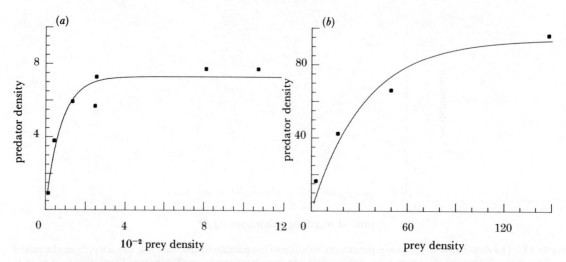

FIGURE 15. Numerical responses of two generalist predators described by equation (17), fitted by nonlinear least squares. (a) *Peromyscus maniculatus* in relation to the density of larch sawfly (*Neodiprion setifer*) cocoons (per thousand acres) (1 acre = 4046.8564 m²) (data from Holling 1959a). (b) The bay-breasted warbler (*Dendroica fusca*) (nesting pairs per 100 acres) in relation to larvae of the spruce budworm (*Choristoneura fumiferana*) numbers per 10 square feet (1 foot = 0.3048 m) of foliage (data from Mook 1963). Estimated parameter values ($\pm 95\%$ confidence limits); (a) $h = 7.30 \pm 1.07$, $b = 76.87 \pm 49.16$. (b) $h = 94.32 \pm 42.21$, $b = 32.97 \pm 42.27$. (After Hassell & May (1986).)

Here $a'$, $T_h'$ and $k'$ are the parameters of the generalists' type II functional response, as in (2). Locally stable equilibria can occur (figure 17) owing to the density dependence in equation (20a), and are made more likely by small handling times, high searching efficiency, a 'strong' numerical response (large $h$, small $b$) and low net host rates of increase. The same parameters also maximize the degree of depression in the host equilibrium.

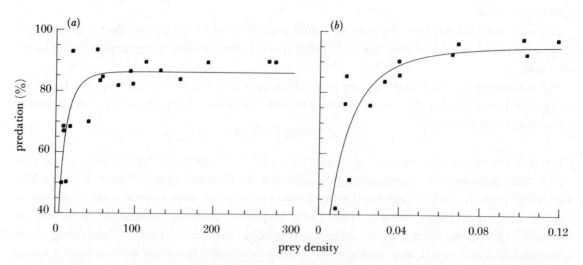

FIGURE 16. Examples of density-dependent predation of soil-pupating Lepidoptera, ascribed primarily to predation by carabid and staphylinid beetles. Data described by equations (18) and (19), fitted by nonlinear least squares. (a) Mortality of winter moth pupae per square metre; $a'h = 1.99 \pm 0.18$ (s.e.), $b = 15.94 \pm 3.17$, $k \to \infty$ (data from Varley et al. 1973). (b) Mortality of *Pardia tripunctatana* pupae per 0.18 m²; $a'h = 3.08 \pm 1.0$, $b = 0.03 \pm 0.01$, $k \to \infty$ (data from Bauer (1985)). (After Hassell & May (1986).)

[ 42 ]

We now add to this picture by the introduction of a specialist parasitoid (P) as part of a biological control programme:

$$N_{t+1} = FN_t f(P_t) g(N_t f),$$

(20a)

and

$$P_{t+1} = cN_t\{1 - f(P_t)\}.$$

(20b)

Here, the function $f$ is again given by (2). As discussed above, with more than one mortality acting, we need to be explicit on their relative timing in the host's life cycle. Equations (20a, b) are for the case of generalists acting after the specialist; if they act first the model becomes

$$N_{t+1} = FN_t f(P_t) g(N_t),$$

(21a)

and

$$P_{t+1} = cN_t g(N_t) [1 - f(P_t)].$$

(21b)

The following conclusions emerge from an analysis of these models (see Hassell & May (1986) for further details).

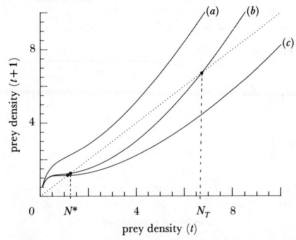

FIGURE 17. Map of prey densities in successive generations, $t$ and $t+1$, from equations (18) and (19). A locally stable equilibrium occurs at $N^*$ and an unstable, 'release' point at $N_T$. (a) $a'h = 3$, $a'bT_h' = 0.04$. (b) $a'h = 2$, $a'bT_h' = 0.04$. (c) $a'h = 3$, $a'bT_h' = 0.08$. $F = 7$ and $k \to \infty$, throughout. (After Hassell & May (1986).)

(1) The introduced parasitoid, P, can invade and coexist more easily if it acts before the generalist in the host's life cycle (figure 18a). This is simply due to the larger pool of hosts available. Conversely, if the host rate of increase, $F$ is too low, or if the generalist's overall efficiency, $a'h$, is too high relative to P, the specialist will be unable to invade and a persistent three-species interaction is impossible. This is broadly the same conclusion as reached by Holt (1977). Specialist egg-parasitoids may thus be easier to establish than larval or pupal ones, particularly if the pest has a relatively low net rate of increase and already suffers significant mortality from generalist natural enemies.

(2) Once again, if the specialist acts before generalists, and if the generalists cause strong over-compensating density dependence, there is the risk of higher host populations than existed before the introduction with only the generalist acting on its own (figure 18b).

(3) After successful establishment, there can either be only one equilibrium point (or stable cycle), or there may be more complex situations with a variety of possible alternative stable

states. Thus there may be two alternative persistent states, one with only the generalist and the other with all three species present, or two alternative three-species states in which the interaction may 'flip' between high and low levels if sufficiently perturbed. These possibilities are illustrated in figure 19.

(4) A stable system with all three species can exist when one or both of the two-species interactions alone would be unstable.

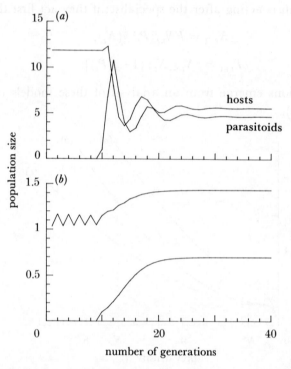

FIGURE 18. Numerical examples from the model in equation (20), where the specialist parasitoids 'invade' the host–generalist interaction in generation 10. Parameter values; $F = 8$, $T_h' = T_h = 0$, $h = 20$, $b = 10$, $k' \to \infty$, $k = 0.8$, $a = 0.8$, and (a) $a' = 0.15$ and (b) $a' = 1$.

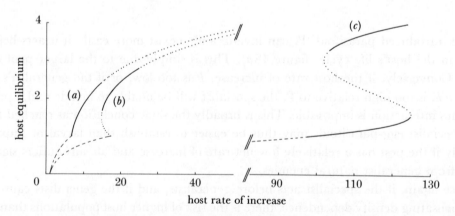

FIGURE 19. Three examples of the dependence of the host equilibrium, $N^*$, on the host rate of increase, $F$, for the model in equation (20). (a): $h = 20$, $b = 10$; (b): $h = 30$, $b = 10$; (c): $h = 5$, $b = 0.4$, $a' = a = 1$ and $k' = k \to \infty$ throughout. The broken lines indicate host–generalist interactions, the solid lines indicate locally stable host–generalist–specialist interactions, and the dotted lines indicate locally unstable ones.

[ 44 ]

In short, unlike the separate pairwise interactions each of which have rather straightforward dynamics, the combined three-species system presents a wider, and in some respects unexpected, range of properties. Not only are such studies of fundamental interest in showing how population dynamics can affect community structure, but also they caution us against formulating biological control strategies purely in terms of two-species interactions.

### (c) Pathogens and parasitoids

Various models for the combined action of a pathogen and a parasitoid or predator upon a target host population have been considered by Carpenter (1981) and Anderson & May (1986).

In general, all such systems may be viewed as specialized studies in two-species competition, in which the pathogen and the parasitoid compete for a common resource (the host species). It is therefore not surprising that basically four situations can arise, depending on the parameters characterizing the interactions (searching efficiency, aggregation, etc. for the parasitoid; virulence, transmissibility, etc. for the pathogen): parasitoid and pathogen may coexist; either parasitoid or pathogen species may regulate the host population to densities below the threshold for maintenance of the other species, thus 'competitively excluding' it; or there may be two alternative stable states, one with parasitoid only and the other with pathogen only, with the initial conditions determining which state is attained in any particular instance. Moreover, given the oscillatory propensities of the individual components of these systems, any one of the above states may be a steady equilibrium, or a stable cycle, or even (in some models) chaotic fluctuations.

It is pedagogically interesting to consider the very simplest such model, for the case of a host population with discrete, non-overlapping generations (R. M. May & M. P. Hassell, unpublished results). Combining the models in (1) and (6), we suppose the adult population in generation $t$, $N_t$, is first attacked by a lethal pathogen spread by direct contact, and then the survivors are attacked by randomly searching parasitoids:

$$N_{t+1} = FN_t S(N_t) f(P_t), \tag{22a}$$

and
$$P_{t+1} = cN_t S(N_t) \{1 - f(P_t)\}. \tag{22b}$$

Here $S(N)$ is the fraction surviving the epidemic, given earlier (see (6)) by the implicit relation $S = \exp[-(1-S)N_t/N_T]$, and $f$ has the Nicholson–Bailey form $f(P) = \exp(-aP)$. For $acN_T(\ln F)/(F-1)$ less than 1, the pathogen excludes the parasitoid (essentially, by maintaining the host population at levels too low to sustain the parasitoid, with its relatively low searching efficiency, $(a)$. For values of $acN_T$ significantly in excess of $(F \ln F)/(F-1)$, a linear analysis might suggest the parasitoid would exclude the pathogen for similar reasons. But a pure Nicholson–Bailey system gives diverging oscillations, and the pathogen can always invade as the hosts cycle to high values. A typical outcome is shown in figure 20, where the 'noisy' curves derive from the simple and purely deterministic equation (22). Figure 20 has a moral: the basic period of the oscillations in host abundance is determined primarily as the Nicholson–Bailey period for parasitoid dynamics; but the stable – if somewhat ragged (chaotic) – oscillations, rather than diverging Nicholson–Bailey cycles, derives from the pathogen. It is thus meaningless to ask whether the dynamics of this system are determined mainly by the parasitoid or by the pathogen. Both are important in different ways. The

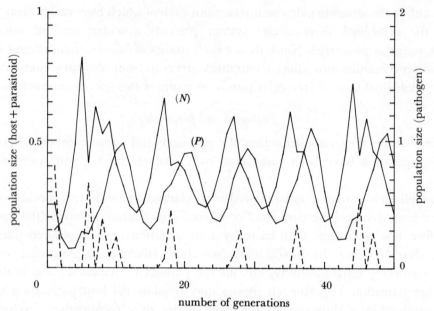

FIGURE 20. A numerical example from the model in equation (22), where $a = F = 2$ (for further details see text). Pathogen populations drawn to half scale.

parasitoid sets average host abundances and oscillatory periods, but the pathogen provides long-term stability, preventing overshoot or crash.

## COMPLEX LIFE CYCLES

For parasitoids, our discussion so far has focused on non-linear difference equations as a means of representing coupled, synchronized interactions with discrete generations. These correspond well to many temperate zone situations, where seasonality often synchronizes the populations and provides a natural interval between the appearance of successive generations. Such models, however, would not seem appropriate to the many host–parasitoid interactions in more tropical climes, where the life cycles of hosts and parasitoids may be of quite different lengths and where one would expect continuous generations with all stages present at the same time. These call for models in continuous time, with the age structure of the populations being explicitly included. A classic study of this kind, using host–parasitoid models framed as delay-differential equations, is that of Auslander *et al.* (1974). Interestingly, they found that discrete generation 'waves' could easily occur in such interactions with suitable parameter combinations.

Recently, Godfray & Hassell (1987) have also demonstrated how cycles whose period is approximately equal to the duration of one host generation period can unexpectedly arise, in this case depending in large measure on the ratio of the lengths of the host and the parasitoid life cycles. They developed a simulation model with a host population having four stages – pre-parasitism (e.g. eggs), susceptible (e.g. larvae), post-parasitism (e.g. pupae) and adults – and with the adults having a constant fecundity per unit time. The parasitoids have a life cycle divided into only two stages: the adults that search for and parasitize hosts, and the immature stages developing on or in parasitized hosts. All the immature stages of host and parasitoid have distributed developmental periods, drawn from an inverse quadratic distribution with specified mean and variance (Sharpe *et al.* 1977). The adults have an exponential survivorship curve. Finally, the rate of parasitism is given again by equation (2). (Note that the model collapses to (1) if the total host and parasitoid life cycles are of the same length, the adult hosts and parasitoids live for only one time unit and if there is no variance in the duration of the immature stages.)

Numerical simulations of this model suggest two distinct types of population behaviour at equilibrium:

(1) constant population sizes with all host and parasitoid age classes present (continuous generations) (figure 21*a*), and

(2) stable cycles of host and parasitoid populations with periods of both being approximately equal to the average duration of one host generation ('discrete' generations) (figure 21*b*).

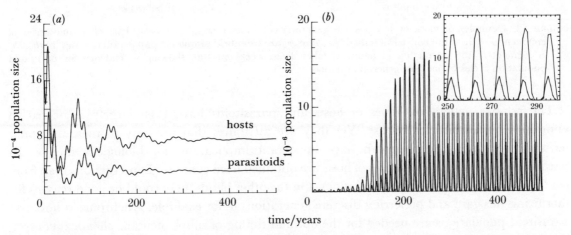

FIGURE 21. Simulations from the age-structured model described in the text. (*a*) Complete overlap of stages at equilibrium; host and parasitoid life cycles of equal length. (*b*) Stable cycles of host and parasitoids with periods of both approximately equal to the duration of one host generation (see inset); parasitoid life cycle half as long as that of the host. Other parameters the same for both examples. (From Godfray & Hassell (1987), in which further details are given.)

The two most important parameters affecting which of these behaviours occurs are (*a*) the degree of aggregation in the distribution of parasitism (*k*) (very small values of *k* promote continuous generations), and (*b*) the ratio of the host and parasitoid life-cycle lengths. It is particularly interesting that discrete generations are most likely when the parasitoid's life cycle is about 0.5 or 1.5 times that of the hosts. Conversely, parasitoid life cycles that are very short, or about the same length as the host's, or about twice as long, promote continuous generations. In a recent theoretical study of a broadly related problem, MacDonald (1986) has shown that delays in regulatory mechanisms affecting prey or predator populations separately, usually cause oscillatory dynamics, but that a stable equilibrium can ensue when such delays are present for both populations and are of approximate equal duration (as is the case in the above models when host and parasitoid life cycles are of similar length).

Some support for these theoretical suggestions comes from examples of time series of laboratory and natural host–parasitoid systems. Interestingly, a tendency for discrete generations in these systems generally occurs when the ratio of the lengths of host and parasitoid life cycles is approximately two to one (figure 22). Such unequal generation times appear to be typical of many lepidopteran host–parasitoid systems in the tropics.

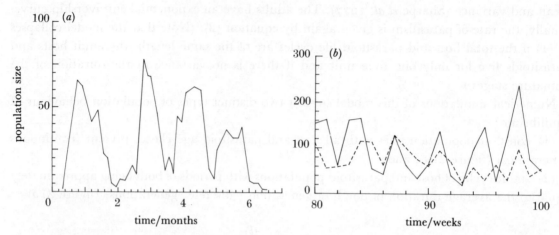

FIGURE 22. Examples of more or less discrete generations in insect populations. (*a*) Part of a time series of emergences of the adult coffee leaf miner *Leucoptera caffeina* from field samples of pupae (after Notley 1956). (*b*) A segment of the interaction in figure 4, taken from weeks 80–100, showing a tendency for parasitoid population cycles of one host generation period.

The relative generation times of hosts and parasitoids have been largely neglected in appraising parasitoids for release. Yet they are attributes that are easy to measure under natural conditions and they can have important implications for biological control. In particular, lower average densities of hosts are obtained from continuous interactions than from comparable ones with discrete generations. On the other hand, there could be good reasons for sacrificing this gain and preferring discrete generations if, for example, synchronized host and parasitoid populations are needed for the optimal timing of supplementary chemical control. Some problems of integrating chemical and biological methods of control are considered in the next section.

### PESTICIDES AND NATURAL ENEMIES

Modern pest management aims at integrating a variety of chemical, biological and cultural methods of pest control. A recurrent problem in this, however, has been the antagonistic effects of biological and chemical control methods, because pesticides in general have an adverse effect on natural enemies, often to a greater degree than on the target pest population. In some cases this has even led to 'resurgence' of the pest population to levels higher than occurred before the application of the pesticide (DeBach 1974).

### (*a*) Pesticides and parasitoids

In this subsection we explore the effects of a regular application of insecticide to the host–parasitoid system described by equation (1) (with $g(fN_t)$ equal to 1), focusing in particular on the timing of insecticide application relative to parasitism. A much fuller treatment, with details of the model, is given in Hassell (1984) and Waage *et al.* (1985). Some comparable models in continuous time are discussed by Barclay & van den Driessche (1977) and Barclay (1982).

There are four obvious possibilities for the relative timing of insecticides and parasitism:
(1) insecticides act after parasitism and only kill hosts;
(2) insecticides act before parasitism and only kill hosts;

[ 48 ]

(3) insecticides act after parasitism and also kill parasitized hosts, or

(4) insecticides act before parasitism and also kill adult parasitoids.

The effects of these different strategies can be viewed as the depression ($q$) of the host equilibrium caused by the insecticides:

$$q = N^*_{(+I)}/N^*_{(-I)}. \qquad (23)$$

Here $N^*_{(+I)}$ and $N^*_{(-I)}$ are the equilibrium host populations with and without insecticides, respectively. Values of $q$ less than 1 thus indicate a net benefit from insecticide application (figure 23$a$), whereas $q$ greater than 1 indicates a perverse increase in host abundance compared with the insecticide-free level (figure 23$b$).

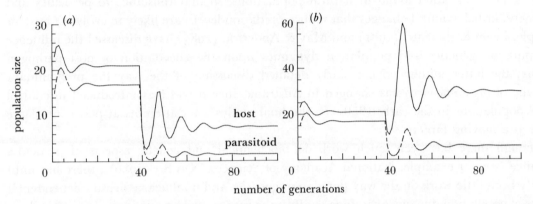

FIGURE 23. Examples of supression and 'resurgence' from the model in equations (1) and (2) with the addition of insecticides in generation 40 onwards, affecting both hosts and adult parasitoids ($I_h$ and $I_p$ are the fraction of hosts and parasitoids surviving insecticides, respectively). ($a$) Insecticides compliment the parasitoids in reducing host populations; $I_h = 0.4$, $I_p = 1$. ($b$) Insecticides also affecting the parasitoids and causing resurgence; $I_h = 0.4$, $I_p = 0.35$. Other parameters the same for both examples; $a = 1$, $T_h = 0.05$, $k = 0.6$, $F = 5$. (See Waage *et al.* (1985) for further details.)

An obvious conclusion from the models is that insecticides that have no effect on the parasitoids always contribute to reduced host population levels ($q$ less than 1). However, if the insecticides also kill adult or immature parasitoids this depression is reduced to the point that pest resurgence may occur ($q$ greater than 1). This problem is accentuated by adult parasitoids often being more susceptible to insecticides than the host stage which they attack (Abdelrahman 1973; Croft & Brown 1975; Croft 1977), and this only increases the likelihood of pest resurgence.

### (b) Pesticides and pathogens

Carpenter (1981) has documented the fact that 'disease is implicated in the natural regulation of invasions of the aquatic nuisance *Myriophyllum spicatum* (L.), yet harvested and herbicide-treated stands sometimes persist long after decimation of neighbouring stands'. He has gone on to explore the combined effects of pathogens and control measures (such as pesticides or harvesting) upon the dynamics of the target pest population, by using the basic framework developed above for the host–pathogen interactions.

Carpenter (1981) concludes that pesticides, or other interventions that increase the pest death rate can, on the one hand, permit a less virulent pathogen to control the population (the criterion $\alpha > r$ is easier to meet if $r$ is reduced by an elevated death rate). On the other hand, such pesticides will usually increase the threshold pest population necessary for the pathogen to spread, and also will lengthen the time required for the pathogen to reduce pest population levels. In contrast, Carpenter (1981) notes that supplementary control measures that decrease the pest birth rate (such as release of sterile males) do not usually exhibit such antagonistic interactions with control by pathogens.

### POPULATION DYNAMICS AND THE EVOLUTION OF PESTICIDE RESISTANCE

Up to this point, we have dealt exclusively with dynamical aspects of the interactions between pests and the pathogens, parasitoids, and/or pesticides used in control programmes. In reality, the introduction of such agents of control inevitably alters the selective forces acting on the genetic variation found in natural populations, so that resistance to pesticides and pathogens, or behavioural changes that reduce predation levels, are likely to evolve. Thus, for example, Levin & Pimentel (1981) and May & Anderson (1983) have discussed the influence of population genetics and population dynamics upon the coevolution of host–pathogen systems; the latter authors give a fairly detailed discussion of the way the predominant genotype of myxoma virus has changed in Australia since it was first introduced to control rabbit populations in the early 1950s. In the final analysis, all attempts at pest control are aimed at a moving target.

Although there has been much work on biochemical and genetic aspects of pesticides resistance (see, for example, National Academy of Sciences (N.A.S.) (1986)), there has until recently been little work on the way population genetics and nonlinear ('density dependent') aspects of population dynamics combine to affect the rate at which pesticide resistance evolves. Comins (1977 a, b, 1984) has studied some of these problems in the absence of natural enemies, and Tabashnik & Croft (1982) and Tabashnik (1986) have made numerical studies of the characteristically different rates at which pesticide resistance evolves among orchard pests and their natural enemies. May & Dobson (1986) have recently reviewed this subject, and outlined a more general analysis of the evolution of pesticide resistance in interacting systems of pests and natural enemies. What follows is a brief summary of their work.

It is helpful to begin by considering the population genetics of pesticide resistance for a pest species in a region subject to repeated application of the pesticide, but where immigration from untreated regions occurs in each generation. We consider resistance to involve a single diallelic locus (as is indeed sometimes the case), with resistant, heterozygote, and susceptible genotypes denoted by $RR$, $RS$, and $SS$, respectively. Under pesticide application, the three genotypes are assumed to have relative fitnesses $1: 1-hs: 1-s$, respectively. Here $s$ represents the 'selection strength' of the pesticide $(1 > s > 0)$, and $h$ measures the degree to which the resistance allele, $R$, is dominant (for $R$ recessive, $h = 1$; for $R$ dominant, $h = 0$). Suppose that, in each generation, a fraction $m$ of the total gene pool in the treated area derives from susceptible, $SS$, immigrants, with the remaining fraction $(1-m)$ deriving from the previous generation in the treated region. The gene frequency of $R$ in generation $t+1$, $p_{t+1}$, is then given by a standard calculation as

$$p_{t+1} = \frac{(1-m)\{p_t^2 + p_t q_t(1-hs)\}}{(1-m)\{p_t^2 + 2p_t q_t(1-hs) + q_t^2(1-s)\} + m}. \tag{24}$$

Here, as usual, $q$ is the gene frequency of $S$; $q_t = 1 - p_t$. Equilibrium solutions of (24) are obtained by putting $p_{t+1}$ equal to $p_t$ equal to $p$, and solving the resulting algebraic equation.

One solution is always $p = 0$. Other solutions (with 1 less than $q$ less than 0) are given by the quadratic equation

$$(1-2h)q^2 + hq - \varphi = 0. \qquad (25)$$

Here $\varphi$ is a parameter characterizing the relative strengths of migration and selection, $\varphi \equiv m/\{s(1-m)\}$. For $h$ greater than $\frac{2}{3}$, (25) can have two distinct solutions, providing $\varphi$ is small enough (specifically, $\varphi < h^2/\{4(2h-1)\}$); for $h < \frac{2}{3}$, (25) always has at most one sensible solution with 1 less than or equal to $q$ less than or equal to 0.

This simple model gives an illuminating (and surprisingly unfamiliar) metaphor for what can happen when selection is opposed by gene flow. The possibilities are illustrated in figure 24, which shows equilibrium values of the gene frequency of the resistance allele, $R$, as a function of the migration-selection parameter, $\varphi \equiv m/\{s(1-m)\}$, for various values of $h$. If $R$ is not too dominant ($h > \frac{2}{3}$), there are two alternative stable states when migration is neither too large nor too small in relation to the selection strength. The possibility of alternative stable states disappears if resistance is sufficiently dominant ($h < \frac{2}{3}$), in which case the resistance allele always predominates at low enough migration levels. As emphasized by Comins (1977b), in a somewhat more complex treatment, the time taken for resistance to appear can be significantly prolonged by deliberate efforts to keep immigration from untreated regions relatively high, particularly if resistance is a recessive character.

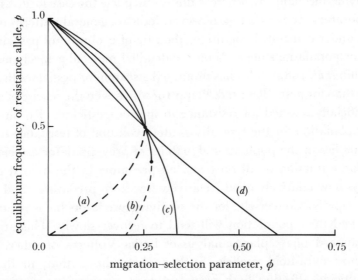

FIGURE 24. The equilibrium frequency, $p$, of the resistant allele, $R$, plotted as a function of the parameter characterizing the relative strengths of migration and selection, $\varphi = m/\{s(1-m)\}$, for the simple model defined by equation (24). The curves labelled (a), (b), (c), (d) are for $h$ (the dominance parameter) equal to 1.00, 0.80, 0.67, 0.40, respectively. The curves labelled (a) and (b) can exhibit two alternative stable states ($p$ large and $p$ equal to 0), divided by an unstable state (dashed curves); for sufficiently large $\varphi$, $p$ equal to 0 is the only stable state.

These remarks about the evolution of resistance in the presence of gene flow assume new significance when they are combined with consideration of the population dynamics of the pest. By definition, pests with undercompensating density dependence tend to recover steadily and monotonically to their original densities after a disturbance (such as application of a pesticide) that reduces population density. Conversely, pest populations with overcompensating density dependence tend to manifest a perverse response to pesticide application: if driven to a low level by pesticide application, such a population tends in the next generation to bounce back to a higher level than would otherwise have been the case. It follows that, for pests with undercompensating density dependence, the population densities of the next generation on average will be lower in treated regions that in untreated ones, making the effects of migration from untreated regions relatively more significant. Conversely, for pests with overcompensating density dependence, the next generation on average will be at higher densities in treated regions than in untreated ones, whence migration is relatively less significant. But we have just seen that resistance tends to evolve faster when migration is relatively unimportant, which prompts the qualitative conclusion that undercompensating density dependence tends to retard the evolution of pesticide resistance, and overcompensating density dependence to accelerate it. These ideas are developed more fully by May & Dobson (1986), who note, *inter alia*, that a pest exhibiting a most pronounced degree of overcompensation in field studies is the colorado potato beetle (*Leptinotarsa decemlineata*), which (perhaps coincidentally) is notorious for the speed with which it has developed resistance to a wide range of pesticides.

The propensity for pest species to evolve resistance more quickly than their natural enemies do has often been noted (Tabashnik 1986; Roush & Croft 1986). One reason might be that the coevolution between plants and phytophagous insects has preadapted the latter to the evolution of detoxifying mechanisms, whereas this is much less the case for the natural enemies of such insects. Laboratory studies do not, however, indicate general patterns of this kind, and it seems likely that under controlled conditions the rate of evolution of pesticide resistance in prey and in predator populations depends on the detailed molecular mechanisms underlying detoxification (Mullin *et al.* 1982). This has prompted a search for pesticides that are less lethal for natural enemies than for pests (Roush & Plapp 1982), or even the release of natural enemies that have been artificially selected for resistance to specific pesticides (Roush & Hoy 1981).

An alternative explanation for the typically swifter evolution of resistance by pests than by their natural enemies lies in the population dynamics of prey–predator associations. Suppose a pesticide kills a large fraction of all prey and all predators in the treated region. For the surviving prey, life is now relatively good (relatively free from predators), and the population is likely to increase rapidly. Conversely, for the surviving predators life is relatively bad (food is harder to find), and their population will tend to recover slowly. This argument can be elaborated by a standard phase plane analysis of Lotka–Volterra or other, more realistic, prey–predator or host–parasitoid models. Such analysis shows that, in the aftermath of application of a pesticide affecting both prey and predator, prey populations will tend to exhibit overcompensating density-dependent effects, whereas predator populations will tend to manifest undercompensation. From the arguments developed earlier in this section, we would expect that, for a given level of migration and pesticide application, pest species (which effectively have overcompensating density dependence) will tend to develop resistance faster than will their natural enemies (which effectively have undercompensating density dependence).

In short, both population genetics and population dynamics must be considered in projecting the long-term consequences of control programmes, particularly if natural enemies are combined with pesticides or other 'artificial' control methods.

## CONCLUSION

Fundamental studies of host–parasitoid and host–pathogen interactions reveal several factors affecting the dynamics both of natural systems, and of manipulated ones arising from biological control. Simple mathematical models can provide a potent tool for gaining rapid insights into population behaviour: insights that would otherwise only accrue gradually, and piecemeal, as examples slowly accumulate where natural and biological control 'case histories' have been analysed in some detail. Unfortunately, almost none of the 300 or so 'successes' in biological control have been studied in the field beyond the relatively short period when natural enemies are actually being released, and then only in a rather superficial way. This is a great opportunity being wasted. Biological control programmes are, in effect, manipulation experiments on a grand scale involving relatively few species. If properly monitored, they would provide invaluable information, for example, on population regulation, on the dynamics of interactions involving predators, parasitoids and pathogens, and on species invasions; ecology and biological control would both benefit greatly.

## REFERENCES

Abdelrahman, I. 1973 Toxicity of malathion to the natural enemies of California red scale *Aonidiella aurantis* (Mask.) (Hemiptera: Diaspididae). *Aust. J. agric. Res.* **24**, 119–133.

Ables, J. R. & Ridgeway, R. L. 1981 Augmentation of entomophagous arthropods to control pest insects and mites. In *Biological control in crop production* (ed. G. C. Papavizas), pp. 273–303. Totowa, New Jersey: Allanheld, Osmun.

Anderson, R. M. & May, R. M. 1980 Infectious diseases and population cycles of forest insects. *Science, Wash.* **210**, 658–661.

Anderson, R. M. & May, R. M. 1981 The population dynamics of microparasites and their invertebrate hosts. *Phil. Trans. R. Soc. Lond.* B **291**, 451–524.

Anderson, R. M. & May, R. M. 1986 The invasion, persistence and spread of infectious diseases within animal and plant communities. *Phil. Trans. R. Soc. Lond.* B **314**, 533–570.

Anon. 1980 *Biological Control Service. 25 years of achievement.* Slough: Commonwealth Agricultural Bureaux.

Auslander, D. M., Oster, G. F. & Huffaker, C. B. 1974 Dynamics of interacting populations. *J. Franklin Inst.* **295**, 345–376.

Bailey, V. A., Nicholson, A. J. & Williams, E. J. 1961 Interactions between hosts and parasites when some host individuals are more difficult to find than others. *J. theor. Biol.* **3**, 1–18.

Barclay, H. J. 1982 Models for pest control using predator release, habitat management and pesticide release in combination. *J. appl. Ecol.* **19**, 337–348.

Barclay, H. & van den Driessche, P. 1977 Predator–prey models with added mortality. *Can. Ent.* **109**, 763–768.

Barclay, H. J., Otrus, I. S. & Thomson, A. J. 1985 Models of periodic inundation of parasitoids for pest control. *Can. Ent.* **117**, 705–716.

Bauer, G. 1985 Population ecology of *Pardia tripunctana* Schiff. and *Notocelia roborana* Den. and Schiff. (Lepidoptera, Tortricidae) – an example of 'equilibrium species'. *Oecologia* **65**, 437–441.

Beddington, J. R., Free, C. A. & Lawton, J. H. 1975 Dynamic complexity in predator–prey models framed in difference equations. *Nature, Lond.* **255**, 58–60.

Beddington, J. R., Free, C. A. & Lawton, J. H. 1978 Modelling biological control: on the characteristics of successful natural enemies. *Nature, Lond.* **273**, 513–519.

Bess, H. A., van den Bosch, R. & Haromoto, F. H. 1961 Fruit fly parasites and their activities in Hawaii. *Proc. Hawaii ent. Soc.* **17**, 367–378.

Box, H. E. 1932 Studies on early larval mortality of *Diatraea saccharalis* in Antigua with special reference to natural parasitism of eggs by *Trichogamma*. *Proc. int. Soc. Sug. Cane Technol.* **122**, 1–6.

Broadhead, E. & Cheke, R. A. 1975 Host spatial pattern, parasitoid interference and the modelling of the dynamics of *Alaphus fusculus* (Hym: Mymaridae), a parasitoid of two *Mesopsocus* species (Psocoptera). *J. Anim. Ecol.* **44**, 767–793.

Carpenter, S. R. 1981 Effect of control measures on pest populations subject to regulation by parasites and pathogens *J. theor. Biol.* **92**, 181–184.

Chesson, P. L. 1981 Models of spatially distributed populations: the effect of within-patch variability. *Theor. Pop. Biol.* **19**, 288–325.

Chesson, P. L. & Murdoch, W. W. 1986 Relationships among host–parasitoid models. *Am. Nat.* **127**, 696–715.

Clausen, C. P. 1978 *Introduced parasites and predators of arthropod pests and weeds: a world review.* Washington: United States Department of Agriculture Agricultural Research Service.

Comins, H. N. 1977a The development of insecticide resistance in the presence of migration. *J. theor. Biol.* **64**, 177–197.

Comins, H. N. 1977b The management of pesticide resistance. *J. theor. Biol.* **65**, 399–420.

Comins, H. N. 1984 The mathematical evaluation of options for managing pesticide resistance. In *Pest and pathogen control: strategic, tactical and policy models* (ed. G. R. Conway), pp. 454–469. New York: John Wiley.

Croft, B. A. 1977 Resistance in arthropod predators and parasites. In *Pesticide management and insecticide resistance* (ed. D. L. Watson & A. W. A. Brown), pp. 377–393. New York: Academic Press.

Croft, B. A. & Brown, A. W. A. 1975 Responses of arthropod natural enemies to insecticides. *A. Rev. Ent.* **20**, 285–335.

DeBach, P. 1974 *Biological control of natural enemies.* Cambridge University Press.

DeBach, P. & Hagen, K. S. 1970 Manipulation of entomophagous species. In *Biological control of insect pests and weeds* (ed. P. DeBach), pp. 429–458. London: Chapman & Hall.

Elliott, J. M. 1982 The life cycle and spatial distribution of the aquatic parasitoid *Agriotypus armatus* (Hymenoptera: Agriotypidae) and its caddis host *Silo pallipes* (Trichoptera: Goeridae). *J. Anim. Ecol.* **51**, 923–941.

Elliott, J. M. 1983 The responses of the aquatic parasitoid *Agriotypus armatus* (Hymenoptera: Agriotypidae) to the spatial distribution and density of its caddis host *Silo pallipes* (Trichoptera: Goeridae). *J. Anim. Ecol.* **52**, 315–330.

Embree, D. G. 1965 The population dynamics of the winter moth in Nova Scotia 1954–1962. *Mem. ent. Soc. Can.* **46**, 1–57.

Embree, D. G. 1966 The role of introduced parasites in the control of the winter moth in Nova Scotia. *Can Ent.* **98**, 1159–1168.

Ewald, P. W. 1987 Pathogen induced cycling of outbreak insect populations. In *Insect outbreaks: ecological and evolutionary processes* (ed. P. Barbosa & J. C. Schultz), pp. 209–286. New York: Academic Press.

Falcon, L. A. 1982 Use of pathogenic viruses as agents for the biological control of insect pests. In *Population biology of infectious diseases* (ed. R. M. Anderson & R. M. May), pp. 191–210. Springer-Verlag: New York.

Godfray, H. C. J. & Hassell, M. P. 1987 Natural enemies can cause discrete generations in tropical insects. *Nature, Lond.* **327**, 144–147.

Griffiths, K. L. 1969 Development and diapause in *Pleolophus basizonus* (Hymenoptera: Ichneumonidae). *Can. Ent.* **101**, 907–914.

Griffiths, K. J., Cunningham, J. C. & Otvos, I. S. 1984 *Neodiprion sertifer* (Geoffroy), European pine sawfly (Hymenoptera: Diprionidae). In *Biological control programmes against insects and weeds in Canada 1969–1980* (ed. J. S. Kelleher & M. A. Hulme) pp. 331–340. Slough: Commonwealth Agricultural Bureaux.

Gross, H. R., Lewis, W. J., Jones, R. L. & Nordlund, D. A. 1975 Kairomones and their use for management of entomophagous insects: III Stimulation of *Trichogramma achaeae*, *T. pretiosum* and *Microplitis croceipes* with host seeking stimuli at the time of release to improve efficiency. *J. chem. Ecol.* **1**, 431–438.

Hassell, M. P. 1968 The behavioural response of a tachinid fly *Cyzenis albicans* (Fall.) to its host, the winter moth, *Operophtera brumata* (L.). *J. Anim. Ecol.* **37**, 627–639.

Hassell, M. P. 1969a A study of the mortality factors acting upon *Cyzenis albicans* (Fall.), a tachinid parasite of the winter moth *Operophtera brumata* (L.). *J. Anim. Ecol.* **38**, 329–339.

Hassell, M. P. 1969b A population model for the interaction between *Cyzenis albicans* (Fall.) (Tachinidae) and *Orthophtera brumata* (L.) (Geometridae) at Wytham, Berkshire. *J. Anim. Ecol.* **38**, 567–576.

Hassell, M. P. 1978 *The dynamics of arthrod predator–prey systems.* Princeton University Press.

Hassell, M. P. 1980 Foraging strategies, population models and biological control: a case study. *J. Anim. Ecol.* **49**, 603–628.

Hassell, M. P. 1982a Patterns of parasitism by insect parasites in patchy environments. *Ecol. Ent.* **7**, 365–377.

Hassell, M. P. 1982b What is searching efficiency? *Ann appl. Biol.* **101**, 143–203.

Hassell, M. P. 1984 Parasitism in patchy environments: inverse density dependence can be stabilizing. *I.M.A. J. math. appl. med. Biol* **1**, 123–133.

Hassell, M. P. & Anderson, R. M. 1984 Host susceptibility as a component in host–parasitoid systems. *J. Anim. Ecol.* **53**, 611–621.

Hassell, M. P. & May, R. M. 1973 Stability in insect host–parasite models. *J. Anim. Ecol.* **42**, 693–726.

Hassell, M. P. & May, R. M. 1974 Aggregation in predators and insect parasites and its effect on stability. *J. Anim. Ecol.* **43**, 567–594.

Hassell, M. P. & May, R. M. 1985 From individual behaviour to population dynamics. In *Behavioural ecology. Ecological consequences of adaptive behaviour* (ed. R. M. Sibly & R. H. Smith), pp. 3–32. Oxford: Blackwell Scientific Publications.

Hassell, M. P. & May, R. M.  1986  Generalist and specialist natural enemies in insect predator–prey interactions. *J. Anim. Ecol.* **55**, 923–940.

Hassell, M. P. & Waage, J. K.  1984  Host–parasitoid population interactions. *A. Rev. Ent.* **29**, 89–114.

Hassell, M. P., Waage, J. K. & May, R. M.  1983  Variable parasitoid sex ratios and their effect on host–parasitoid dynamics *J. Anim. Ecol.* **52**, 889–904.

Holling, C. S.  1959a  The components of predation as revealed by a study of small mammal predation of the European pine sawfly. *Can. Ent.* **91**, 293–320.

Holling, C. S.  1959b  Some characteristics of simple types of predation and parasitism. *Can. Ent.* **91**, 385–398.

Holt, R. D.  1977  Predation apparent competition and the structure of prey communities. *Theor. Pop. Biol.* **12**, 197–229.

Huffaker, C. B., Messenger, P. S. & De Bach, P.  1971  The natural enemy component in natural control and the theory of biological control. In *Biological control* (ed. C. B. Huffaker), pp. 16–67. New York: Plenum.

Jacques, R. P.  1977  Stability of entomopathogenic viruses. *Misc. Publs ent. Soc. Am.* **10**, 99–116.

Kakehashi, N., Suzuki, Y. & Iwasa, Y.  1984  Niche overlap of parasitoids in host–parasitoid systems: its consequence to single versus multiple introduction controversy in biological control. *J. appl. Ecol.* **21**, 115–131.

Kareiva, P. & Odell, G. M.  1987  Swarms of predators exhibit 'preytaxis' if individual predators use area restricted search. *Am. Nat.* **130**, 233–270.

Kermack, W. O. & McKendrick, A. G.  1927  A contribution to the mathematical theory of epidemics. *Proc. R. Soc. Lond.* A **115**, 700–721.

Knipling, E. F.  1972  Simulated population models to appraise the potential for suppressing sugarcane borer populations by strategic releases of the parasite *Lixophaga diatraeae*. *Envir. Ent.* **1**, 1–6.

Knipling, E. F. & McGuire, J. V., Jr.  1968  Population models to appraise the limitations and potentialities of *Trichogramma* in managing host insect populations. *Tech. Bull. U.S. Dept. Agric.* **1387**, 1–44.

Leslie, P. H. & Gower, J. C.  1960  The properties of a stochastic model for the predator–prey type of interaction between two species. *Biometrika* **47**, 219–224.

Lessells, C. M.  1985  Parasitoid foraging: should parasitism be density dependent? *J. Anim. Ecol.* **54**, 27–41.

Levin, S. A. & Pimentel, D.  1981  Selection for intermediate rates of increase in parasite–host systems. *Am Nat.* **117**, 308–315.

Lewis, W. J., Jones, R. L., Nordlund, D. A. & Sparks, A. N.  1975  Kairomones and their use for management of entomophagous insects: I Evaluation for increasing rates of parasitization by *Trichogramma* spp. in the field. *J. chem. Ecol.* **1**, 343–347.

McNamee, P. J., McLeod, J. M. & Holling, C. S.  1981  The structure and behaviour of defoliating insect/forest systems. *Univ. Br. Columb. Inst. Resour. Ecol. Publ.* R-25, 1–89.

MacDonald, D. W.  1986  *Rabies and wildlife: a biologist's perspective.* Oxford University Press.

Magasi, L. P. & Syme, P. D.  1984  *Gilpinia hercyniae* (Hartig), European sawfly (Hymenoptera: diprionidae). In *Biological control programmes against insects and weeds in Canada 1969–1980* (ed. J. S. Kelleher & M. A. Hulme), pp. 295–297. Slough: Commonwealth Agricultural Bureaux.

May, R. M.  1978  Host–parasitoid systems in patchy environments: a phenomenological model. *J. Anim. Ecol.* **47**, 833–843.

May, R. M.  1985  Regulation of populations with nonoverlapping generations by microparasites: a purely chaotic system. *Am. Nat.* **125**, 573–584.

May, R. M. & Anderson, R. M.  1983  Epidemiology and genetics in the coevolution of parasites and hosts. *Proc. R. Soc. Lond.* B **219**, 281–313.

May, R. M. & Dobson, A. P.  1986  Population dynamics and the rate of evolution of pesticide resistance. In *Pesticide resistance: strategies and tactics for management*, pp. 170–193. Washington D.C.: National Academy Press.

May, R. M. & Hassell, M. P.  1981  The dynamics of multiparasitoid-host interactions. *Am. Nat.* **117**, 234–261.

May, R. M., Hassell, M. P., Anderson, R. M. & Tonkyn, D. W.  1981  Density dependence in host–parasitoid models. *J. Anim. Ecol.* **50**, 855–865.

Maynard Smith, J.  1974  *Models in ecology.* Cambridge University Press.

Messenger, P. S.  1976  Theory underlying introduction of exotic parasitoids. In *Perspectives in forest entomology* (ed. J. F. Anderson & H. K. Kaya), pp. 191–214. New York: Academic Press.

Metcalfe, J. R. & Breniere, J.  1969  Egg parasites (*Trichogramma* spp.) for control of sugar cane moth borers. In *Pests of sugar cane* (ed. J. R. Williams, J. R. Metcalfe, R. W. Mungomery & R. Mathes), pp. 81–115. Amsterdam: Elsevier.

Metcalfe, J. R. & van Whervin, L. W.  1967  Studies on liberated and naturally occurring egg parasites of moth borer (*Diatraea saccharalis* (F.)) in Barbados. *Proc. int. Soc. Sug. Cane Technol.* **12**, 1420–1434.

Mook, L. J.  1963  Birds and the spruce budworm. In *The dynamics of epidemic spruce budworm populations* (ed. R. F. Morris) (*Mem. ent. Soc. Can.* **31**, 268–271).

Mullin, C. A., Croft, B. A., Strickler, K., Matsumura, F. & Miller, J. R. 1982 Detoxification enzyme differences between a herbivorous and predatory mite. *Science, Wash.* **217**, 1270–1272.

Murdoch, W. W. 1969 Switching in general predators: experiments on predator and stability of prey populations. *Ecol. Monogr.* **39**, 355–354.

Murdoch, W. W., Chesson, J. & Chesson, P. L. 1985 Biological control in theory and practice. *Am. Nat.* **125**, 344–366.

Murdoch, W. W. & Oaten, A. 1975 Predation and population stability. *Adv. ecol. Res.* **9**, 2–131.

Myers, J. G. 1929 Some recent work on parasites of the small moth borers. (*Diatraea*) of sugar cane. *Trop. Agric., Trin.* **6**, 310–312.

N.A.S. 1986 *Pesticide resistance: strategies and tactics for management.* (National Academy of Sciences Committee on Strategies for the Management of Pesticide Resistant Pest Populations) Washington D.C.: National Academy Press.

Nicholson, A. J. 1933 The balance of animal populations. *J. Anim. Ecol.* **2**, 132–178.

Nicholson, A. J. & Bailey, V. A. 1935 The balance of animal populations. Part 1. *Proc. Zool. Soc. Lond.* **3**, 551–598.

Notley, F. B. 1955 The *Leucoptera* leaf miners of coffee on Kilimanjaro. *Bull. ent. Res.* **46**, 899–912.

Perry, J. N. & Taylor, L. R. 1986 Stability of real interacting populations in space and time: implications, alternatives and the negative binomial kc. *J. Anim. Ecol.* **55**, 1053–1068.

Pickles, A. 1936 Observations on the early larval mortality of certain species of *Diatraea* (Lep., Pyralidae) under canefield conditions in Trinidad. *Trop. Agric., Trin.* **13**, 155–160.

Pielou, E. C. 1969 *An introduction to mathematical ecology.* New York: John Wiley.

Reuter, O. M. 1913 *Lebensgewohnheiten und Instinkte den Inseckten bis zum Erwachen der Socialoen Instinkte.* Berlin: Friedlander.

Roush, R. T. & Croft, B. A. 1986 Experimental population genetics and ecological studies of pesticide resistance in insects and mites. In *Pesticide resistance: strategies and tactics for management,* pp. 257–270. Washington D.C.: National Academy Press.

Roush, R. T. & Hoy, M. A. 1981 Laboratory, glasshouse and field studies of artificially selected carbaryl resistance in *Metaseiulus occidentalis. J. econ. Entomol.* **74**, 142–147.

Roush, R. T. & Plapp, F. W. 1982 Biochemical genetics of resistance to aryl carbamate insecticides in the predaceous mite, *Metaseiulus occidentalis. J. econ. Entomol.* **75**, 304–307.

Royama, T. 1970 A comparative study of models of predation and parasitism. *Res. Pop. Ecol.* **1**, 1–91.

Sabelis, M. W. & Laane, W. E. M. 1986 Regional dynamics of spider mite populations that become extinct locally because of food source depletion and predation by phytoseiid (Acarina: Tetranychidae, Phytoseiidae). In *Dynamics of physiologically structured populations* (ed. J. A. J. Metz & O. Diekmann), pp. 345–376. Berlin: Springer-Verlag.

Sabelis, M. W. & van der Meer, J. 1986 Local dynamics of the interaction between predatory mites and two-spotted spider mites. In *Dynamics of physiologically structured populations* (ed. J. A. J. Metz & O. Diekmann), pp. 322–344. Berlin: Springer-Verlag.

Sharpe, P. J. H., Curry, G. L., DeMichele, D. W. & Cole, C. L. 1977 Distribution model of organism developmental times. *J. theor. Biol.* **66**, 21–38.

Southwood, T. R. E. & Comins, H. N. 1976 A synoptic population model. *J. Anim. Ecol.* **45**, 949–965.

Stinner, R. E. 1977 Efficacy of inundative releases. *A. Rev. Ent.* **22**, 515–531.

Stinner, R. E., Ridgway, R. L., Coppedge, J. R., Morrison, R. K. & Dickerson, W. A. 1974 Parasitism of *Heliothis* eggs after field releases of *Trichogramma pretiosum* in cotton. *Envir. Ent.* **3**, 497–500.

Tabashnik, B. E. 1986 Computer simulation as a tool for pesticide resistance management. In *Pesticide resistance: strategies and tactics for management,* pp. 194–206. Washington D.C.: National Academy Press.

Tabashnik, B. E. & Croft, B. A. 1982 Managing pesticide resistance in crop-arthropod complexes: interactions between biological and operational factors. *Envir. Ent.* **11**, 1137–1144.

Tinsley, T. W. 1979 The potential of insect pathogenic viruses as pesticide agents. *A. Rev. Ent.* **24**, 63–87.

Tinsley, T. W. & Entwhistle, P. F. 1974 The use of pathogens in the control of insect pests. In *Biology in pests and disease control* (ed. D. Price-Jones & M. E. Solomon), pp. 115–129. Oxford: Blackwell Scientific Publications.

Tucker, R. W. E. 1934*a* A contribution towards the solution of the problem of control of *Diatraea saccharalis* in cane through a mathematical evaluation of the real mortality of *D. saccharalis* due to egg parasites, egg predators, natural larval mortality, larval parasitism and other factors. *Agric. J. Dep. Sci. Agric. Barbados* **3**, (1) 59–80.

Tucker, R. W. E. 1934*b* A further contribution to the analysis of field data on *Diatraea saccharalis* in Barbados. *Agric. J. Dep. Sci. Agric. Barbados* **3**, (4) 26–32.

Turnbull, A. L. & Chant, P. A. 1961 The practice and theory of biological control of insects in Canada. *Can. J. Zool.* **39**, 697–753.

van den Bosch, R. & Messenger, P. S. 1973 *Biological control.* New York: Intext Press.

van Hamburg, H. & Hassell, M. P. 1984 Density dependence larval mortality and the augmentative release of egg parasitoids against graminaceous stalkborers. *Ecol. Ent.* **9**, 101–108.

Varley, G. C., Gradwell, G. R. & Hassell, M. P. 1973 *Insect population ecology.* Oxford: Blackwell Scientific Publications.

Waage, J. K. & Hassell, M. P. 1982 Parasitoids as biological control agents – a fundamental approach. *Parasitology* **84**, 241–268.

Waage, J. K., Hassell, M. P. & Godfray, H. C. J. 1985 The dynamics of pest–parasitoid–insecticide interactions. *J. appl. Ecol.* **22**, 825–838.

Wang, Y. H. & Gutierrez, A. P. 1980 An assessment of the use of stability analyses in population ecology. *J. Anim. Ecol.* **49**, 435–452.

Watt, K. E. F. 1965 Community stability and the strategy of biological control. *Can. Ent.* **97**, 887–895.

Zwolfer, H. 1979 Strategies and counterstrategies in insect population systems competing for space and food in flower heads and plant galls. *Fortschr. Zool.* **25**, 331–353.

## APPENDIX 1

This appendix derives the dynamical properties of equation (12), as summarized in the text.

Possible equilibrium values of the host and parasitoid populations are obtained by putting $N_{t+1} = N_t = N^*$ and $P_{t+1} = P_t = P^*$, respectively. For $g$ equal to 1, (12a) gives $P^*$ from

$$Ff(P^*) = 1. \tag{A 1}$$

Equation (A 1) says that the equilibrium parasitoid density is equal to that obtained in the absence of any inundative release (i.e. for $R$ equal to 0). If $f(P)$ has the form of equation (2), with $T_h$ equal to 0, (A 1) gives

$$P^* = (k/a)\,(F^{\frac{1}{k}} - 1). \tag{A 2}$$

Equation (12b) gives simply

$$N^* = (P^* - R)/(1 - 1/F). \tag{A 3}$$

Clearly, no equilibrium is possible, and the host population will be eradicated, if sustained release of parasitoids is made at a rate $R$ greater than $P^*$.

For $R$ less than $P^*$, the linearized stability properties of the system may be obtained in the usual way by writing $N_t = N^* + x_t$ and $P_t = P^* + y_t$, neglecting nonlinear terms, and writing $x_t, y_t \sim \Lambda^t$, to obtain for the eigenvalues $\Lambda$ the quadratic equation

$$\Lambda^2 - (1 + \zeta/F)\,\Lambda + \zeta = 0. \tag{A 4}$$

Here $\zeta$ is defined in general by

$$\zeta = -FN^*(\mathrm{d}f/\mathrm{d}P)^*. \tag{A 5}$$

The equilibrium state will be locally stable iff both eigenvalues $\Lambda$ have modulus less than unity, which is to say iff

$$\zeta < 1. \tag{A 6}$$

This criterion (A 6) is, in general, increasingly easy to satisfy as $R$ increases from zero to the critical value $P^*$.

In particular, if $f(P)$ is given by (2) (with $T_h = 0$), we have

$$\zeta = F^{\frac{-1}{k}}\{k(F^{\frac{1}{k}} - 1) - aR\}/\{1 - 1/F\}. \tag{A 7}$$

That is, the equilibrium state is stable to small disturbances iff

$$aR > F^{\frac{1}{k}}\{k(1 - F^{\frac{-1}{k}}) - (1 - F^{-1})\}. \tag{A 8}$$

This requirement is always satisfied if $k < 1$, and for $k > 1$ it is increasingly easily satisfied as $aR$ increases. Even for the randomly-searching parasitoids of the original Nicholson–Bailey model (which corresponds to $k \to \infty$ in (A 8)), the familiar diverging oscillations can be replaced by a stable equilibrium if inundative release rates are large enough that $aR > (\ln F - 1 + 1/F)$; the critical rate of release for eradication is yet higher at $aR > \ln F$.

*Discussion*

P. NEUENSCHWANDER (*International Institute of Tropical Agriculture, Ibadan, Nigeria*). Professor Hassell's presentation implies that on the basis of simulation models simple introduction of the most efficient parasitoid is superior over multiple introductions, under conditions where strong density-dependent factors are already at work. Practical experience does not bear this out. Could you tell us what differences in host densities are involved in the different examples. This answer is of considerable importance for the practitioner in the field who has to justify introduction without being able to document efficiency beforehand.

M. P. HASSELL. On the contrary, our analytical models suggest that multiple introductions of parasitoids are a sound biological control strategy, even in the presence of additional density dependence affecting the host population. Additional releases will usually lead to further depression of the host population, and where this is not the case, the effect is very slight, so that two parasitoid species perform almost as well as the most efficient on its own. As discussed in our paper, Kakehashi *et al.* (1984) show that there are situations where a single introduction of the most efficient parasitoid is the better strategy for reducing the host population. Their model, however, requires all the parasitoid species to respond in the same behavioural way to the spatial distribution of hosts, which we believe to be unrealistic.

D. J. ROGERS (*Department of Zoology, University of Oxford, U.K.*). Professor Hassell's paper mentions an inverse relation between a host's effective rate of increase and the degree of suppression that a parasitoid can achieve (i.e. lower rates of increase are associated with greater degrees of suppression).

Bearing in mind the large amount of suppression recorded by Beddington *et al.* (1978) in cases of successful biological control would Professor Hassell like to comment on the very low rates of increase of the pest species that this result implies, i.e. do pests really have such low rates of increase? If so, why do they become pests?

Could this explain the mediocre success rate of 'classical biological control' and are failures attributable to host species having relatively higher rates of increase?

M. P. HASSELL. The examples that I showed of parasitoids reducing host populations, but not to the low levels characteristic of classical biological control successes, come from laboratory interactions where parasitism is the only major mortality suffered by the host population. Insect populations in the field will normally have a net rate of increase very much lower than their *per capita* fecundity due to the many other factors affecting their natality or mortality. Experience has shown that insects with very low net rates of increase can easily become pests if divorced from their usual complement of natural enemies. A pest species with a high net rate of increase will clearly require a more efficient natural enemy to cause a given level of depression. I know of no good evidence indicating that the failures in classical biological control are correlated with high rates of increase.

T. R. E. SOUTHWOOD, F.R.S. (*Department of Zoology, University of Oxford, U.K.*). In the previous paper Dr Wagge and Dr Greathead indicated how the specificity of potential biological control agents could be tested by a 'centrifugal technique': testing them against other potential hosts of decreasing relatedness to the target species. Does Professor Hassell think, in the light of his emphasis on search pattern, that this and other behavioural characters should (or could) also be taken into account in assessing potential control agents before release?

M. P. HASSELL. Several behavioural characters of natural enemies that are highly relevant to biological control could well be studied before release, particularly when comparing a number of potential biological control agents. For example, the ability of natural enemies to locate isolated patches of hosts, their maximum attack rates within such patches, whether or not they host feed (therefore affecting longevity), all affect the overall efficiency of a natural enemy and thus its ability to depress the host population. Behavioural characters such as these are all amenable to careful study under controlled conditions as part of evaluating candidates for a biological control programme. They may also provide useful pointers to the specificity of a natural enemy, because highly evolved behavioural adaptations for locating host individuals are much more likely to occur in relatively specific natural enemy species than in polyphagous ones.

*Phil. Trans. R. Soc. Lond.* B **318**, 171–182 (1988)

*Printed in Great Britain*

# Management of the environment for the control of pathogens

By R. J. Cook

*United States Department of Agriculture Agricultural Research Service, Root Disease and Biological Control Research Unit, Washington State University Department of Plant Pathology, Pullman, Washington 99164-6430, U.S.A.*

Pathogens can be controlled by management of the environment of (1) the host plant, to maximize resistance, (2) nonpathogens associated with the pathogen, to enhance antagonisms, and (3) the pathogen itself, to limit its activity or longevity directly. Each can be illustrated with controls developed for root diseases of Pacific Northwest wheat. For example: management of plant water potentials to minimize water stress in the host controls *Fusarium* foot rot; root-colonizing fluorescent pseudomonads, with ability to inhibit *Gaeumannomyces graminis* by antibiosis, achieve highest populations on roots and provide best control of take-all at rhizosphere matric water potentials of $-0.3$ to $-0.7$ bar (1 bar $= 10^5$ Pa) and rhizosphere pH values below 7.0; and infection of wheat seedlings by *Pythium* spp., being directly limited by soil matric water potentials drier than $-0.4$ to $-0.5$ bar, is controlled by sowing in early autumn while the seed zone is still well-drained or by burning surface residues to expose the soil to drying, and possibly also killing propagules by heat-treatment of the soil. Depending on the host–pathogen–nonpathogen interaction, tillage can maximize host plant resistance, intensify antagonism of pathogens by nonpathogens, and directly limit inoculum potential of the pathogen in soil.

## 1. Plant disease: an outcome of host–pathogen–nonpathogen interactions

The development of a plant disease is the outcome of a succession of biological interactions involving host, pathogen, and nearly always one or more nonpathogens coexisting on, or in, the host with the pathogen. The nonpathogens may be weakly parasitic to the plant or strictly saprophytic, and they may be related (e.g. a strain or a species of the same genus) or unrelated (e.g. nonpathogenic bacteria with a pathogenic fungus) to the pathogen. These nonpathogens occur in diverse and commonly dense populations on plant surfaces and in the courts of infection and may well provide the initial defence of plants against pathogens. Nonpathogens also become secondary colonists of lesions, where they compete with or parasitize (in special cases) the pathogen; these effects may retard lesion development and production of inoculum by the pathogen. Some nonpathogens, as cohabitants with pathogens, may increase disease severity, but examples of this outcome are rare compared with the converse. Of course, the living host has its own succession of defence mechanisms against ingress by the pathogen, and some resistance responses may be induced by the presence of a nonpathogen (Kuć 1982).

In considering the influence of environment on plant disease development (and ultimately the use of environment to control plant pathogens) we must keep all three of these interacting biological systems in mind and not just the host and pathogen as done so often in the past.

## 2. Definitions of cultural and biological controls

'Cultural control' is used broadly in this paper to include any control of a pathogen achieved by a cultural practice. Cultural controls generally work by bringing about a change in the environment unfavourable to the pathogen, favourable to the host, favourable to antagonists, or some combination of these three possibilities. The controls discussed in this paper for soil-borne pathogens of wheat in the Pacific Northwest U.S.A. are of these types, designed to change the environment so as to favour the host, nonpathogens, or both relatively more than the pathogen and thereby minimize disease severity. Some cultural practices control pathogens entirely through direct effects of the modified environment on the pathogen, for example soil that is too dry for pathogen growth at the time of sowing. In most cases, however, the practice works through effects on the outcome of biological interactions involving host and nonpathogens as well as the pathogen.

'Biological control' is also used broadly in this paper to include any pathogen control accomplished through one or more organisms (antagonists, host, or pathogen used against itself) other than man (Cook & Baker 1983). Any adjustment in the environment that decreases inoculum density or suppresses disease-producing activities of a pathogen but is achieved through greater host-plant resistance or increased antagonistic effects of the nonpathogens is an example of biological control.

An important point not commonly recognized is that often only the slightest change in the environment will bring about a major change in disease severity. For example, soft rot of potatoes, caused by *Erwinia carotovora*, develops in tubers at $-6.5$ bar† matric water potential but not in tubers at $-7.5$ to $-8.0$ bar (Pérombelon & Kelman 1980). The difference in severity of soft rot over this narrow range of water potentials seems too dramatic to be explained simply on the basis of a higher and hence more favourable turgor potential for growth of the bacterial cells at $-6.5$ than at $-7.5$ to $-8.0$ bar. Host-susceptibility factors almost certainly are involved. A slight change in pH or temperature can have equally dramatic effects on the interactions between a pathogen and nonpathogens on the phylloplane or rhizoplane (Cook & Baker 1983). In the case of host factors, the different reactions (e.g. resistant or susceptible) under the different environments may be near instantaneous, requiring only that the host tissues or cells achieve the water potential, temperature, oxygen status, or other environmental conditions required for maximal expression of resistance. In the case of interactions between a pathogen and associated nonpathogens, the outcome is usually decided over a longer time, more typical of interacting populations in an ecosystem.

## 3. Rationale for use of the environment to bring about biological control of plant pathogens

It is sometimes stated that plant pathologists have been relatively unsuccessful in developing biological controls for plant pathogens. This statement can be made only with reference to the narrowest possible definition of biological control, namely the introduction or application of an antagonist, probably a single antagonist, to control the pathogen. Baker (1987) refers to this approach as the 'one-on-one' syndrome that seems to dominate the thinking in biological

† 1 bar = $10^5$ Pa.

control and to parallel our use of single genes and single chemicals for pathogen control. Obviously, many successes can be cited for the single-agent approach to pathogen control. The use of *Agrobacterium radiobacter* var. *radiobacter* strain K84 to control crown gall (Kerr 1980) and *Phlebia gigantea* to control *Heterobasidion* root rot of pine (Rishbeth 1979) are excellent examples of single, introduced antagonists effective in the field. However, most of the biological controls in plant pathology have involved manipulations of the environment to manage host-plant susceptibility together with a myriad of resident, nonpathogenic and potentially antagonistic microorganisms on the host and in host residues and thereby to relegate the pathogen to a lesser position in its ecological niche. In this approach, our science has been quite successful.

Biological control achieved through management of the environment brings to bear the combined effects of many antagonists or potential antagonists, all adapted to the niche or replaced by those that are adapted. Suppressive soils, defined as those soils where the pathogen does not establish, establishes but causes little or no disease, or causes disease at first but then declines (Baker & Cook 1974), are mostly examples of environments relatively more favourable to a community of resident antagonists than to some pathogen that otherwise would cause severe disease. Detailed studies of a suppressive soil (or of other pathogen-suppressive environments) may, on occasion, produce a single antagonist or group of related antagonists responsible for the effect. This antagonist can then be isolated and reintroduced to enhance the effect. One example is *Trichoderma harzianum* obtained from a Colombian soil suppressive to *Rhizoctonia solani* (Chet & Baker 1981), and another is the fluorescent *Pseudomonas* species obtained from wheat-field soils that have undergone take-all decline, and used to control take-all (Weller & Cook 1983). In some cases, the quality of the microbial community is the key, in other cases the quantity (total numbers or mass of microorganisms active at a time critical to the pathogen) is more important. Generally, however, the quality and quantity of nonpathogenic microorganisms are both important. 'The greater the complexity of the biological community, the greater is its stability.' At the very least, cultural practices should be selected that do not environmentally upset the suppressive communities of microorganisms that help defend plants against pathogens.

### 4. Control of *Fusarium* foot rot of wheat in the low- to intermediate-rainfall areas of the Pacific Northwest U.S.A.

Fusarium foot rot of wheat, caused by *Fusarium culmorum*, is a problem in the Pacific Northwest, U.S.A., mainly on winter wheat subjected to severe plant water stress (Papendick & Cook 1974; Cook 1980). The pathogen had been noted on wheat for decades (Sprague 1950), but acute foot rot typified by crown rot, premature plant blight, and a chocolate-brown discolouration extending one to two internodes up the stem, did not become important until the 1960s (Cook 1968). The appearance of the severe form of the disease coincided with the use of the high-yielding, semi-dwarf cultivars of winter wheat. Moreover, those who noted the first outbreaks of this disease also noted that it was most serious for the 'best' farmers in the low- to intermediate-rainfall areas (25–40 cm annual precipitation) of Washington State. Papendick & Cook (1974) related the occurrence of severe plant water stress to excessive nitrogen fertilization. The so-called better farmers were fertilizing for yields greater than possible for the available water. Wheat plants are remarkably resistant to foot rot caused by

*F. culmorum*, provided their mid-day plant water potentials go no lower than −28 to −32 bar, but they become extremely susceptible to the disease if their mid-day plant water potentials go below −32 to −35 bar (Cook 1973). Some plants developed water potentials as low as −40 to −50 bar.

The control, now widely practised in the dryland Pacific Northwest of the U.S.A., is to fertilize for a yield no greater than can be expected for available water (Cook 1986). This exemplifies the use of cultural practices to manage the environment of a pathogen. The environment, in this case, is the water potential of the host tissue occupied by the pathogen. Nonpathogenic (strictly saprophytic) fusaria related to *F. culmorum* are commonly present as secondary colonists of wheat roots and basal stem tissues occupied by *F. culmorum*, but whether they play any role in this disease control on non-stressed plants is unknown.

Field surveys done over a ten year period, approximately 1965–75, revealed that populations of *F. culmorum* sufficient to produce disease (greater than 100 propagules per gram dry mass of soil) occurred almost exclusively in the low- and intermediate-rainfall areas and not in the high-rainfall areas (greater than 45–50 cm precipitation annually) such as near Pullman. Large populations of *F. culmorum* established naturally or experimentally in the Pullman area were observed to disappear from the soil in only 1–2 years. This raised the possibility that soils around Pullman were suppressive, of the type that did not allow the pathogen to establish (Baker & Cook 1974). However, Inglis & Cook (1986) showed that chlamydospores of this pathogen die faster in the dry, harsh soil environment in the low- than in the high-rainfall areas. They proposed that the higher frequency of infested fields in the low- than in the high-rainfall areas was the result of conditions more favourable to disease, and hence replenishment of inoculum of the pathogen, and not of differences in conditions required for survival of the pathogen between susceptible crops. The presence of *F. culmorum* in wheat-field soils of the Pacific Northwest is therefore thought to be a function of its parasitic (pathogenic) activities and not of its ability as a soil saprophyte.

Cook & Bruehl (1968) similarly concluded that the presence of *F. culmorum* in fragments of wheat stubble after harvest was the result of parasitism, i.e. the establishment of the fungus in the lower internodes as a parasite while the plant was still alive, rather than of saprophytic colonization of the straw after harvest. Those portions of standing stubble not occupied by *F. culmorum* as a parasite become quickly colonized by airborne saprophytes, and these pre-empt *F. culmorum* as a colonist once the stubble is mixed with soil infested with this pathogen (Cook 1970).

By managing plant water potentials, the parasitic activities of *F. culmorum* are virtually prevented. By leaving the stubble standing to become mouldy after harvest, the saprophytic activities of this fungus are virtually prevented. Because chlamydospores gradually die out in soils of the region (Inglis & Cook 1986), the pathogen without recourse to either parasitism or saprophytism has ceased to be a factor in wheat production in the region.

5. CONTROL OF *PYTHIUM* ROOT ROT OF WHEAT IN THE INTERMEDIATE-
TO HIGH-RAINFALL AREAS

*Pythium* root rot of wheat is caused by several *Pythium* species (Chamswarng & Cook 1985), with *P. ultimum* and *P. irregulare* being the most widespread and thought to be the most important. These fungi existed in association with roots and residues of the prairie grasses

(Sprague 1950) long before wheat farming began in the region in the late 19th century. The disease can be divided into two phases: a generally non-lethal infection of the embryos of seeds during the first 1–2 d after sowing that results in stunted, twisted leaves, and spindly appearance (in severe cases) of seedlings (Hering *et al.* 1987); and infection of root hairs and the cortical tissues of roots and rootlets that may continue during the life of the plant (Cook & Haglund 1982; Cook *et al.* 1987). Adult wheat plants affected by *Pythium* root rot are generally 3–5 cm and sometimes up to 10 cm shorter, have 15–25 % fewer tillers, and head 3–5 days later than plants of the same age but grown in soil freed of *Pythium* spp. by either heat treatment (e.g. solarization) or fumigation (Cook *et al.* 1987).

Although *Pythium* spp. pathogenic to wheat are ubiquitious, and *Pythium* root rot occurs across all major wheat-management systems in the region, control is needed only in the intermediate- to high-rainfall areas (35–40 cm of available water or more, annually). The disease occurs in the drier areas, probably during October–March when most rainfall occurs, and elimination of inoculum of *Pythium* spp. from soil by fumigation invariably produces an early increased-growth response for wheat in the drier areas. However, available water and not *Pythium* root rot is almost always the yield-limiting factor in areas of the region with less than 35–40 cm (Cook 1986; Cook *et al.* 1987). For this reason, all efforts to date aimed at control of *Pythium* root rot have been focused in the higher rainfall areas of the far-eastern edge of Washington State, northeastern Oregon, and northern Idaho.

The most effective controls at present for damage to wheat caused by *Pythium* spp. are those combinations of practices that: (1) minimize the amount of wheat straw (especially the chaff) at the soil surface or mixed with the top 10–15 cm of soil (Chamswarng 1984); (2) keep the soil surface exposed to drying winds and the sun, especially during emergence and early seedling growth (R. J. Cook, unpublished results); and (3) keep the soil matric potentials in the top 10–15 cm of soil drier than −0.4 to −0.5 bar (Hering *et al.* 1987). These three factors determine whether the soil environment will be suitable to activity of *Pythium* spp. and are not mutually exclusive.

The benefits of a well-drained seedbed and removal of potential foodbases for control of *Pythium* spp. are perhaps best illustrated by noting that *Pythium* root rot is most severe for winter wheat when direct-drilled through a layer of straw into wet soil late in the autumn (e.g. mid-October or later). Average daily temperatures are dropping during this period and the chance is very low that the soil will dry during establishment of the stand. In this situation, final grain yields are commonly only 50–75 % of what they could be with the moisture available to the crop (Cook 1986). Infection of germinating wheat seeds is maximal at −0.1 bar matric water potential but is virtually prevented in soils at −0.4 to −0.5 bar or drier (Hering *et al.* 1987). Most wheat seedlings emerge in spite of embryo infections, but fewer seedlings emerge and those that do are distinctly spindly in straw- (or chaff-) amended soils, and the addition of nitrogen with the straw does not correct the problem (Ingram 1987). All evidence indicates that the chaff and other straw fragments are used by *Pythium* spp. as a foodbase, unless the straw is already colonized by other fungi (Rush *et al.* 1986). The straw can be eliminated (and damage from *Pythium* spp. is almost always reduced accordingly) by burning, deep burial with a plough (i.e. deeper than 10–15 cm), or rotation with a crop such as dry peas or lentils (which leaves the soil surface relatively bare).

The benefits of straw removal are apparent from the results of a field experiment conducted in eastern Washington during the 1985–86 crop year. Winter wheat direct-drilled in the autumn of 1985 into standing stubble of a 1985 spring wheat crop averaged (five replicates)

4.5 t ha$^{-1}$†. Injection of chloropicrin 10–12 cm below the soil surface (about 10 l ha$^{-1}$ 5–7 cm below and 5–7 cm to one side of the seed) with the fertilizer at the time of sowing reduced the population of *Pythium* spp. by nearly 50%, produced a typical increased-growth response of the wheat, and resulted in an average yield of 5.2 t ha$^{-1}$. However, winter wheat that was direct-drilled the same day at the same site but with stubble removed by burning averaged 5.8 t ha$^{-1}$, and injection of chloropicrin into these plots resulted in about the same yield (5.9 t ha$^{-1}$). The adult plants in the burned, non-fumigated plots showed no evidence of *Pythium* root rot and their yield probably was the maximum possible for available water at that site (Cook 1986) and therefore could not be increased by fumigation. Differences in initial inoculum density of *Pythium* spp. cannot account for the growth and yield differences of the wheat in the stubble-standing and stubble-burned sites. Complete removal of the straw to produce a black soil surface was obviously of great benefit, possibly because the fungus was denied access to a foodbase, or possibly because of a greater opportunity for the soil to dry below the critical (−0.4 to −0.5 bar) matric water potential. The response of wheat to fumigation in the standing stubble supports our findings in glasshouse studies that, although surface crop residues are a contributing factor to the stunting of wheat associated with direct drilling, it is the soil and not the straw that must be fumigated to eliminate the microorganisms responsible for the effect.

Burning wheat straw on the soil surface may also reduce the population of *Pythium* spp. by a heat or possibly also by a smoke effect. At Pullman, wheat straw placed as a layer on bare fallow (surface already black and the soil drained) at 0, 3, 6 and 12 t ha$^{-1}$ and burned resulted in average yields of 5.1, 5.8, 5.9 and 6.2 t ha$^{-1}$ for winter wheat grown in the replicated plots (Cook *et al.* 1987). In another experiment, burning a layer of straw (12–15 t ha$^{-1}$) on the soil surface was nearly as effective as solar heating of the soil in reducing the *Pythium* population in the top 5–10 cm of soil, and the wheat yields were 15–20% greater than where no treatment or where straw ash only was applied (Cook *et al.* 1987). The temperature of moist soil needs to be elevated to only 42–43 °C for 10 min virtually to eliminate the population of *Pythium* in these soils (Cook *et al.* 1987; W.-h. Tang, unpublished results). Moreover, a 10 min exposure of *Pythium*-infested soil to smoke-filled air, produced by burning wheat straw, was sufficient to render the population of *Pythium* spp. undetectable when the soil was returned to clean air and dilution-plate counted (W.-h. Tang, unpublished results).

Pythium root rot of winter wheat is also limited by seeding early in the autumn, while the soils are still well drained or are not likely to be wet for a prolonged period. The chances for adequate drainage and improved control of *Pythium* root rot are greatly increased if the soil has no tillage pan (plough-sole layer) formed by prior tillage operations (R. R. Allmaras and J. M. Kraft, unpublished results). Even a slight difference in the soil matric potential during times critical to the saprophytic or parasitic activities of *Pythium* spp. in the spermosphere and rhizosphere of wheat can greatly affect the amount of damage caused by this fungus.

## 6. CONTROL OF TAKE-ALL IN CONSECUTIVE CROPS OF WHEAT IN THE HIGH-RAINFALL AND IRRIGATED AREAS

Take-all, caused by *Gaeumannomyces graminis* var. *tritici*, is easily controlled in most areas of the world by not growing wheat or barley in the same field more than every other year (minimum of a two year rotation). The pathogen survives in fragments of root and basal stem

† 1 hectare = 10$^4$ m$^2$.

tissues colonized through parasitism, while the fragments were still part of the living host. Rotation to non-host crops is effective because the pathogen either depletes its nutrient supply in these fragments or is displaced by more competitive microorganisms within a few months in most biologically active soils. The disease can also be managed with consecutive crops of wheat or barley. Biological control is also involved in this approach, and is thought to include the combined effects of competition from fungi and bacteria in the foodbase (inoculum source), which reduce the inoculum potential of the pathogen, and antagonistic microorganisms in the rhizoplane and in young lesions, which prevent infection or limit the secondary spread of the pathogen by runner hyphae (Cook & Weller 1987).

The competitive effects of fungi and bacteria with *G. graminis* var. *tritici* in fragments of infested crop residue is a continuous process that probably begins as the lesions age but intensifies once the host dies. Garrett (1976, 1985) has done extensive studies of the factors affecting longevity of *G. graminis* var. *tritici* in tiller bases as a means of saprophytic survival and as a foodbase for this pathogen. The importance of competition from fungi, in particular, was demonstrated by W.-h. Tang (unpublished results) using a benomyl-resistant strain of the pathogen; the infection efficiency (number of root lesions produced per unit mass of inoculum (Wilkinson *et al.* 1985)) was 25–50 % greater when benomyl was infused (5 parts in $10^6$ by mass) into the pathogen-infested (inoculum) fragments. The increase was equivalent to that achieved by moist heat treatment of the soil at 60 °C for 30 min (Wilkinson *et al.* 1985; Cook *et al.* 1986). Experiments with the pasteurized soil revealed only that soil microorganisms have a suppressive effect on the infection efficiency of this pathogen, but experiments with benomyl infused into the particles indicated that the suppressive agent(s) is (are) benomyl-sensitive. Subsequent experiments indicated that nonpathogenic (saprophytic) *Fusarium* spp. are partly or largely responsible for the suppression; a strain of *F. oxysporum* reduced the infection efficiency for the take-all pathogen when added with inoculum of the benomyl-resistant pathogen to pasteurized soil, but not if benomyl was present in the fragments of inoculum.

From a practical standpoint, the competitive effects of microorganisms on *Gaeumannomyces graminis* var. *tritici* in its foodbase can be maximized by tillage (Moore & Cook 1984) together with a delayed seeding date (Taylor *et al.* 1983). Tillage is well known to promote temporary bursts in microbial activity and to accelerate breakdown of organic matter in soil. The response is thought to result from a combination of the fresh surfaces on fragments of residue made available for microbial colonization and the temporary improvement in soil aeration. In Washington State, some tillage is essential for take-all control in consecutive crops of wheat (Moore & Cook 1984). Delayed seeding is also beneficial, possibly because the extra 1–2 weeks between harvest of one crop and sowing the next crop allows more time for the nonpathogens to displace the pathogen.

The suppression of take-all by antagonistic bacteria on the roots of wheat is also a common phenomenon but intensifies or becomes more effective with any of the following practices: (1) the use of ammonium rather than nitrate fertilizer (Smiley 1978); (2) growing consecutive crops of wheat (Cook & Rovira 1976; Weller 1985); and (3) introducing the bacteria with the wheat seed (Weller & Cook 1983).

Workers in Idaho (Huber *et al.* 1968), Oregon (Christensen *et al.* 1981), and Washington (Smiley & Cook 1973) all have reported that the use of ammonium nitrogen results in less take-all on wheat than occurs with the use of nitrate nitrogen. The ammonium effect is apparently the result of a lower pH in soil around roots taking up this form of nitrogen (Smiley & Cook

1973). However, the lower rhizosphere pH cannot, by itself, account for the disease suppression because the effect did not occur in soil fumigated with methyl bromide. Smiley (1978) showed that the frequency of fluorescent pseudomonads inhibitory to G. graminis var. tritici is significantly greater in the rhizosphere of wheat treated with ammonium compared with nitrate fertilizers. Howie (1985) presents evidence that this effect is also the result of a lower rhizosphere pH; both the indigenous population of fluorescent pseudomonads and the population of P. fluorescens strain 2-79 introduced with the seed tended to be higher at rhizosphere pH values of 6.0 to 6.5 than at 7.0. Rouatt & Katznelson (1961) noted that pseudomonads are commonly favoured in the rhizosphere by slightly acidic conditions.

Manipulation of the rhizosphere pH with form of applied nitrogen illustrates the potential practical value of managing environmental factors in specific courts of infection, namely microsites such as the root–soil interface, rather than more generally in the bulk of the soil. Manipulation of rhizosphere pH may not be sufficient itself, but when combined with tillage and the presence of certain nonpathogens, e.g. fluorescent pseudomonads inhibitory to the pathogen, the additional degree of disease control can be significant.

Populations of fluorescent pseudomonads inhibitory to G. graminis var. tritici also tended to increase spontaneously with consecutive crops of wheat and in the presence of the take-all fungus. The evidence of Weller (1985, in Cook & Baker 1983) points to a qualitative as well as quantitative change towards higher populations of fluorescent Pseudomonas sp. inhibitory to the take-all pathogen. Indeed, this phenomenon is thought to contribute to or be responsible for the well-known take-all decline phenomenon (Cook & Weller 1987). Certain strains of the bacteria are also now providing modestly effective control against take-all under field conditions when introduced as a living seed treatment; the average yield compared with appropriate checks was 7.6% (400 kg ha$^{-1}$) greater for ten experiments done in naturally-infested commercial fields over a 5 year period (R. J. Cook, D. M. Weller & E. N. Bassett, unpublished results).

Both the indigenous population of fluorescent pseudomonads and the population of P. fluorescens strain 2-79 introduced with the seed were consistently 1–2 $\log_{10}$ units larger on roots of wheat seedlings that were 28 days in the presence than in the absence of the take-all fungus (Howie 1985). This response of fluorescent pseudomonads to the take-all fungus was also observed by Weller (1984), with a marked strain monitored in the field, and is thought to result from response of the bacteria to root lesions caused by the pathogen. Several workers have noted the proliferation of Gram-negative bacteria in root lesions caused by G. graminis var. tritici (Vojinović 1973; Cook & Rovira 1976). By establishing in root lesions, the bacteria are then ideally positioned both to inhibit further spread of the pathogen on the roots and to carry over as cohabitants with the pathogen in host-plant fragments after the crop is harvested (Cook et al. 1986). Thus, as the incidence and severity of take-all increases, the populations of fluorescent pseudomonads (and possibly other bacteria) increase in response to the amount of infected root tissue. Cook & Weller (1987) have proposed that after one or two severe outbreaks of take-all, an equilibrium may develop between populations of bacteria, which is sufficient to limit future outbreaks of severe take-all, but which also allows enough lesions to maintain populations of the bacteria. This hypothesis can account for why, after take-all decline, the pathogen can still be readily isolated from wheat roots and is fully virulent in a conducive rooting medium but is prevented from causing severe disease in the field (Asher 1980; Cook & Naiki 1982).

In addition to the presence of the take-all pathogen, and pH of the rhizosphere, any source of inorganic nitrogen (either ammonium or nitrate) added to a nitrogen-impoverished soil resulted in $1$–$2$ $\log_{10}$ unit larger populations of P. fluorescens strain 2-79 than occurred on roots of plants in the soil with no added nitrogen. Nitrogen deficiencies are well-known to favour take-all and many reasons have been proposed for the effect. This list of proposed reasons can now be extended to include larger populations of potentially antagonistic bacteria in the rhizosphere, possibly brought about by greater root exudation from the better-nourished plants.

Another major factor is rhizosphere water potential. Populations of P. fluorescens strain 2-79 introduced on wheat seeds achieved largest populations when the water potential of the rhizosphere was $-0.5$ to $-0.7$ bar, and oxygen entry into the soil and turgor potential of the bacterial cells both presumably are maximal (Howie et al. 1987). The optimal water potential for the take-all pathogen is also in this range of soil water potentials (Cook et al. 1972); as such, the pathogen is maximally exposed to fluorescent pseudomonads and probably other Gram-negative bacteria. This may explain why the environmental factors that affect activity of the bacteria have such an effect on the activity of this pathogen.

The suppression of take-all on wheat in soils fertilized with ammonium nitrogen, and after wheat monoculture and one or two outbreaks of the disease, is associated not only with larger populations of fluorescent pseudomonads but also with a greater frequency of types inhibitory to the pathogen (Weller, in Cook & Baker 1983). P. fluorescens strain 2-79 produces a phenazine-type antibiotic inhibitory to G. graminis var. tritici at only $1$ µg ml$^{-1}$ of medium (Gurusiddaiah et al. 1986). Antibiotic-negative mutants, produced by inactivating single genes by Tn5 mutagenesis, were significantly less suppressive to take-all than the parent when introduced with the seed (Thomashow et al. 1986). Restoration of phenazine-producing ability, by complementation with a fragment of wild-type DNA introduced using a cosmid vector, also restored ability of the mutant to suppress take-all (L. S. Thomashow and D. M. Weller, unpublished results). This evidence makes clear that antibiotic-producing ability is important for biocontrol with this strain of P. fluorescens and justifies seeking this trait in either natural or engineered strains. However, the stage is also now set for studies of ways to enhance antibiotic production through manipulation of the rhizosphere environment. Rhizosphere pH, oxygen supply, redox potential and nutrient availability are among the many factors that could influence either production or activity of the antibiotic, and can also be studied experimentally in finding ways to control this pathogen by management of the environment.

## REFERENCES

Asher, M. J. C. 1980 Variation in pathogenicity and cultural characters in Gaeumannomyces graminis var. tritici. Trans. Br. Mycol. Soc. 75, 213–220.

Baker, K. F. 1987 Developing concepts in biological control of plant pathogens. A. Rev. Phytopath. 25, 67–85.

Baker, K. F. & Cook, R. J. 1974 (original edn) Biological control of plant pathogens. San Francisco: W. H. Freeman. Reprinted edn, 1982. St Paul, Minnesota: American Phytopathology Society.

Chamswarng, C. 1984 Etiology and epidemiology of pythium root rot of wheat. Ph.D. thesis, Washington State University, Pullman.

Chamswarng, C. & Cook, R. J. 1985 Identification and comparative pathogenicity of Pythium species from wheat roots and wheat-field soils in the Pacific Northwest. Phytopathology 75, 821–827.

Chet, I. & Baker, R. 1981 Isolation and biocontrol potential of Trichoderma hamatum from soil naturally suppressive to Rhizoctonia solani. Phytopathology 71, 286–290.

180     R. J. COOK

Christensen, N. W., Taylor, R. G., Jackson, T. L. & Mitchell, B. L. 1981 Chloride effects on water potentials and yield of winter wheat infected with take-all root rot. *Agron. J.* **73**, 1053–1058.

Cook, R. J. 1968 Fusarium root and foot rot of cereals in the Pacific Northwest. *Phytopathology* **58**, 127–131.

Cook, R. J. 1970 Factors affecting saprophytic colonization of wheat straw by *Fusarium roseum* f. sp. *cerealis* 'Culmorum'. *Phytopathology* **60**, 1672–1676.

Cook, R. J. 1973 Influence of low plant and soil water potentials on diseases caused by soilborne fungi. *Phytopathology* **63**, 451–458.

Cook, R. J. 1980 Fusarium foot rot of wheat and its control in the Pacific Northwest. *Pl. Dis.* **64**, 1061–1066.

Cook, R. J. 1986 Wheat management systems in the Pacific Northwest. *Pl. Dis.* **70**, 894–898.

Cook, R. J. & Baker, K. F. 1983 *The nature and practice of biological control of plant pathogens.* (539 pages.) St Paul, Minnesota: American Phytopathological Society.

Cook, R. J. & Bruehl, G. W. 1968 Relative significance of parasitism versus sparophytism in colonization of wheat straw by *Fusarium roseiu* 'Culmorum' in the field. *Phytopathology* **58**, 306–308.

Cook, R. J. & Haglund, W. A. 1982 Pythium root rot: a barrier to yield of Pacific Northwest wheat. *Wash. State Univ. Agric. Res. Centr. Res. Bull.* No. XB0913. (20 pages.)

Cook, R. J. & Naiki, T. 1985 Virulence of *Gaeumannomyces graminis* var. *tritici* from fields under short-term and long-term wheat cultivation in the Pacific Northwest, USA. *Pl. Path.* **31**, 201–207.

Cook, R. J., Papendick, R. I. & Griffin, D. M. 1972 Growth of two root-rot fungi as affected by osmotic and matric water potentials. *Proc. Soil Sci. Soc. Am.* **36**, 78–82.

Cook, R. J. & Rovira, A. D. 1976 The role of bacteria in the biological control of *Gaeumannomyces graminis* by suppressive soils. *Soil Biol. Biochem.* **8**, 267–273.

Cook, R. J., Sitton, J. W. & Haglund, W. A. 1987 Influence of soil treatments on growth and yield of wheat and implications for control of Pythium root rot. *Phytopathology* **77**, 1192–1198.

Cook, R. J. & Weller, D. M. 1987 Management of take-all in consecutive crops of wheat or barley. In *Innovative approaches to plant disease control* (ed. I. Chet), Wiley, pp. 41–76.

Cook, R. J., Wilkinson, H. T. & Alldredge, J. R. 1986 Evidence that microorganisms in suppressive soil associated with wheat take-all decline do not limit the number of lesions produced by *Gaeumannomyces graminis* var. *tritici*. *Phytopathology* **76**, 342–345.

Garrett, S. D. 1976 Influence of nitrogen on cellulolysis rate and saprophytic survival in soil of some cereal foot rot fungi. *Soil Biol. Biochem.* **8**, 229–234.

Garrett, S. D. 1985 Effect of soil texture on microbial abbreviation of saprophytic survival of the take-all fungus of wheat. *Proc. Indian Acad. Sci. (Pl. Sci.)* **94**, 85–90.

Gurusiddaiah, S., Weller, D. M., Sarkar, A. & Cook, R. J. 1986 Characterization of an antibiotic produced by a strain of *Pseudomonas fluorescens* inhibitory to *Gaeumannomyces graminis* var. *tritici* and *Pythium* spp. *Antimicrob. Ag. Chemother.* **29**, 488–495.

Hering, T. F., Cook, R. J. & Tang, W.-h. 1987 Infection of wheat embryos by *Pythium* species during seed germination and the influence of seed age and soil matric potential. *Phytopathology* **77**, 1104–1108.

Howie, W. J. 1985 Factors affecting colonization of wheat roots and suppression of take-all by pseudomonads antagonistic to *Gaeumannomyces graminis* var. *tritici*. Ph.D. thesis, Washington State University, Pullman.

Howie, W. J., Cook, R. J. & Weller, D. M. 1987 Effects of soil matric potential and cell motility on wheat root colonization by fluorescent pseudomonads suppressive to take-all. *Phytopathology* **77**, 286–292.

Huber, D. M., Painter, C. G., MacKay, H. C. & Peterson, D. L. 1968 Effect of nitrogen fertilization on take-all of winter wheat. *Phytopathology* **58**, 1470–1472.

Ingram, D. 1987 Pathogenicity of *Pythium* species on major crops in the Palouse. Ph.D. thesis, Washington State University, Pullman.

Inglis, D. A. & Cook, R. J. 1986 Persistence of chlamydospores of *Fusarium culmorum* in wheat field soils of eastern Washington. *Phytopathology* **76**, 1205–1208.

Kerr, A. 1980 Biological control of crown gall through production of agrocin 84. *Pl. Dis.* **64**, 25–30.

Kuć, J. 1982 Induced immunity to plant disease. *BioScience* **32**, 854–860.

Moore, K. J. & Cook, R. J. 1984 Increased take-all of wheat with direct drilling in the Pacific Northwest. *Phytopathology* **76**, 1044–1049.

Papendick, R. I. & Cook, R. J. 1974 Plant water stress and development of Fusarium foot rot in wheat subjected to different cultural practices. *Phytopathology* **64**, 358–363.

Pérombelon, M. C. M. & Kelman, A. 1980 Ecology of the soft rot erwinias. *A. Rev. Phytopath.* **18**, 361–387.

Rishbeth, J. 1979 Modern aspects of biological control of *Fomes* and *Armillaria*. *Eur. J. For. Path.* **9**, 331–340.

Rouatt, J. W. & Katznelson, H. 1961 A study of the bacteria on the root surface and in the rhizosphere soil of crop plants. *J. appl. Bact.* **24**, 164–171.

Rush, C. M., Ramig, R. E. & Kraft, J. M. 1986 Effects of wheat chaff and tillage on inoculum density of *Pythium ultimum* in the Pacific Northwest. *Phytopathology* **76**, 1330–1332.

Smiley, R. W. 1978 Antagonists of *Gaeumannomyces graminis* from the rhizoplane of wheat in soils fertilized with ammonium- or nitrate-nitrogen. *Soil Biol. Biochem.* **10**, 169–174.

Smiley, R. W. & Cook, R. J. 1973 Relationship between take-all of wheat and rhizosphere pH in soils fertilized with ammonium vs. nitrate-nitrogen. *Phytopathology* **63**, 882–890.

Sprague, R. 1950 *Diseases of cereals and grasses in North America.* (538 pages.) New York: Ronald Press.

Taylor, R. G., Jackson, T. L., Powelson, R. L. & Christensen, W. W. 1983 Chloride nitrogen form, lime, and planting date effects on take-all root rot of winter wheat. *Pl. Dis.* **67**, 1116–1120.

Thomashow, L. S., Weller, D. M. & Cook, R. J. 1986 Molecular analysis of phenazine antibiotic synthesis by *Pseudomonas fluorescens* strain 2-79. Third International Symposium on the Molecular Genetics of Plant-Microbe Interactions. July 27–31, McGill University, Montreal, Canada.

Vojinović, Z. D. 1973 The influence of microorganisms following *Ophiobolus graminis* Sacc. on its further pathogenicity. *Org. Eur. Med. Prot. Plantes Bull.* **9**, 91–101.

Weller, D. M. 1983 Colonization of wheat roots by a fluorescent pseudomonad suppressive to take-all. *Phytopathology* **73**, 1548–1553.

Weller, D. M. 1984 Distribution of a take-all suppressive strain of *Pseudomonas fluorescens* on seminal roots of winter wheat. *Appl. envir. Microbiol.* **48**, 897–899.

Weller, D. M. 1985 Application of fluorescent pseudomonads to control root diseases. In *Ecology and management of soilborne plant pathogens* (ed. A. A. Parker, A. D. Rovira, K. J. Moore, P. T. W. Wong & J. F. Kollmorgen), pp. 137–140. St. Paul, Minnesota: American Phytopathological Society.

Weller, D. M. & Cook, R. J. 1983 Suppression of take-all of wheat by seed treatments with fluorescent pseudomonads. *Phytopathology* **73**, 463–469.

Wilkinson, H. T., Cook, R. J. & Alldredge, J. R. 1985 Relation of inoculum size and concentration to infection of wheat roots by *Gaeumannomyces graminis* var. *Phytopathology* **75**, 98–103.

## Discussion

G. Défago (*Swiss Federal Institute of Technology, Zürich, Switzerland*). Can I ask Dr Cook for more information on the location of his rhizobacteria? Are they on the root surface or inside the roots? We have some evidence that in the case we are studying it is necessary that the rhizobacteria are inside the roots to suppress disease.

R. J. Cook. According to results of my associate, Dr D. M. Weller, about 90 % of the bacteria are in the rhizosphere and 10 % are on the rhizoplane. This is the distribution found on and around wheat roots after introduction of an antibiotic-resistant strain on the seed. However, I have seen results from my own earlier experiments that indicate a portion of the bacteria on roots are either attached very tightly (cannot be washed off by standard techniques) or they are inside root tissues. A portion of the cells are immersed in or beneath the mucilage of roots.

R. R. M. Paterson (*C.A.B. International Mycological Institute, Kew, U.K.*). A number of years ago there were reports about the use of fungal spores (e.g. *Penicillium*) to coat seeds in a manner that sounds similar to that described for the bacterium that was mentioned. Does Dr Cook know what has happened to the work?

R. J. Cook. This work has been, and continues to be, done by Dr T. Kommedahl and his students at the University of Minnesota. No patent was ever obtained on the effective organisms (or on their use as seed treatments) and without the prospects of an exclusive licence, private companies generally are not interested in developing these agents for commercial use. However, Dr Kommedahl's best strains are as good as standard chemical seed treatments.

J. M. Lynch (*Glasshouse Crops Research Institute, Littlehampton, U.K.*). About the effects of *Pythium* and *Fusarium*, Dr Cook also recognized that phytotoxins produced in the microbial degradation of straw could contribute to the total reduction in yield. Growth-inhibitory pseudomonads can also contribute to the yield reduction (Elliott & Lynch 1985). These effects could be synergistic in reducing yield. Does Dr Cook envisage that a single biological control agent could be applied to counteract these various effects or does he see more prospect in the use of a microbial 'cocktail' consisting of two or more antagonists?

*Reference*

Elliott, L. F. & Lynch, J. M. 1985 Plant growth-inhibitory pseudomonads colonizing winter wheat (*Triticum aestivum* L.) roots. *Pl. Soil* **84**, 57–65.

R. J. COOK. We know from results with selective treatments applied in both greenhouse and field experiments that the poor-growth syndrome for wheat sown into a trashy seed bed (e.g. direct-drill or conservation tillage) is associated mainly, if not entirely, with soil-inhabiting microorganisms and not the microorganisms present as a natural component of the straw microbiota. *Pythium* spp. are a major component of this deleterious microbiota, along with possibly *Rhizoctonia* spp., inhibitory pseudomonads, and other pathogens. Knowing this leads me to believe that a good seed and root protectant would go far to solve the problem. However, I am not so encouraged to believe that a single antagonist around the seeds and roots would be sufficient. We may need a mixture of antagonists or seed-treatment chemicals plus antagonists.

D. HORNBY (*Rothamsted Experimental Station, Harpenden, U.K.*). Would Dr Cook say in what proportion of tests in commercial fields he has obtained biological control of natural epidemics of take-all? How was this assessed: by yield increases, or by actual measurements of the disease?

R. J. COOK. As of 1986, we have completed ten replicated trails in cooperation with growers in fields with natural infestations of the take-all fungus. These fields were all seeded with the grower's own drill. Each field was second- or third-year wheat and in each case, take-all turned out to be the main yield-limiting factor. Root ratings, plant heights (a highly sensitive indicator of take-all) and yields were measured in each trial. Evidence of efficacy was obtained by one or more of these three measurements in at least five of the nine trials. Root ratings were nearly always lower with than without the treatment, but owing to variation, these differences were significant in only two or three cases. Differences were easiest to demonstrate statistically by measurement of plant heights. Yields were greater by only 1.5–5% in five trials (not significant) and 9.6–22.0% in four trials (significant at $p$ equal to 0.05 or 0.01). The average for the nine trials was 7.6% greater yield (0.4 t ha$^{-1}$). Where the treatment worked, it was obvious. However, independent assessments in these trails indicated that complete control of take-all would have elevated yields by 20–25%, on the average. Thus we have some way to go. Nevertheless, we are encouraged by the results obtained thus far. We think of our strains as prototypes of strains still to come.

*Phil. Trans. R. Soc. Lond.* B **318**, 183–201 (1988)

*Printed in Great Britain*

# The potential for managing indigenous natural enemies of aphids on field crops

By H. F. van Emden

*Departments of Horticulture, and Pure and Applied Zoology, University of Reading, Reading RG6 2AT, U.K.*

The co-evolution of aphids and their indigenous natural enemies means that, on field crops, biological control to a grower-acceptable level will occur only sporadically in the absence of manipulative interventions. Such interventions should focus on raising the natural enemy:aphid ratio. This ratio is far more important than the absolute number of natural enemies present. The main interventions for improving the ratio are habitat modifications, advancing in time the activity of natural enemies on the crop, reducing aphid multiplication through genetically based or induced partial plant resistance, and ingenious use of pesticide to build in relative selectivity of kill. The interactions between biological control and some of the other interventions offer exciting opportunities for managing natural enemies.

## 1. Introduction

The gardener who collects ladybirds from around his garden to place them on his roses for aphid control is exemplifying the underlying principle of managing indigenous natural enemies; he is increasing the natural enemy:aphid ratio. He is also aware that, without such intervention, he cannot rely on biological control being timely and effective.

The literature is generally not encouraging about the value of indigenous natural enemies for the control of aphids. Thus Jones & Jones (1984) state that aphid 'capacity for increase outstrips their enemies and is almost exponential', and in a major review of over 400 papers Hagen & van den Bosch (1968) found it striking 'that this great mass of literature has produced so little tangible evidence on the impact of these enemies'. At the end of the five-year International Biological Programme research effort on *Myzus persicae*, Mackauer & Way (1976) concluded 'No immediate improvement is apparent that would drastically increase the impact of natural enemies on the green peach aphid'. Shands *et al.* (1965) reported a maximum of only 0.63 % parasitization of potato aphids in northeastern Maine over 12 years.

Southwood *et al.* (1974) analysed the life tables of 32 different insects, and from this Southwood (1975) proposed a synoptic model of the relation between population growth and population density along the *r*–*K* continuum. This model included the important concept of the 'natural enemy ravine', where many insects may be kept at stable populations by natural enemies (held on the 'endemic ridge') until or unless some enviromental disturbance (e.g. a change in host plant condition) allows the population to escape towards a much greater density (onto the 'epidemic' ridge). Should the population escape past the 'release point' on the far side of the natural enemy ravine, natural enemies can no longer exert a significant check on population growth. Southwood (1977) cites aphids as typical of pests near the *r*-end of the continuum which escape the ravine most frequently. Aphid workers frequently smooth out the population growth curve early in the season, yet inspection of the original data points frequently suggests a 'natural enemy ravine' may have been crossed, e.g. Dean & Luuring's (1970) graph of aphid populations on wheat. When the time-scale of population growth is slower, as with *Brevicoryne brassicae* (van Emden 1965), the ravine is very apparent and was identified as representing stabilization by predators until a change in host-plant condition in late summer. All this suggests that the natural enemy restraint is usually inadequate, but nevertheless often adequate enough for attempting magnification by intervention.

Even though it is possible to find several reports of predators controlling aphid populations (examples are Minoranskii 1967; Tamaki *et al.* 1967; Chambers *et al.* 1982; Holmes 1984), it is clear that such control is too unpredictable and sporadic for practical utilization without some additional measures to enhance the predictability. A measure of this unpredictability is found in the International Biological Programme analyses of *Myzus persicae* populations on potatoes on 35 occasions, over three years and in five countries in the northern hemisphere (37°–56° N). A summary of these analyses (Mackauer & Way 1976) showed that predation was theoretically able to contain the measured potential increase rate of the aphid population on half the occasions, and succeeded in preventing an increase of the aphid population on all but two of these. Shands *et al.* (1972) had similar results in northeastern Maine; predators were responsible for decreasing only 45% of 31 aphid populations on potatoes.

It is perhaps not surprising that the natural enemies of aphids have such an unpredictable impact. By many centuries of co-evolution, one would expect predators and parasites of such a mobile and erratically abundant food source to have evolved the capacity to harvest the interest without digging too deeply into the capital! Even classical biological control using imported natural enemies very often involves some intervention to forestall the natural enemy:prey ratio declining to its indigenous equilibrium level. The elimination of natural enemy mortality by pathogens and parasitoids during quarantine is an important intervention of this kind. With natural enemies of aphids, co-evolution would seem to have led to a delay in the arrival of predators and parasites after aphid immigration, and their functional and numerical responses are geared to follow rather than overtake the high innate capacity for increase of aphid populations (van Emden 1966; Dixon 1985). Interventions to improve biological control of aphids by indigenous natural enemies need to address themselves to one or both of these co-evolved responses. Resolving the co-evolved poor synchronization of predators and parasites involves creating an 'unnaturally' high natural enemy:aphid ratio, particularly early in the season. This will be reviewed under the headings of direct augmentation of natural enemies and habitat modification. Early enhancement of parasite activity in crops has recently been reviewed by Powell (1986). The problem of functional and numerical responses needs tackling by interventions which probably reduce numbers of both natural enemies and aphids, but which disproportionately maximize the natural enemy:aphid ratio. This will be reviewed under the headings of plant resistance and use of pesticides.

## 2. DIRECT AUGMENTATION
### (a) *Releases*

Predator releases have had some success, though with doubtful economic viability. Massive releases of the ladybird *Hippodamia convergens* were attempted in North America as early as 1908 for the control of *Aphis gossypii* on canteloupes, but failed because the beetles dispersed rapidly within three days of release (Hagen 1962). Cooke (1963) made four releases (40000–150000 beetles per release) of *H. convergens* on lucerne in Washington State, but any reduction in aphids was uneconomic compared with the costs of release. Again, the beetles dispersed rapidly, even if previously fed on protein hydrolysate. However, Iperti (in Hodek 1973) found that starving the coccinellids inhibited dispersion. Shands *et al.* (1972) released laboratory bred chrysopid and coccinellid larvae in small (0.1 ha†) potato plots and obtained a maximum of 60% aphid control with the release of 30200 coccinellid larvae and 85100 chrysopid larvae. In other experiments (Shands & Simpson 1972) 13500 coccinellid eggs were applied in an agar solution, but satisfactory aphid control was not obtained. Ankersmit (1983) has reported failure of attempts to increase parasitoid numbers in cereals early in the season by releasing them with aphids.

### (b) Synomones and kairomones

These are naturally produced chemicals influencing insect behaviour. Synomones emanate directly from the plant whereas kairomones emanate from insects or their feeding activity. The most well-known example of the use of kairomones in aphid control is the spraying of 'artificial honeydew' in California to increase numbers of *Hippodamia* spp. and *Chrysoperla carnea* in lucerne fields. These predators respond positively to the odour of a breakdown product of tryptophane, probably indole acetaldehyde (van Emden & Hagen 1976), emanating from aphid honeydew. Both types of predator remained in the treated area even if aphids were absent; the chrysopids even oviposited in the absence of prey. Enough aphid control to prevent economic damage was achieved with artificial honeydew consisting of a mixture of cheap commercial yeast hydrolysate, sucrose and water (Hagen *et al.* 1971). More recently, Hagen (1986) has concluded that *C. carnea* must receive a synonome from the crop in order to respond to the kairomone.

With parasitoids, Schlinger & Dietrick (1960) reported that enhancement early in the season by synomones associated with strip-cutting lucerne required the presence of hosts, unlike the use of yeast hydrolysate sprays for predators. Although some parasitoids of aphids are strongly responsive to aphid and honeydew odours and do not react to the odour of the host plant, it seems more usual that parasitoids respond to host-plant produced synonomes before any response to aphids or honeydew. *Aphidius nigripes* appears to be in the former category; it responds to a wide range of aphid species and their honeydew, but not to potato, the host plant of these aphids (Bouchard & Cloutier 1985). Read *et al.* (1979) first demonstrated the attraction to a synonome (mustard oil in crucifers) of a parasitoid of aphids (*Diaretiella rapae* parasitizing *Brevicoryne brassicae*). There have since been similar reports for parasitoids of cereal aphids (Schuster & Starks 1974; Powell & Zhi-Li 1983) and at Reading University, M. G. V. Wickremasinghe (unpublished results) has also detected strong host-plant odour versus aphid odour attraction in several parasitoid and aphid combinations, including some on non-crop hosts such as nettles, oak and sycamore (figure 1).

The behaviour of natural enemies of aphids in relation to plant-derived odours is still a new research area, and the practical possibilities are still to be determined. Presumably, the crop odour could be enhanced artificially or by crop cultivars that produce such volatiles to a greater degree. The need to test the synonomes of crop cultivars has been stressed by van Emden (1978), who reported the failure of biological control of *B. brassicae* by *D. rapae* on the Brussels sprout cultivar Early Half Tall related to its lower levels of mustard oils.

† One hectare = $10^4$ m$^2$.

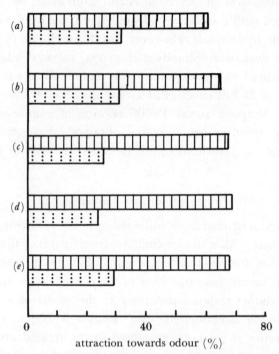

attraction towards odour (%)

FIGURE 1. The percentage response of aphid parasitoids to plant odours (barred line) versus odours of their host
   aphids (dotted line). Order of listing is aphid host-plant, aphid, parasitoid (data of M. G. V. Wickremasinghe,
   unpublished results). (*a*) Nettle, *Microlophium carnosum*, *Aphidius ervi*; (*b*) wheat, *Rhopalosiphum padi*, *Aphidius
   rhopalosiphi*; (*c*) Dock, *Aphis fabae*, *Lysiphlebus fabarum*; (*d*) oak, *Tuberculoides annulatus*, *Praon* sp.; (*e*) Sycamore,
   *Drepanosiphum platanoides*, *Aphelinus flavus*.

## 3. HABITAT MODIFICATION

### (*a*) Overwintering conditions

The provision of shelter adjacent to crop fields to promote an increase and earlier occurrence
of coccinellids on crops has been demonstrated for sugar beet (Bombosch 1965), potatoes
(Fenjves 1945) and recommended in Czechoslovakia to compensate for increased areas of
monoculture (Hodek *et al.* 1962). Iperti (1966) found that coccinellids migrating from crops in
the autumn to form aggregations in the hills around the cultivated plains of southeastern
France could suffer over 60% mortality from the fungus *Beauveria* over winter. In ladybird
aggregations on plants below 1000 m altitude, the fungus became a serious threat. Mortality
was much reduced above 1000 m, or in aggregations in rock cracks. Iperti (1966) was able to
demonstrate that coccinellids both preferred and survived better (less than 15% mortality) in
artifically created rock-piles. He devised a special trap for coccinellid aggregations (Hodek
1973); this trap facilitated the transport of vast numbers of coccinellids to high altitudes and
later return to the crop areas.

### (*b*) Alternative prey

The provision of suitable non-crop plants to host alternative aphid prey for parasitoids has
been extensively studied by Stary (1983, 1986) in Czechoslovakia. He regarded aphids on
perennial stinging nettle (*Urtica dioica*) as a useful source of *Aphidius ervi*, which parasitizes

several crop aphid pests including *Sitobion avenae* and *Acyrthosiphon pisum*. *Cirsium arvense* carries large populations of *Aphis fabae cirsiliacanthoides*. Unfortunately, the dominant parasitoid on this aphid is *Lysiphlebus cardui* and not *L. fabarum*, which is the important parasitoid for *Aphis fabae*. Eikenbary & Rogers (1974) reported that *Schizaphis graminum* on cereals was more parasitized when sunflowers infested with *Aphis helianthi* were growing nearby. The parasitoid *Lysiphlebus testaceipes* was able to maintain itself on large populations of *A. helianthi* during two critical periods of the year when *S. graminum* was scarce or absent on the cereal crop.

However, some doubt has been cast on the value of such reservoirs. Although in the last example the parasitoid appeared to switch aphid hosts successfully, this is not always the case. Cameron *et al.* (1984) found that *A. ervi* reared on several other aphid species parasitized few *Sitobion avenae* on wheat. That this was not just a plant synomone effect was indicated by a change in parasitoid esterase bands shown in electrophoretic analysis when the parasitoid was switched from *Acyrthosiphon pisum* to *S. avenae*. Powell (1986) found mummy production by *Aphidius rhopalosiphi* much reduced when switched to *S. avenae* after several generations on *Metopolophium dirhodum*, though the reverse switch resulted in an increase in parasitization.

An interesting recent development has been the acceptance by many cereal farmers in the U.K. of the proposal to leave an edge area of the crop unsprayed by pesticides, including herbicides. As yet, there is no evidence that this provides a reservoir of aphid predators and parasitoids, but it could lead to an increase of the natural enemy restraint on aphids in the central area of the crop.

### (c) Flowers

Pollen and nectar are particularly required by the adults of adult syrphids, but also by coccinellids when aphid prey is missing (Hodek 1973). The provision of plant sources of pollen and nectar for syrphids has been recommended in the Rhône valley in France (Mackauer & Way 1976). One of few studies identifying increased predation on the crop associated with adjacent flowers is by van Emden (1965), who planted flowers along parts of two edges of a Brussels sprout crop and found significantly more syrphid eggs laid on the crop near these flowers than elsewhere. This was associated with 65–70 % predation mortality of *Brevicoryne brassicae* near the edges with flowers, compared with under 50 % at other edges and the centre. With the high mobility of most adult predators, it is unlikely that mortality from predation in any part of the field (0.7 ha) was totally unrelated to the presence of flowers. This is one of the problems of experimentally showing the impact of without-crop habitat modification, and it has led to many unwarranted negative conclusions in the literature. After all, Jacobson (1946) showed that damage to wheat by a pentatomid bug originating from a patch of the weed *Salsola* sp. at the edge of the field extended for at least 3 km into the crop, i.e. a square field would have to be over 1000 ha in area for the centre to be free of such edge effects!

### (d) Crop background

The work of Smith (1969a, b) offers considerable opportunities for manipulating the natural enemy:aphid ratio, but has hardly been followed up. Smith compared populations of *B. brassicae* and its natural enemies in clean and weedy Brussels sprout plots. Aphid populations remained negligible on plants in the weedy plots, but reached over 100 aphids per plant on the clean plots by late September. Many fewer immigrant aphids were trapped over the weedy plots, but additionally, several predator species (particularly the syrphid *Melanostoma* spp.

ovipositing and *Anthocoris nemorum*) were more numerous on the weedy plots early in the season. Syrphids in the genus *Platycheirus*, however, laid more eggs on plants in the clean plots.

There has been a little subsequent work on the same theme. Powell *et al.* (1981) compared the numbers of polyphagous predators caught in pitfall traps in unweeded and clean plots of winter wheat (figure 2). Of the 12 significant effects among the 14 combinations of 7 beetles and 2 years, 7 indicated greater beetle numbers in the weedy plots. The other 5 showed more beetles in the clean plots. However, this is the expected result given equal numbers because the hindrance of horizontal movement by the weeds would result in a reduced chance of capturing beetles by pitfall trapping in weedy plots (Greenslade 1964).

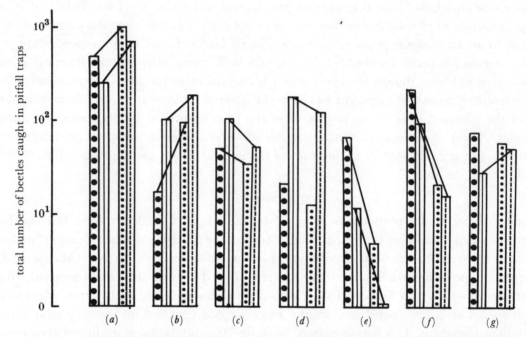

FIGURE 2. Numbers of different beetle species (*a–g*) caught in pitfall traps in clean (small dots or broken line) versus weedy (large dots or continuous line) cereal plots in 1980 (dots) and 1981 (lines). Bold lines join statistically significant within-year differences (data of Powell *et al.* 1981). (*a*) *Pterostichus melanarius*; (*b*) *P. madidus*; (*c*) *Loricera pilicornis*; (*d*) *Agonum dorsale*; (*e*) *Amara* spp.; (*f*) *Philonthus cognatum*; (*g*) *Tachyporus* spp.

Andow *et al.* (1986) found reduced populations of *B. brassicae* on cabbages grown with living mulches of grasses or clover, but did not investigate how far this was due to any enhancement of biological control. Powell (1983) released *Myzus festucae* with the parasitoid *Aphidius uzbekistanicus* onto rye grass undersown or as strips in wheat. Summer *Sitobion avenae* populations on wheat were smallest in plots that had developed the largest populations of *M. festucae* in the spring.

The effect on the biological control of aphids of increasing crop plant density has also received some attention. Increasing crop density in itself tends to reduce the number of immigrant alate aphids (see, for example, Way & Heathcote 1966), both by changing the crop background and by influencing the physiology of the crop plants and their suitability for the aphids. However, Honek (1983) showed that the ladybird *Propylaea quattordecimpunctata*, as well as syrphids, preferred dense plant stands; *Coccinella* spp. preferred less dense stands.

TABLE 1. THE EFFECT OF STRIP-HARVESTING AND NORMAL HARVESTING ON THE AVERAGE NUMBER OF NATURAL ENEMIES OF *THERIOAPHIS TRIFOLII* (DATA FROM SCHLINGER AND DIETRICK (1960))

| natural enemies | thousands per hectare | |
| --- | --- | --- |
| | normal harvesting | strip-harvesting |
| coccinellid adults | 114 | 507 |
| coccinellid larvae | 27 | 573 |
| chrysopid larvae | 482 | 509 |
| hymenopterous parasitoids | 173 | 709 |
| 'big-eyed' Heteroptera | 492 | 991 |
| aphidophagous spiders | 259 | 2703 |
| totals | 1547 | 5992 |

Schlinger & Dietrick (1960) spectacularly demonstrated the disadvantages for biological control of harvesting lucerne fields completely compared with leaving refuges for natural enemies by strip-harvesting. The density of natural enemies of *Therioaphis trifolii* was nearly four times greater in strip-harvested than in totally harvested lucerne (table 1).

## 4. PLANT RESISTANCE

### (a) *Plant resistance and biological control*

Plant resistance decreases aphid numbers, particularly by slowing the growth of the aphid population in time. If predators and parasitoids show a less than proportional response to the reduction in the number of their prey, an improved natural enemy:aphid ratio will result and therefore the impact of biological control should be magnified. Two recent publications have discussed the interactions of plant resistance and biological control for plant pests in general. The review by Herzog & Funderburk (1985) stresses the reductions in biological control that might occur from (a) lower prey numbers and (b) anatomical and chemical barriers of the resistant varieties discouraging natural enemies directly; the review also includes some examples of a beneficial interaction. A whole book on the interaction (Boethel & Eikenbary 1986) emphasizes the potential benefits.

None of Herzog & Funderburk's examples (1985) of reduced biological control on resistant varieties concern aphids. Obrycki & Tauber (1984, 1985) studied biological control of aphids on potato cultivars with dense glandular hairs, a very strong resistance mechanism against aphids. No adverse effects of this pubescence on predators and parasitoids was found in the field, and large numbers of aphid mummies were recorded. Any less active movement by predator larvae seemed cancelled out by the preferred oviposition by predators on pubescent varieties. Karner & Manglitz (1983) investigated whether the feeding activity of *Hippodamia convergens* was reduced on a resistant lucerne cultivar (Baker) compared with a susceptible one (Vermal). They placed the same number of *Acyrthosiphon pisum* on both cultivars, and measured the proportion of aphids consumed by different instars of the ladybird at three different temperatures. With 8 of 12 instar–temperature combinations, the proportion of aphids consumed was greater on the resistant cultivar.

van Emden & Wearing (1965) used a simple model to propose that partial plant resistance should enhance biological control of a multivoltine pest such as an aphid. This was confirmed experimentally in the glasshouse by Starks *et al.* (1972) with *Schizaphis graminum* on two barley varieties ('Rogers', susceptible; 'Will', partly resistant) with the parasitoid *Lysiphlebus testaceipes* (figure 3). Without parasitoids, the number of aphids on Rogers was never more than 1.5 times the number on Will; with parasitoids, however, there was a 2.5-fold increase by the third week. With chrysanthemums, Wyatt (1970) reported that biological control of *Myzus persicae* by *Aphidius matricariae* was only effective if the variety used was partly aphid resistant.

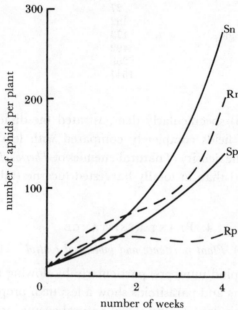

FIGURE 3. Population growth of *Schizaphis graminum* on the susceptible barley variety Rogers (S) and the partly resistant variety Will (R) in the presence (p) and absence (n) of the parasitoid *Lysiphlebus testaceipes* (Starks *et al.* 1972).

Dodd (1973) compared two Brussels sprout varieties in field trials. Over a five day interval, predation on the cultivar Winter Harvest (susceptible) was just over 30%, but was 55% on the cultivar Earley Half Tall (very little resistance). In this example, the potential increase rate of the aphids over the same time period was 1.33 on the susceptible and 1.30 on the partly resistant cultivar. With cereals, Lykouressis (1982) found that peak populations of *Sitobion avenae* on Pamena oats in the glasshouse were only 1.25-fold greater than on a barley cultivar. Yet in the presence of the parasitoid *Aphelinus abdominalis*, aphid numbers on barley did not rise above 20 per plant, but peaked at about 70 per plant on the oats.

van Emden (1986) has run a simple population model with built-in density dependence of parasitoid impact (Hassell 1975) to simulate the interaction between partial plant resistance and biological control. Figure 4*a* shows the output of the model, as well as two additional curves for a partly resistant variety with biological control. One of these (RP) assumes that percentage mortality on the two cultivars is not affected by the differing prey densities and is identical on both, whereas the other line (RA) assumes the same numerical mortality on both cultivars (representing a large percentage mortality on the resistant cultivar). Figure 4*b* illustrates how the output of the model is reflected in the apparent difference between populations of aphids on the two varieties. The apparent resistance of the partly resistant variety increases with each generation as the growth rates of the two populations diverge, and of course is identical whether biological control is absent (R) or proportionally the same (RP)

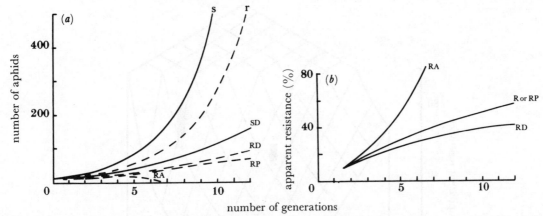

FIGURE 4. The effect of biological control on change in time of the apparent resistance (*b*) of a partly resistant variety given various aphid population growth curves (*a*). s, Susceptible variety and r, partly resistant variety, both in the absence of biological control; SD, RD, the same varieties with biological control assumed to show density dependence; RP, resistant variety with same percentage mortality from biological control between generations as on the susceptible variety; RA, resistant variety with same numerical mortality between generations as on the susceptible variety.

on both varieties. Any tendency for apparent resistance to be magnified in relation to this R or RP line, i.e. greater percentage mortality on the resistant than on the susceptible cultivar, moves the line towards RA (the same numerical mortality on both cultivars).

Figure 5 shows a response surface generated on the 'RA' assumption, i.e. higher percentage mortality on the resistant cultivar to the extent of matching the mortality on the susceptible numerically. This is, of course, across a generation with differing increase rates on the two varieties; it is therefore the apparent phenomenon and not a true quantitative estimate of mortality. The response surface shows the apparent resistance under the equal numerical mortality assumption of combinations of different percentage plant resistance with different percentage biological control occurring on the susceptible variety. A, B and C mark the data of respectively Starks *et al.* (1972), Dodd (1973) and Lykouressis (1982), the three examples quoted earlier where the level of plant resistance (in the absence of parasitoids), the degree of biological control on the susceptible variety and the final apparent resistance were all measured independently.

Figure 5 indicates that percentage biological control on the partly resistant plants in all three examples was greater than on the susceptible plants; in Dodd's (1973) work it considerably exceeded the assumption of an equal numerical impact. Possible explanations for the increase in percentage biological control on resistant plants are that host plants can be more attractive to parasitoids than aphids (see §2*b*) and also the colonial habit of aphids and the rather predictable distribution on the plant of the colonies. Rabbinge *et al.* (1984) have modelled how clustering increases the impact of parasitoids of aphids.

Nothing is yet known about the longer-term effects on predators and parasitoids when being reared on aphids on resistant varieties. Kuo (1986) has pointed out that, as resistant plants may make aphids smaller, this could affect the fecundity of natural enemies, particularly parasitoids. With parasitoids there is also the possibility that a greater proportion of males might be produced.

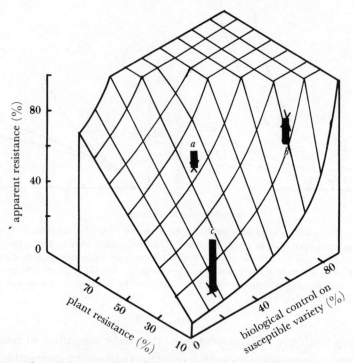

FIGURE 5. Response surface of the apparent resistance of varieties with different levels of resistance (in comparison
with a susceptible variety) with varying biological control mortalities on the latter and assuming the same
numerical mortality on both varieties. (a) Data of Starks *et al.* (1972); (b) data of Lykouressis (1982); (c) data
of Dodd (1973).

### (b) *Use of pesticides in relation to biological control*

Pesticides are normally considered likely to damage biological control, yet can be a potent
intervention for increasing the natural enemy:aphid ratio. The early example of integrated
control of *Therioaphis trifolii* on alfalfa in California (Stern *et al.* 1959) was based on the concept
that a reduced dosage of pesticide would enhance this ratio to give satisfactory control in a
situation where biological control in the absence of pesticide was ineffective. Raising the
natural enemy:aphid ratio is the consequence of any treatment that selectively kills aphids,
even if such selectivity is only partial.

### (i) *Selective pesticides*

The carbamate insecticide pirimicarb is well known for being selective against aphids and
many Diptera, including Syrphidae; it is non-toxic at normal doses to coccinellids, anthocorids,
chrysopids and parasitoids of aphids. Powell *et al.* (1981) compared pitfall trap catches of
predators in cereal plots treated with pirimicarb and dimethoate. Pirimicarb had very little
effect on Carabidae, Staphylinidae and spiders, but dimethoate immediately reduced numbers
of these predators, although immigrants caused some increase after a week. The selectivity of
pirimicarb has made it especially valuable because, despite limited persistance, one application
may be enough for natural enemies, which have accumulated on the aphid population, to
maintain control.

Less selective pesticides still have the potential of raising the natural enemy:aphid ratio, though less dramatically than pirimicarb. Appropriate screening of a range of pesticides will usually show differences in pesticide impact on aphids versus predators and parasitoids. For example, Croft & Brown (1975) reviewed the available data on the relative toxicity (as $LC_{50}$ or $LD_{50}$) of pesticides to pests and natural enemies. Coccinellidae seem generally more resistant to pesticides than their prey. Of 29 pesticide–coccinellid combinations, 26 showed selectivity in favour of coccinellids. For chrysopids and nabids respectively, 2 out of 3 and 2 out of 2 combinations similarly showed greater toxicity to the aphid than to the predator. With parasitoids, however, only 1 of 4 combinations showed greater toxicity to the aphid than the parasitoid.

Bartlett (1964) catalogued the toxicity of 60 insecticides and fungicides to natural enemies. For natural enemies of aphids he identified only seven insecticides as showing low toxicity to coccinellids, three to parasitoids and three to syrphids. Zeleny (1966) found malathion far less toxic than sumithion to all stages of *Coccinella septempunctata*. Sotherton & Moreby (1984), in response to increasing evidence that foliar applied fungicides were damaging polyphagous predator populations, did laboratory bioassays of seven such fungicides at field application rates with three beetle predators common in cereal fields: *Agonum dorsale*, *Demetrias atricapillus* and *Tachyporus chrysomelinus*. The species varied in their response, but pyrazophos caused 100 % mortality of all. The other fungicides caused less mortality, especially carbendazim and tridimefon.

### (ii) *Selective placement*

Systemic insecticides, particularly when applied to the soil rather than foliage, are likely to cause relatively little kill of natural enemies on the plants (see, for example, Zeleny 1966; Saharia 1985), although not necessarily of ground-dwelling polyphagous predators.

Little work appears to have been done on restricting pesticide, as far as possible, to parts of the plants where aphids are most abundant. Modern controlled droplet application makes possible accurate placement of the majority of the pesticide, so targeting toxin specifically to the sites occupied by aphids would appear practicable for raising the natural enemy:aphid ratio. For example, electrostatic sprayers offer the possibility of largely restricting insecticide deposits for the control of *Sitobion avenae* on the ears of cereals.

An interesting placement technique developed for tree fruit in the U.S.A. (Lewis & Hickey 1964) has potential for aphid control in field crops. It relies on the selectivity inherent in reduced dosages (see below). This is the 'alternative row middle' technique, translatable to field crops as 'band spraying'. The swathes (or boom spans) are so arranged that there are narrow unsprayed bands between sprayed swathes that only receive spray on a subsequent spraying occasion when different bands remain unsprayed. Reduced concentrations of pesticide can be used because the pesticide deposit is renewed over most of the field after a relatively short interval. The system has been found to increase the natural enemy:prey ratio on apples in the U.S.A. and is being used for 95 % of all applications to apples in Pennsylvania (Hull *et al.* 1983).

### (iii) *Selective timing*

There are very few references to timing of pesticides to improve selectivity of kill. Bartlett (1964) discussed the general principle of avoiding pesticide treatments destructive to natural enemies as far as possible during periods of effective predator and parasitoid activity.

Early in the season before parasitoid generations overlap, it may be possible to time sprays to coincide with a high proportion of parasitoids pupated within aphid mummies (Bartlett 1964). However, emerging adult parasitoids can be killed by contact with residual insecticide on the mummies. Saharia (1985) recommended that granular systemic insecticides against *Lipaphis erysimi* should be applied to mustard crops before *Coccinella repanda* enters the crop.

### (iv) *Dosage reductions*

Hull & Beers (1985) have reviewed the numerous cases where reduced doses have been used successfully in commercial control of various pests, to give double savings; first, in the amount of pesticide applied per spray and secondly, in the saving of repeat sprays where valuable natural enemy action was conserved (see §4*b* (i) for the relative toxicities of pesticides to aphids and their predators and parasitoids).

As mentioned previously (§4*b*), reduced doses of organophosphate insecticide were used successfully on lucerne in California (Stern *et al.* 1959) to raise the natural enemy:aphid ratio and give control of populations of organophosphate resistant *Therioaphis trifolii*. Reduced damage to natural enemy populations and subsequent natural enemy multiplication more than offset the initially poorer kill of the pest (Bartlett 1964).

The selectivity of reduced doses stems from the fact that dose response curves of many natural enemies are steeper than those of their prey (figure 7); Dodd (1973), for example, has shown this for coccinellids and *Diaeretiella rapae* (a parasitoid of *Brevicoryne brassicae*). The difference in slope of the response may well stem from the armoury of detoxifying enzymes needed by a herbivore to deal with plant compounds but not needed by a carnivore (Plapp 1981).

The use of a partly resistant crop variety benefits biological control besides magnifying the impact of natural enemies. This additional benefit is the possibility of further raising the

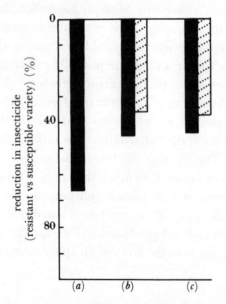

FIGURE 6. Reduction in concentration of insecticide as $LC_{50}$ (solid line) and $LD_{50}$ (dotted line) possible on partly resistant varieties in comparison with susceptible ones. (*a*) Data of Selander *et al.* (1972) on susceptibility to parathion of *Myzus persicae* on chrysanthemums; (*b*) data of Bin Muid (1977) on susceptibility to malathion of *M. persicae* on Brussels sprouts; (*c*) data of Attah (1984) on susceptibility to malathion of *Metopolophium dirhodum* on wheat.

natural enemy: aphid ratio by reducing insecticide dose. After the work of Selander *et al.* (1972) on the susceptibility to parathion of *Myzus persicae* on resistant chrysanthemum cultivars (figure 6), Bin Muid (1977) and Attah (1984) have shown enhanced susceptibility to malathion of organophosphate resistant *Myzus persicae* and of *Metopolophium dirhodum* on partly resistant varieties of Brussels sprouts and wheat respectively. The varieties studied by Bin Muid and Attah had only low levels of resistance (the Brussels sprout varieties used by Bin Muid were those used by Dodd (1973); see §4a), yet in each case $LC_{50}$ values were reduced by nearly one half (figure 6). Aphids on the resistant varieties were smaller, but their increased susceptibility to insecticide was mostly physiological in nature because correction for body mass did not account for the differences. The possibility of using reduced doses on partly resistant varieties has implications on selectivity far greater than are at first apparent, because it is unlikely that the dose–response curve of natural enemies is affected by the plant resistance to the aphid (figure 7). Thus a two thirds dose on a partly resistant variety gives kill of aphids equivalent to full dose on a susceptible variety, yet remains only a two thirds dose for the parasitoid or predator. The increased selectivity of kill (see figure 7) is likely to be dramatic and result in considerable amplification of the natural enemy: aphid ratio.

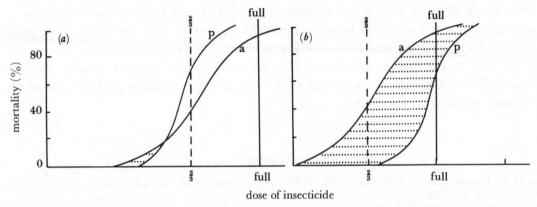

FIGURE 7. Theoretical selectivity of pesticide application on a resistant variety (*b*) compared with on a susceptible variety (*a*). a, Dose mortality curve of pest aphid; p, dose mortality curve of predator or parasitoid. Doses ($\frac{2}{3}$ or full) above graphs are relevant to the aphid, doses below graphs are relevant to predator or parasitoid. Selectivity 'window' is stippled.

The argument is often raised that advocating reduced doses carries the danger of promoting insecticide resistance in the pest by allowing the survival of individuals carrying genes for resistance in the heterozygous condition. However, if such dose reduction is advocated in pest management, then survivors of a pesticide application become the prey of the natural enemies that the dose reduction has preserved.

### (c)  *The pest management triad*

Although plant resistance and use of pesticides to improve the natural enemy: aphid ratio have been given separate headings in this account, it is clear that, with biological control, a three-way interaction exists which has been called the 'pest management triad' (van Emden 1983). The introduction of a variety partly resistant to the aphid pest enhances the ratio directly because its effect on aphid population size exceeds any similar effect on the natural enemies, and by lowering the tolerance of the pest to pesticide. This in turn allows the ratio to be built up still further by the selectivity of kill inherent in the relation described above between the response curves to pesticide of the aphids and their natural enemies. The ratio can then be further enhanced by using a selective pesticide.

## 5. Conclusions

In spite of the pessimism in much of the literature about the potential of indigenous natural enemies of aphids in field crops, adequate biological control for the farmer does occur sporadically and, where it does not, there is much evidence that the aphids have suddenly or temporarily escaped the natural enemy restraint rather than that restraint is insignificant.

There are many ways in which the natural enemy: aphid ratio can be raised by intervention to hinder the escape of the aphid population from the natural enemy restraint. These have so far largely been studied in isolation, and the degree of intervention necessary to achieve effective aphid control is usually uneconomic or unacceptable to the farmer in his management of the crop system. However, the few examples where such interventions have been integrated demonstrate a combined impact on the efficiency of biological control far higher than would have been predicted from what is known about the effect of each intervention on its own.

It appears that it is interaction between interventions, rather that the potential of those interventions in themselves, that holds the key to managing indigenous natural enemies of aphids in field crops. Adequate impact of indigenous natural enemies should often be attainable and should encourage us to seek to develop pest management packages out of the ideas already available as components.

## References

Andow, D. A., Nicholson, A. G. & Willson, H. R. 1986 Insect populations on cabbage grown in living mulches. *Envir. Ent.* **15**, 293–299.

Ankersmit, G. W. 1983 Aphidiids as parasites of the cereal aphids *Sitobion avenae* and *Metopolophium dirhodum*. In *Aphid antagonists* (ed. R. Cavalloro), pp. 42–49. Rotterdam: Balkema.

Attah, P. K..1984 An investigation of the host plant modification of malathion tolerance of *Metopolophium dirhodum* (Walker) on wheat. Ph.D. thesis, University of Reading.

Bartlett, B. R. 1964 Integration of chemical and biological control. In *Biological control of insect pests and weeds* (ed. P. De Bach), pp. 489–511. London: Chapman and Hall.

Bin Muid, M. 1977 Host plant modification of insecticide resistance in *Myzus persicae*. Ph.D. thesis, University of Reading.

Boethel, D. J. & Eikenbary, R. D. 1986 *Interactions of plant resistance and parasitoids and predators of insects*. Chichester: Ellis Horwood.

Bombosch, S. 1965 Untersuchungen über die Dispersion und Abundanz von Blattläusen und deren natürlichen Feinden. In *Proceedings of the 12th International Congress of Entomology, London, 1964*, pp. 578–580.

Bouchard, V. & Cloutier, C. 1985 Role of olfaction in host finding by aphid parasitoid *Aphidius nigriceps* (Hymenoptera: Aphidiidae). *J. chem. Ecol.* **11**, 801–808.

Cameron, P. J., Powell, W. & Loxdale, H. D. 1984 Reservoirs for *Aphidius ervi* Haliday (Hymenoptera: Aphididae), a polyphagous parasitoid of cereal aphids (Hemiptera: Aphididae). *Bull. ent. Res.* **74**, 647–656.

Chambers, R. J., Sunderland, K. D., Stacey, D. L. & Wyatt, I. J. 1982 A survey of cereal aphids and their natural enemies in winter wheat in 1980. *Ann. appl. Biol.* **101**, 175–178.

Cooke, W. C. 1963 Ecology of the pea aphid in the Blue Mountain area of eastern Washington and Oregon. *Tech. Bull. U.S. Dep. Agric.* **1287**, 1–48.

Croft, B. A. & Brown, A. W. A. 1975 Responses of arthropod natural enemies to insecticides. *A. Rev. Ent.* **20**, 285–335.

Dean, G. J. & Luuring, B. B. 1970 Distribution of aphids in cereal crops. *Ann. appl. Biol.* **66**, 485–496.

Dixon, A. F. G. 1985 *Aphid ecology*. Glasgow: Blackie.

Dodd, G. D. 1973 Integrated control of the cabbage aphid (*Brevicoryne brassicae* (L.)). Ph.D. thesis, University of Reading.

Eikenbary, R. D. & Rogers, C. E. 1974 Importance of alternative hosts in establishment of introduced parasites. *Proc. Tall Timbers Conf. ecol. Anim. Contr. Habitat Mgmt* **5**, 119–133.

van Emden, H. F. 1965 The effect of uncultivated land on the distribution of the cabbage aphid (*Brevicoryne brassicae*) on an adjacent crop. *J. appl. Ecol.* **2**, 171–196.

van Emden, H. F. 1966 The effectiveness of aphidophagous insects in reducing aphid populations. In *Ecology of aphidophagous insects* (ed. I. Hodek), pp. 227–235. Prague: Academia.

van Emden, H. F. 1978 Insects and secondary plant substances – an alternative viewpoint with special reference to aphids. In *Biochemical aspects of plant and animal co-evolution* (ed. J. B. Harborne), pp. 309–323. London: Academic Press.

van Emden, H. F. 1983 Pest Management – routes and destinations. *Antenna* **7**, 163–168.

van Emden, H. F. 1986 The interaction of plant resistance and natural enemies: Effects on populations of sucking insects. In *Interactions of plant resistance and parasitoids and predators of insects* (ed. D. J. Boethel & R. D. Eikenbary), pp. 138–150. Chichester: Ellis Horwood.

van Emden, H. F. & Hagen, K. S. 1976 Olfactory reactions of the green lacewing, *Chrysopa carnea*, to tryptophan and certain breakdown products. *Envir. Ent.* **5**, 469–473.

van Emden, H. F. & Wearing, C. H. 1965 The role of the host plant in delaying economic damage levels in crops. *Ann. appl. Biol.* **56**, 323–324.

Fenjves, P. 1945 Beiträge zur Kenntnis der Blattlaus *Myzus* (*Myzodes*) *persicae* Sulz., Überträgerin der Blattrollenkrankheit der Kartoffel. *Mitt. schweiz. ent. Ges.* **19**, 489–611.

Greenslade, P. J. M. 1964 Pitfall trapping as a method for studying populations of Carabidae (Coleoptera). *J. Anim. Ecol.* **33**, 301–310.

Hagen, K. S. 1962 Biology and ecology of predaceous Coccinellidae. *A. Rev. Ent.* **7**, 289–326.

Hagen, K. S. 1986 Ecosystem analysis: plant cultivars (HPR), entomophagous species and food supplements. In *Interactions of plant resistance and parasitoids and predators of insects* (ed. D. J. Boethel & R. D. Eikenbary), pp. 151–197. Chichester: Ellis Horwood.

Hagen, K. S. & van den Bosch, R. 1968 Impact of pathogens, parasites, and predators on aphids. *A. Rev. Ent.* **13**, 325–384.

Hagen, K. S., Sawall, E. F. Jr. & Tassan, R. L. 1971 The use of food sprays to increase effectiveness of entomophagous insects. *Proc. Tall Timbers Conf. ecol. Anim. Contr. Habitat Mgmt* **3**, 59–81.

Hassell, M. P. 1975 Density-dependence in single-species populations. *J. Anim. Ecol.* **44**, 283–295.

Herzog, D. C. & Funderburk, J. E. 1985 Plant resistance and cultural practice interactions with biological control. In *Biological control in agricultural IPM systems* (ed. M. A. Hoy & D. C. Herzog), pp. 67–88. London: Academic Press.

Hodek, I. 1973 *Biology of Coccinellidae*. Prague: Academia.

Hodek, I., Stary, P. & Stys, P. 1962 The natural enemy complex of *Aphis fabae* and its effectiveness in control. *Proc. 11th int. Congr. Ent., Vienna, 1960*, **2**, 747–749.

Holmes, P. R. 1984 A field study of the predators of the green aphid, *Sitobion avenae* (F.) (Hemiptera: Aphididae), in winter wheat in Britain. *Bull. ent. Res.* **74**, 623–631.

Honek, A. 1983 Factors affecting the distribution of larvae of aphid predators (Col., Coccinellidae and Dipt., Syrphidae) in cereal stands. *Z. angew. Ent.* **95**, 336–345.

Hull, L. A. & Beers, E. H. 1985 Ecological selectivity: modifying chemical control practices to preserve natural enemies. In *Biological control in agricultural IPM systems* (ed. M. A. Hoy & D. C. Herzog), pp. 103–122. London: Academic Press.

Hull, L. A., Hickey, K. D. & Kanour, W. W. 1983 Pesticide usage patterns and associated pest damage in commercial apple orchards of Pennsylvania. *J. econ. Ent.* **76**, 577–583.

Iperti, G. 1966 Protection of coccinellids against mycosis. In *Ecology of aphidophagous insects* (ed. I. Hodek), pp. 189–190. Prague: Academia.

Jacobson, L. A. 1946 The effect of Say stinkbug on wheat. *Can. Ent.* **77**, 200.

Jones, F. W. G. & Jones, M. G. 1984 *Pests of field crops*. London: Edward Arnold.

Karner, M. A. & Manglitz, G. R. 1985 Effects of temperature and alfalfa cultivar on pea aphid (Homoptera: Aphididae) fecundity and feeding activity of the covergent lady beetle (Coleoptera: Coccinellidae). *J. Kans. ent. Soc.* **58**, 131–136.

Kuo, H.-L. 1986 Resistance of oats to cereal aphids: effects on parasitism by *Aphelinus asychis* (Walker). In *Interactions of plant resistance and parasitoids and predators of insects* (ed. D. J. Boethel & R. D. Eikenbary), pp. 125–137. Chichester: Ellis Horwood.

Lewis, F. H. & Hickey, K. D. 1964 Pesticide application from one side on deciduous fruit trees. *Penn. Fruit News* **43**, 13–24.

Lykouressis, D. 1982 Studies under controlled conditions on the effects of parasites on the population dynamics of *Sitobion avenae* (F.). Ph.D. thesis, University of Reading.

Mackauer, M. & Way, M. J. 1976 *Myzus persicae* Sulz. an aphid of world importance. In *Studies in biological control* (ed. V. L. Delucchi), pp. 51–119. Cambridge University Press.

Minoranskii, V. A. 1967 Über die Faktoren, die die Massenvermehrung der Rübenblattlaus (*Aphis fabae* Scop.) im Süden der UdSSR verhindern. *Arch. PflSchutz* **3**, 101–114.

Obrycki, J. J. & Tauber, M. J. 1985 Seasonal occurrence and relative abundance of aphid predators and parasitoids on pubescent potato plants. *Can. Ent.* **117**, 1231–1237.

Plapp, F. W. Jr 1981 Ways and means of avoiding or ameliorating resistance to insecticides. *Proc. Symp. 9th Int. Congr. Pl. Prot., Wash., 1979* **2**, 244–249.

Powell, W. 1983 The role of parasitoids in limiting cereal aphid populations. In *Aphid antagonists* (ed. R. Cavalloro), pp. 50–56. Rotterdam: Balkema.

Powell, W. 1986 Enhancing parasite activity in crops. In *Insect parasitoids* (ed. J. Waage & D. Greathead), pp. 319–340. London: Academic Press.

Powell, W., Dean, G. J., Dewar, A. & Wilding, N. 1981 Towards integrated control of cereal aphids. *Proc. Br. Crop Prot. Conf., Brighton, 1981* **1**, 201–206.

Powell, W. & Zhi-Li, Z. 1983 The reactions of two cereal aphid parasitoids, *Aphidius uzbekistanicus* and *A. ervi* to host aphids and their food. *Physiol. Ent.* **8**, 439–443.

Rabbinge, R., Kroon, A. G. & Driessen, H. P. J. M. 1984 Consequences of clustering on parasite-host relations of the cereal aphid *Sitobion avenae*: a simulation study. *Neth. J. agric. Sci.* **32**, 237–239.

Read, D. P., Feeney, P. P. & Root, R. B. 1970 Habitat selection by the aphid parasite *Diaretiella rapae* (Hymenoptera: Braconidae) and hyperparasite *Charips brassicae* (Hymenoptera: Cynipidae). *Can. Ent.* **102**, 1567–1578.

Schlinger, E. I. & Dietrick, E. J. 1960 Biological control of insect pests aided by stripfarming alfalfa in experimental program. *Calif. Agric.* **14**, 8–9, 15.

Schuster, D. J. & Starks, K. J. 1974 Response of *Lysiphlebus testaceipes* in an olfactometer to a host and a non-host insect and to plants. *Envir. Ent.* **3**, 1034–1035.

Saharia, D. 1985 Field evaluation of some granular systemic insecticides on *Lipaphis erysimi* (Kltb.) and its predator *Coccinella repanda* Theob. *J. Res. Assam afric. Univ.* **3**, 181–185.

Selander, J. M., Markkula, M. & Tiittanen, K. 1972 Resistance of the aphids *Myzus persicae* (Sulz.), *Aulacorthum solani* (Kalt.) and *Aphis gossypii* Glov. to insecticides and the influence of the host plant on this resistance. *Annls agric. fenn.* **11**, 141–145.

Shands, W. A. & Simpson, G. W. 1972 Insect predators for controlling aphids on potatoes. 7. A pilot test of spraying eggs of predators on potatoes in plots separated by bare fallow land. *J. econ. Ent.* **65**, 1383–1387.

Shands, W. A., Simpson, G. W., Muesebeck, C. F. & Wave, H. E. 1965 Parasites of potato-infesting aphids in northeastern Maine. *Bull. Me agric. Exp. Stn, tech. Ser.* **19**, 1–77.

Shands, W. A., Simpson, G. W., Wave, H. E. & Gordon, C. C. 1972 Importance of arthropod predators in controlling aphids on potatoes in northeastern Maine. *Tech. Bull. Univ. Maine* **54**, 1–49.

Smith, J. G. 1969*a* Some effects of crop background on populations of aphids and their natural enemies on Brussels sprouts. *Ann. appl. Biol.* **63**, 326–330.

Smith, J. G. 1969*b* Effects of crop background on populations of brassica aphids and their natural enemies. Ph.D. thesis, University of London.

Sotherton, N. W. & Moreby, S. J. 1984 Contact toxicity of some foliar fungicide sprays to three species of polyphagous predators found in cereal fields. *Tests Agrochem. Cultivars* **5**, 16–17.

Southwood, T. R. E. 1975 The dynamics of insect populations. In *Insects, science and society* (ed. D. Pimentel), pp. 151–199. New York: Academic Press.

Southwood, T. R. E. 1977 Entomology and mankind. In *Proceedings of the 15th International Congress of Entomology, Washington, D.C., 1976*, pp. 36–51.

Southwood, T. R. E., May, R. M., Hassell, M. P. & Conway, G. R. 1974 Ecological strategies and population parameters. *Am. Nat.* **108**, 791–804.

Starks, K. J., Muniappan, R. & Eikenbary, R. D. 1972 Interaction between plant resistance and parasitism against the greenbug on barley and sorghum. *Ann. ent. Soc. Am.* **65**, 650–655.

Stary, P. 1983 The perrenial stinging nettle (*Urtica dioica*) as a reservoir of aphid parasites (Hymenoptera, Aphidiidae). *Acta ent. Bohemoslov.* **80**, 81–86.

Stary, P. 1986 Specificity of parasitoids (Hymenoptera, Aphidiidae) to the black bean aphid, *Aphis fabae* complex, in agroecosystems. *Acta ent. Bohemoslov.* **83**, 24–29.

Stern, V. M., Smith, R. F., van den Bosch, R. & Hagen, K. S. 1959 The integration of chemical and biological control of the spotted alfalfa aphid. The integrated control concept. *Hilgardia* **29**, 81–101.

Tamaki, G., Landis, B. J. & Weeks, R. E. 1967 Autumn populations of green peach aphid on peach trees and the role of syrphid flies in their control. *J. econ. Ent.* **60**, 433–436.

Way, M. J. & Heathcote, G. D. 1966 Interactions of crop density of field beans, abundance of *Aphis fabae* Scop., virus incidence and aphid control by chemicals. *Ann. appl. Biol.* **57**, 409–423.

Wyatt, I. J. 1970 The distribution of *Myzus persicae* (Sulz.) on year-round chrysanthemums. II. Winter season: the effect of parasitism by *Aphidius matricariae* Hal. *Ann. appl. Biol.* **65**, 31–42.

Zeleny, J. 1966 The effect of four organophosphorous insecticides on coccinellids and chrysopids. In *Ecology of aphidophagous insects* (ed. I. Hodek), pp. 337–340. Prague: Academia.

## Discussion

M. J. WAY (*Imperial College at Silwood Park, Ascot, U.K.*). Professor van Emden has dealt primarily with the role of naturally occurring biological control agents against pests on the crop. Could he please reflect on their value against pests where the latter are not on crops, especially because many pests spend most of the year in the non-crop environment?

H. F. VAN EMDEN. I certainly accept that, particularly in the case of many aphids, the most important biological control in terms of the population dynamics of the species occurs in the non-crop environment. However, I particularly titled my paper in such a way as not to get involved with the practical possibilities for farmer-acceptable control of aphids based on interventions in the non-crop environment, because as yet there is little practical guidance that can be given. I certainly believe that the possibility does exist.

T. LEWIS (*Rothamsted Experimental Station, Harpenden, U.K.*). Are the slightly aphid-resistant cultivars Professor van Emden suggests also economically attractive to farmers?

H. F. VAN EMDEN. One of the advantages that partly aphid-resistant cultivars have is that they are indeed available among the cultivars grown by farmers and growers. Very few cultivars have been bred for such resistance, but nevertheless there is considerable variation among the cultivars currently available commercially. By concentrating on commercially available cultivars, the system can be used without the need for a preliminary long term breeding programme.

T. LEWIS. How does Professor van Emden propose to encourage farmers to take up the approaches to control which he has described?

H. F. VAN EMDEN. The question requires a different answer for intensive agriculture and developing agriculture. In developing agriculture, reliance on pesticides for control is usually uneconomic. By maximizing indigenous biological control, it is possible to raise yields considerably with the addition of perhaps a single pesticide spray. This could still be economically feasible, although yields may still be below what might be obtained by a more blanket use of insecticide.

In intensive agriculture, the situation is different. Clearly, the combination of other restraints with pesticides, if successful in protecting yields, is going to give the farmer a saving in pesticide costs. However, I have doubts that this would present sufficient motive for farmers to take up such systems unless they became forced into it by the failure of reliance on pesticides due to insect resistance to them. The history of integrated control measures suggests that even successful integrated systems, almost invariably introduced to deal with the insecticide resistance crisis, fail to survive once an effective insecticide again becomes available.

K. D. SUNDERLAND (*Institute of Horticultural Research, Littlehampton, U.K.*). Are the calculations Professor van Emden has made based only on the antibiosis component of resistance or do they include antixenosis? I ask because there are reasons to believe that antixenotic varieties could improve pest control by, for example, increasing the pests' movement and their exposure to contact pesticides. They could also synergize with natural enemies, which are often vertically stratified in crops; antixenosis and the resulting increased aphid movement could increase aphid–natural enemy encounter rates and thus improve control.

H. F. VAN EMDEN. The calculations are indeed based on the antibiosis component. It is much harder to model the antixenosis component, and it may well be that the surprisingly large improvement of biological control on partly resistant varieties may partly be due to the fact that antixenosis and antibiosis often occur together in a variety. The kind of relations you suggest may therefore account for the field effect of the resistance being so much greater than what one would predict from a density-dependent model.

I am also sure Dr Sunderland is right that antixenotic varieties may well improve the pests' exposure to contact pesticides, but this is of course a little outside the scope of this meeting.

J. K. WAAGE (*C.A.B. International Institute of Biological Control, Ascot, U.K.*). In Professor van Emden's models for the interaction of resistance and biological control, resistance is modelled as affecting the intrinsic growth rate of the pest. How does this really occur, and could it involve mortalities or changes in hosts which could actually interfere with natural enemy survival or reproduction (e.g. lower survival of parasitoids in the smaller aphids on resistant plants)?

H. F. VAN EMDEN. The main effect of resistance is probably to reduce fecundity of the pest, though it may also affect pre-adult mortality if the resistance is high and may also increase development rate. My model excludes any effects on survival, but otherwise includes both fecundity and development rate. Certainly the insects on partly resistant varieties are smaller than those on susceptible ones, and it is to be expected that this could affect the fecundity of parasitoids and even perhaps their sex ratio. This is something that needs further investigation; all I can say at the moment is that the levels of plant resistance used do not give a very dramatic decrease in pest size, and that any deleterious effects on parasitoids have not yet shown themselves within the single seasons when we have done the studies. However, it is still possible that, if such systems using biological control and plant resistance were to be used on a very wide scale and over a large area, effects of the kind on parasitoids Dr Waage suggests might well show in time.

R. J. COOK (*United States Department of Agriculture Agricultural Research Service, Washington State University, Pullman, U.S.A.*). Professor van Emden describes the benefits of what he referred to as 'plant resistance' combined with 'biological control' for management of aphid populations. Without wanting to divert our discussion to a review of terminology. I would submit that both are biological control. I believe a broad concept (i.e. the use of any living organism, plants included, for control of a pathogen or pest species has many advantages. The broad definition is certainly more futuristic. For example, the *Bt* gene for endotoxin production has now been transferred from *Bacillus thuringiensis* to the root bacterium *Pseudomonas fluorescens* and also to tobacco. The expression of this gene in tobacco is a form of host-plant resistance (antibiosis, to use entomological terminology). Our concept of biological control should not be so narrow that expression of a gene in an insect pathogen qualifies as 'biological control', but the same gene expressed in a plant as a defence against insects does not qualify as biological control.

H. F. VAN EMDEN. I certainly take the point that many methods of pest control other than the use of predators, parasitoids and insect pathogens can be regarded as biological control and I would accept your definition as justifiable. However, rightly or wrongly, the word biological control has (certainly in the entomological world) been associated with a narrower definition and it is hard to think of an appropriate alternative for its meaning in that more restricted sense. I hope it doesn't matter terribly, provided that confusion does not result.

*Phil. Trans. R. Soc. Lond.* B **318**, 203–211 (1988)

*Printed in Great Britain*

# Integrating use of beneficial organisms with chemical crop protection

By J. A. Pickett

*AFRC Institute of Arable Crops Research, Rothamsted Experimental Station,*
*Harpenden, Hertfordshire AL5 2JQ, U.K.*

The selectivity of insecticides, particularly of pyrethroids, is described and possibilities are proposed for further development of selectivity. The production of beneficial organisms resistant to pesticides by techniques including genetic manipulation is discussed. Preliminary studies on the use of semiochemicals to improve the efficiency of entomophagous pathogens in controlling pest infestations, and for monitoring and manipulating populations of beneficial insects, are described. The prospects for genetic manipulation of crop plants to improve predation and parasitism of pests are also discussed.

## Introduction

Although broad-spectrum pesticides are likely to remain the major means of crop protection for the next 15 years (Finney 1986), increased use of biological agents will be necessary to overcome problems of pesticide resistance and to reduce possible hazards to the environment. For the most part, more efficient use of biological agents will involve protecting and manipulating the natural populations of beneficial insects and pathogens of pests. This will necessitate improving the selectivity of chemical crop protection agents between pests and beneficial organisms and devising ways of manipulating beneficial organisms to enable them to function more effectively.

## Selectivity of insecticides

Four main groups of insecticides are currently used in crop protection: the organochlorines, organophosphates, carbamates and pyrethroids. The pyrethroids are quickly replacing the earlier groups, and the more recent ones are generally the most selective in terms of relative activity between pest and beneficial organism. One of the most selective and yet most active is deltamethrin (**1**) (Elliott *et al.* 1974), and early bioassay studies using house flies and honey

1. Deltamethrin.

bees show the improvement in relative toxicity as successive pyrethroids were discovered (table 1) (Smart & Stevenson 1982). This difference in relative toxicity was subsequently found to be true for a moth and its parasite: for deltamethrin, the relative toxicity to the lepidopteran pest *Ephestia kuhniella* and its hymenopteran parasite *Venturia canescens* is 12:1 (Elliott *et al.* 1983). In the case of the predatory lacewing *Chrysoperla carnea*, the ability to hydrolyse pyrethroids selectively (Bashir & Crowder 1983) confers a considerable advantage over aphid pests, and makes these insecticides very much more selective than most organophosphorus compounds (table 2) (Stevenson *et al.* 1984). In the field, the pyrethroid cypermethrin causes less damage to hymenopteran aphid parasitoids than the organo-phosphorus compound, demeton-S-methyl (figure 1) (L. E. Smart, J. H. Stevenson &

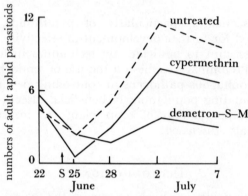

FIGURE 1. Numbers of adult aphid parasitoids caught by suction sampler, before and after insecticide application. (S = date of application.)

TABLE 1. TOXICITY OF PYRETHROIDS TO PEST AND BENEFICIAL INSECTS

| pyrethroid | discovery date | relative toxicity | |
| --- | --- | --- | --- |
| | | house fly | honey bee |
| bioresmethrin | 1967 | 100 | 100 |
| permethrin | 1973 | 60 | 5 |
| deltamethrin | 1974 | 1700 | 11 |

TABLE 2. TOXICITY OF INSECTICIDES TO AN APHID AND ITS PREDATOR

| insecticide | $LD_{50}$ micrograms per insect | | approximate selectivity factor |
| --- | --- | --- | --- |
| | *Myzus persicae* (adult apterae) | *Chrysoperla carnae* (2nd-instar larvae) | |
| demeton-S-methyl | 0.0011 | 0.045 | 10 |
| permethrin | 0.00037 | 0.077 | 40 |
| cypermethrin | 0.000085 | 0.039 | 100 |
| deltamethrin | 0.0000038 | 0.029 | 1500 |

J. H. H. Walters, unpublished results), and a mustard crop sprayed with deltamethrin produced only 127 dead honey bees compared with 2968 dead bees when the crop was sprayed with the organophosphorus compound, dimethoate, even though active foraging continued (Garnier & Baumeister 1985). Further modification to the pyrethroid molecule, for example **2** (NRDC 200 (Elliott 1985)), may give even more selective compounds in this group.

Of the wide range of other insecticides now finding minor use or under development, several show promise for selectivity. For example, the formamidines and acylureas can be less toxic to

2

beneficial insects than most conventional insecticides, and although only in restricted use, the juvenoids and *Bacillus thuringiensis* endotoxins are highly selective in their activity. As these endotoxins are naturally occurring proteins, they can be targets for genetic manipulation studies resulting, for example, in crop plants that produce these materials in their leaves as a defence against chewing insects (Schell 1986). Highly selective, new insecticides may also be developed from the study of insect neuropeptides. These substances are effective at extremely low levels (less than $10^{-10}$ M) and are involved in the regulation of muscle, endocrine and metabolic activity, e.g. the muscle neurotransmitter proctolin and the adipokinetic hormone (AKH) (Menn & Henrick 1985). The baculoviruses currently being developed as biological control agents (Payne, this symposium) could be genetically modified to produce such neuropeptides within the target organism. The resulting disruption of the processes on which they act could have a more immediate effect than the gradual destruction caused by infection with the natural baculovirus.

### PESTICIDE RESISTANCE IN BENEFICIAL ORGANISMS

Pesticide resistance is currently causing considerable concern in agriculture (Jackson 1986). However, if this resistance could be transferred to beneficial organisms, the advantages would be substantial. Some work has been done in selecting insecticide-resistant beneficial organisms (Croft & Morse 1979) and, as has been mentioned above, the lacewing *Chrysoperla carnea* is inherently tolerant to certain insecticides. Already, resistance genes from pest species have been, or are being, cloned, such as the genes responsible for producing high levels of detoxifying esterases in mosquitoes (Mouchès *et al.* 1986) and in aphids (Devonshire *et al.* 1986). Although it is not yet possible to transfer these genes into beneficial insects, the notable success with the transposable P elements in *Drosophila* (Rubin 1985) suggests that this will become feasible.

### SEMIOCHEMICALS TO IMPROVE THE EFFICIENCY OF ENTOMOPHAGOUS PATHOGENS

Semiochemicals (behaviour-controlling chemicals) such as the insect pheromones are already being developed for use in agriculture (Pickett 1984). These materials, by influencing the movement of pest organisms, may be used to bring them more efficiently into contact with biological control agents such as the spores of entomophagous fungal pathogens. Pathogens such as *Verticillium lecanii* are employed against resistant aphids in glasshouses in the U.K., but it is extremely important that the spores are picked up by the pest during the brief period in which they remain viable. The aphid alarm pheromone, (*E*)-β-farnesene (**3**) which

**3.** (*E*)-β-farnesene.

causes dispersal of aphids when they are attacked, can improve pick-up of *V. lecanii* spores by increasing aphid mobility: on plots which were untreated, treated with *V. lecanii*, and treated with *V. lecanii* plus pheromone, numbers of live aphids remaining were in the ratio 9:3:1 (Hockland *et al.* 1986). Attempts are being made to develop another fungal pathogen, *Erynia neoaphidis*, for use against aphids on arable crops (Wilding 1983) and preliminary laboratory results have shown that the alarm pheromone is again successful in improving the infection of aphids with this organism (N. Wilding, personal communication). The sex attractant pheromones of moths are currently being used commercially to control populations of pest species by interfering with mating (Reece 1985). An alternative use of these sex pheromones would be to attract moths to a source of an entomophagous pathogen held in the protected environment of a trap so that the moths, after becoming infected, could transfer the pathogen throughout the rest of the population during their normal mating and aggregation behaviour (E. D. M. Macaulay, personal communication).

## SEMIOCHEMICALS FOR MONITORING BENEFICIAL INSECTS

Although natural predator and parasitoid populations can be responsible for controlling pest infestations, their effects are erratic. However, with accurate monitoring of these populations, their value could be estimated and insecticide treatments planned accordingly. Semiochemicals such as aggregation pheromones could prove invaluable in providing accurate monitoring systems. The identification of such pheromones in the case of coleopteran pests has proved relatively simple, for example, the recent identification of the aggregation pheromone of the pea and bean weevil, *Sitona lineatus* (Blight *et al.* 1984). There is therefore considerable promise for use of aggregation pheromones to monitor beneficial coleopteran insects. Also, many hymenopteran parasitoids are attracted to plant compounds, and respond to oviposition stimulants and attractants produced by their host organisms (Powell & Zhang 1983; Decker & Powell 1985), which could provide the basis for monitoring systems.

## MANIPULATION OF BENEFICIAL INSECTS BY SEMIOCHEMICALS

Honey bees are valuable pollinators of crops and their behaviour is readily manipulated by pheromones; for example, the recently characterized Nasonov pheromone (Pickett *et al.* 1980) can be used to attract honey bees to flowers (Williams *et al.* 1981) and could be used to attract them away from crops being sprayed with insecticide; also, it has been shown that the sting gland and mandibular gland pheromones of the honey bee, which contain isopentyl acetate and 2-heptanone respectively, can act as repellents when applied to food sources (Ferguson & Free 1979). Oil-seed rape treated with a slow release formulation of this chemical attracts fewer foraging honey bees, but the effect is short-lived (table 3) (Free *et al.* 1985). However, by producing precursors that release the active material in sunlight, when honey bees are foraging, more persistence may be obtained (scheme 1) (Liu *et al.* 1984). Such materials could then be formulated with an insecticide to reduce hazard to foraging honey bees.

Hymenopterous parasitoids of aphids such as *Aphidius* spp. are known to make a significant contribution to the control of cereal aphid populations in certain conditions (Powell 1986). As parasitism by *Aphidius* has most impact early in the year, when parasitoid:aphid ratios are large, the aphid–host and plant attractants mentioned above may be useful in attracting and

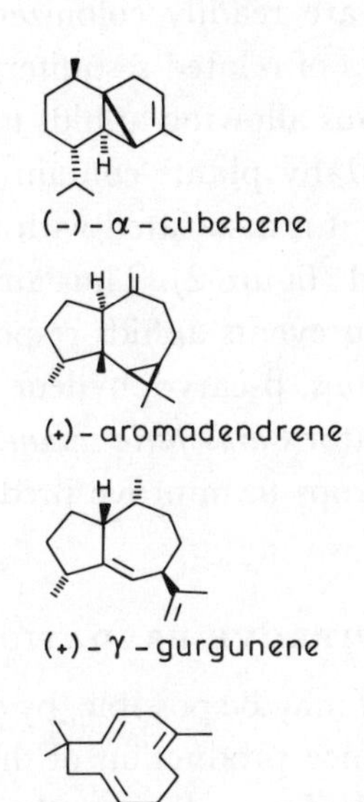

| sesquiterpene | relative concentration (EBF=1) | difference from control (EBF alone) P |
|---|---|---|
| (–) – α – cubebene | 30 | not active |
| (+) – aromadendrene | 30 | not active |
| (+) – γ – gurgunene | 3 | <0·01 |
| α – humulene | 3 | <0·01 |
| (–) – β – caryophyllene | 0·03 | <0·05 |

FIGURE 2. Inhibition of aphid alarm pheromone activity: lowest relative concentration of some hop sesquiterpenes causing inhibition of activity of (E)-β-farnesene (EBF).

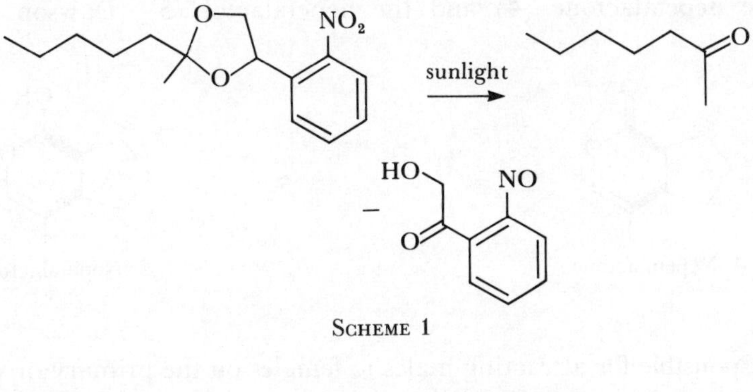

SCHEME 1

TABLE 3. REDUCTION IN NUMBERS OF HONEY BEES FORAGING ON RAPE AFTER TREATMENT WITH THE PHEROMONAL REPELLENTS, ISOPENTYL ACETATE AND 2-HEPTANONE

| time after treatment min | reduction in no. of bees relative to untreated plots (%) |
|---|---|
| 0–30 | 85 |
| 36–60 | 67 |
| 60–90 | 34 |

retaining parasitoids in the crop at the most strategic stage. The aphid alarm pheromone, (E)-β-farnesene, is a component of hop plants, which are readily colonized by aphids. In investigating this anomaly, it was discovered that a series of related sesquiterpenes present in plants (figure 2) acted as inhibitors of the pheromone, thus allowing aphids to colonize plants that contained (E)-β-farnesene (Dawson *et al.* 1984). Many plants contain this compound, although at lower levels than found in hops, and usually it is associated with a larger amount of β-caryophyllene, the most active inhibitory compound (figure 2). Thus air from above the leaves of certain plants, particularly potatoes and hops, prevents aphids responding to (E)-β-farnesene (Pickett *et al.* 1984). Under laboratory conditions, β-caryophyllene is also shown to lower the dispersal of aphids, when attacked by the predator *Chrysoperla carnea*, by about 50%. This compound could therefore be applied directly to crops to improve predation of aphids.

### GENETIC MANIPULATION OF CROP PLANTS TO IMPROVE PREDATION OF PESTS

Because β-caryophyllene is produced by many plants, it may be possible, by employing plant breeding programmes or genetic modifications, to enhance production of this compound in crop plants. This may improve predation of aphids by reducing their dispersal. β-Caryophyllene is also an attractant for predatory lacewings (Flint *et al.* 1979), so could be used to increase numbers of predators on the crop.

Some predators and parasitoids locate their insect hosts by detecting compounds released from plants during feeding by the pests. It is possible that crop plants could be genetically manipulated to produce more of these compounds without the need for prior damage. This might attract predators and parasitoids into the crop at a more timely stage.

The sex pheromone for a number of aphids has recently been shown to comprise two compounds, the nepetalactone (**4**) and the nepetalactol (**5**) (Dawson *et al.* 1987). This

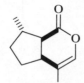

4. Nepetalactone.                                        5. Nepetalactol.

pheromone is responsible for attracting males to females on the primary or winter host. These compounds are closely related to known lacewing attractants (Sakan *et al.* 1970), and may act as kairomones in enabling lacewings to locate populations of aphids during periods when these are scarce. Because these compounds are also produced in plants, particularly those in the *Nepeta* genus, the possibility exists for transferring genes into crop plants to attract lacewing predators.

### REFERENCES

Bashir, N. H. H. & Crowder, L. A. 1983 Mechanisms of permethrin tolerance in the common green lacewing (Neuroptera: Chrysopidae). *J. econ. Entomol.* **76**, 407–409.
Blight, M. M., Pickett, J. A., Smith, M. C. & Wadhams, L. J. 1984 An aggregation pheromone of *Sitona lineatus*. *Naturwissenschaften* **71** S, 480.
Croft, B. A. & Morse, J. G. 1979 Research advances on pesticide resistance in natural enemies. *Entomophaga* **24**, 3–11.

Dawson, G. W., Griffiths, D. C., Pickett, J. A., Smith, M. C. & Woodcock, C. M. 1984 Natural inhibition of the aphid alarm pheromone. *Entomologia exp. appl.* **36**, 197–199.

Dawson, G. W., Griffiths, D. C., Janes, N. F., Mudd, A., Pickett, J. A., Wadhams, L. J. & Woodcock, C. M. 1987 Identification of an aphid sex pheromone. *Nature, Lond.* **325**, 614–616.

Decker, U. M. & Powell, W. 1985 *Rothamsted report for 1985*, 96–97.

Devonshire, A. L., Searle, L. M. & Moores, G. D. 1986 Quantitative and qualitative variation in the mRNA for carboxylesterases in insecticide-susceptible and resistant *Myzus persicae* (Sulz). *Insect Biochem.* **16**, 659–665.

Elliott, M., Farnham, A. W., Janes, N. F., Needham, P. H. & Pulman, D. A. 1974 Synthetic insecticide with a new order of activity. *Nature, Lond.* **248**, 710–711.

Elliott, M., Janes, N. F., Stevenson, J. H. & Walters, J. H. H. 1983 Insecticidal activity of the pyrethrins and related compounds. Part XIV. Selectivity of pyrethroid insecticides between *Ephestia kuhniella* and its parasite *Venturia canescens*. *Pestic. Sci.* **14**, 423–426.

Elliott, M. 1985 Lipophilic insect control agents. In *Recent advances in the chemistry of insect control, Royal Society of Chemistry monograph* (ed. N. F. Janes), pp. 73–102. London: Royal Society of Chemistry.

Ferguson, A. W. & Free, J. B. 1979 Production of a forage marking pheromone by the honeybee. *J. Apicult. Res.* **18**, 128–135.

Finney, J. 1986 The future of the pesticide industry. Paper presented at SCI Meeting 'Novel Approaches in Agrochemical Research', December 1986.

Flint, H. M., Salter, S. S. & Walters, S. 1979 Caryophyllene: an attractant for the green lacewing. *Envir. Ent.* **8**, 1123–1125.

Free, J. B., Pickett, J. A., Ferguson, A. W., Simpkins, J. R. & Smith, M. C. 1985 Repelling foraging honeybees with alarm pheromones. *J. agric. Sci., Camb.* **105**, 255–260.

Garnier, P. & Baumeister, R. 1985 Results obtained in France in 1983 and 1984 in the experimentation on bees with *Decis* on cereals and crucifers. In *International Commission for Bee Botany report: Third symposium on the harmonization of methods for testing the toxicity of pesticides to bees, March 1985*, A17. 1–2.

Hockland, S. H., Dawson, G. W., Griffiths, D. C., Marples, B., Pickett, J. A. & Woodcock, C. M. 1986 The use of aphid alarm pheromone (*E*-β-farnesene) to increase effectiveness of the entomophilic fungus *Verticillium lecanii* in controlling aphids on chrysanthemums under glass. In *Fundamental and applied aspects of invertebrate pathology* (ed. R. A. Samson, J. M. Vlak & D. Peters), Wageningen: Foundation of the Fourth International Colloquium of Invertebrate Pathology, pp. 252.

Jackson, G. J. 1986 Insecticide resistance – what is industry doing about it? In *Proceedings of the British Crop Protection Conference – Pests and Diseases*, pp. 943–949. Croydon: BCPC Publications.

Liu, X., Macaulay, E. D. M. & Pickett, J. A. 1984 Propheromones that release pheromonal carbonyl compounds in light. *J. chem. Ecol.* **10**, 809–822.

Menn, J. J. & Henrick, C. A. 1985 Newer chemicals for insect control. In *Agricultural chemicals of the future* (*BARC symposium 8*) (ed. J. L. Hilton), pp. 247–265. Totowa: Rowman & Allanheld.

Mouchès, C., Pasteur, N., Bergé, J. B., Hyrien, O., Raymond, M., Vincent, B. R. de St., Silvestri, M. de & Georghiou, G. P. 1986 Amplification of an esterase gene is responsible for insecticide resistance in a California *Culex* mosquito. *Science, Wash.* **233**, 778–780.

Pickett, J. A., Williams, I. H., Martin, A. P. & Smith, M. C. 1980 Nasonov pheromone of the honeybee, *Apis mellifera* L. (Hymenoptera: Apidae). Part I. Chemical characterization. *J. chem. Ecol.* **6**, 425–434.

Pickett, J. A. 1984 Prospects for new chemical approaches to insect control. *Chemy. Ind., Lond.* 657–660.

Pickett, J. A., Dawson, G. W., Free, J. B., Griffiths, D. C., Powell, W., Williams, I. H. & Woodcock, C. M. 1984 Pheromones in the management of beneficial insects. In *Proceedings of the British Crop Protection Conference – Pests and Diseases*, pp. 247–254. Croydon: BCPC Publications.

Powell, W. & Zhang, Z. 1983 The reactions of two cereal aphid parasitoids, *Aphidius uzbekistanicus* and *A. ervi* to host aphids and their food-plants. *Physiol. Ent.* **8**, 439–443.

Powell, W. 1986 Enhancing parasitoid activity in crops. In *Insect Parasitoids – Proceedings 13th Symposium of the Royal Entomological Society of London* (ed. D. J. Greathead & J. K. Waage), pp. 319–340. London: Academic Press.

Reece, C. H. 1985 The role of the chemical industry in improving the effectiveness of agriculture. *Phil. Trans. R. Soc. Lond.* B **310**, 201–213.

Rubin, G. M. 1985 P transposable elements and their use as genetic tools in *Drosophila*. *Trends Neurosci.* **8**, 231–233.

Sakan, T., Isoe, S. & Hyeon, S. B. 1970 The chemistry of attractants for Chrysopidae from *Actinidia polygama* Miq. In *Control of insect behaviour by natural products* (ed. D. L. Wood, R. M. Silverstein & M. Nakajima), pp. 237–247. New York: Academic Press.

Schell, J. St. 1986 The development and use of gene transfer systems and efficient expression vectors for the genetic engineering of plants. Paper presented at SCI Meeting 'Novel Approaches to Agrochemical Research', December 1986.

Smart, L. E. & Stevenson, J. H. 1982 Laboratory estimation of toxicity of pyrethroid insecticides to honeybees: relevance to hazard in the field. *Bee Wld* **63**, 150–152.

Stevenson, J. H., Smart, L. E. & Walters, J. H. H. 1984 Laboratory assessment of insecticide selectivity – practical relevance. In *Proceedings of the British Crop Protection Conference – Pests and Diseases*, pp. 355–358. Croydon: BCPC Publications.

Wilding, N. 1983 The current status and potential of entomogenous fungi as agents of pest control. In *Proceedings of the 10th International Congress of Plant Protection*, pp. 743–750. Croydon: BCPC Publications.
Williams, I. H., Pickett, J. A. & Martin, A. P. 1981 Attraction of honeybees to flowering plants by using synthetic Nasonov pheromone. *Entomologia exp. appl.* **30**, 199–201.

## Discussion

L. P. J. J. NOLDUS (*Department of Entomology, Wageningen Agricultural University, The Netherlands*). I would like to make a point regarding the use of semiochemicals to manipulate the behaviour of noxious or beneficial insects. Aphids, for example, can avoid predation by alarm-pheromone-induced dispersal which, however, can also enhance mortality from contact pesticides. If these responses are important in the population dynamics of the insect, does Dr Pickett think that selection may occur for individuals that no longer react to the alarm pheromone? Please also comment on whether beneficials might become resistant to semiochemicals.

J. A. PICKETT. I think it is certain that such insects could become unresponsive to semiochemical treatments but if, as is becoming the case for pesticides, carefully controlled integrated régimes are employed, this should be avoided.

I. HARPAZ (*Department of Entomology, Hebrew University of Jerusalem, Israel*). Another aspect relevant to the topic in this paper is where pesticides can be used for enhancement of biological control. This is done in the control of prickly pear (a noxious plant in South Africa and Australia) by cochineal scale insects of the genus *Dactylopius*. When the infested prickly pear plants are treated with DDT, the pesticide kills predators and parasites of the scale insect, but not the scale insect itself which is not susceptible to DDT. As a result, the control of prickly pear is significantly improved by this unusual, selective pesticidal treatment. Possibilities of using this particular method of integrating biological and chemical measures should not be overlooked.

J. A. PICKETT. I take note of this interesting point.

J. M. FRANZ (*Gundolfstrasse* 14, 6100 *Darmstadt, F.R.G.*). The recommendation was given to use methods established by the IOBC/WPRS Working Group 'Pesticides and Beneficial Organisms', for tests on the toxicity of established and new pesticides on beneficial athropods. These standard methods would seem to be more realistic than simple relative toxicity studies in the laboratory and are applicable to pesticides in general.

J. A. PICKETT. I am aware of the methods recommended by the Working Group; indeed my own staff were involved in drawing up these protocols, and I agree that these should be used when considering selectivity between pests and beneficial organisms. However, our laboratory studies on selective toxicity provide a good indication of chemical structures likely to be less hazardous to beneficial organisms. In addition, I did report numbers of live parasitoids surviving in the field after use of the more selective pyrethroid cypermethrin compared with the non-selective organophosphorus demeton-S-methyl which is the final test of selectivity.

J. K. WAAGE (*C.A.B. International Institute of Biological Control, Ascot, U.K.*). A problem with the use of semiochemicals to attract natural enemies is that one may thereby force natural enemies to forage where they would not normally, instead of in response to natural kairomones which would presumably bring them to high densities of their pest populations. As a result, the searching efficiency of these natural enemies could be reduced, and consequently their reproduction and future population size. The value of such chemicals may therefore be negative in the long term, unless they were used in conjunction with augmented natural enemies. In these circumstances the chemicals might then be of special value in directing released natural enemies to the target pest population.

J. A. PICKETT. I agree with your general point but although we may have to consider augmentation of natural enemies, I feel that this would best be achieved by cultural means.

M. J. WAY (*Imperial College at Silwood Park, Ascot, U.K.*). It seems inevitable that there will often be problems in rectifying a pest-resistant situation once it has developed. I therefore suggest that you have not given sufficient emphasis to the development and use of natural enemies that are resistant to broad-spectrum pesticides that would otherwise harm them. Surely such natural enemies can play a crucial role by killing residues of resistant pests that might be left after pesticide application, and which would otherwise form the nucleus from which wholly resistant pest populations could develop.

J. A. PICKETT. This is a theoretically sound proposal and we are making efforts in this direction. It would be compatible with my view that we must help the agricultural industry to continue use of chemical control agents in ways that minimize possibly harmful consequences.

P. T. HASKELL (*Department of Zoology, University College, Cardiff, U.K.*). As regards attraction of predators and parasites into a crop by using semiochemicals, is there not a limit to the increase that can be caused by density-dependent inhibitory reactions by the parasites and predators involved?

J. A. PICKETT. I agree that inhibition can occur but comment that semiochemicals could allow the balance to be tipped in favour of control.

H. F. VAN EMDEN (*Departments of Horticulture, and Pure and Applied Zoology, University of Reading, U.K.*). Plant odours will attract parasitoids regardless of presence of prey; if there are few prey they may not all stay, but they would never be any use unless you could get them into the crop in the first place!

J. A. PICKETT. I agree, and that is why the work concentrates on both host and host–plant chemicals.

*Phil. Trans. R. Soc. Lond.* B **318**, 213–224 (1988)

*Printed in Great Britain*

# Pathogens for the control of weeds

By J. M. Cullen and S. Hasan

*Commonwealth Scientific and Industrial Research Organization, Biological Control Unit,*
*335 Avenue Paul Parguel,* 34100 *Montpellier, France*

The potential of pathogens for controlling plant populations has often been underestimated because of the subtle nature of their effects and the fact that only the final population equilibrium is observed. The potential exists for restoring such equilibria by classical biological control where they have become imbalanced, or for manipulating the host–pathogen system by the use of mycoherbicides, i.e. increasing the inoculum load. The use of exotic pathogens in classical control is often limited by considerations of sufficient host specificity for introduction into a new environment, whereas use of mycoherbicides is limited by the need to develop commercially viable systems of production, storage and application. Both approaches are subject to legislative restraints, classical control because of the inherent aim of establishing a new, freely dispersing organism throughout a region and mycoherbicides because they are subject to registration and patenting requirements. Neither the presence of a more variable genome in outbreeding plant species nor the high degree of specialization of obligate parasites are seen as significant restraints in re-establishing population equilibria in new environments. Sufficient effectiveness and safety have now been demonstrated in enough programmes to overcome initial hesitancy and considerable increase in activity in this field can be observed.

## Introduction

Potato late blight, Dutch elm disease, chestnut blight and coffee rust are classic examples of the potential of plant pathogens to cause devastating diseases, yet the ability of pathogens in general to kill large numbers of plants and keep populations in check on a permanent basis is not always readily apparent or accepted. The above cases are examples of reintroductions on to hosts long separated in new areas or on to new hosts, and there is a tendency to consider them as rather exceptional. More commonly, pathogens are regularly observed on a plant or crop species, occasionally building up to significant levels, and most often in the artificial situation of crop monocultures which favour both pathogen increase and selection of new, more virulent strains. Fruit or seed production may be seriously affected, but the impression is seldom given of disease causing significant mortality of established plants.

This brief account will suggest that this impression is deceptive and it will try to demonstrate the potential and degree of progress achieved in the practical use of pathogens for weed control. At present only fungal pathogens and nematodes have been seriously considered, with the vast majority of the work concentrated on the fungi.

*The host–pathogen equilibrium*

Natural systems represent the equilibrium phase of a population interaction between host and parasite, which may shift a little one way or the other according to the environment, the season or perhaps a genetic change in its components. The role of the pathogen may only be seen if it is removed or if for some other reason the plant population increases to a high level and an epidemic is initiated, which brings the population back down again. Crop plant populations are maintained at artificially high levels and are prone to such epidemics unless artificial preventive measures are taken. The relative roles of pathogens in natural and disturbed or agricultural situations has been well reviewed by Burdon & Shattock (1980), who point out the difficulties of observing the controlling effects of pathogens on plant populations, but produce considerable evidence as to the generality of their occurrence. Even when pathogens do cause important mortality, their effects can be cryptic and often only manifested when acting in combination with other stresses. The effect of flower and fruit loss, for example *Senecio vulgaris* infected by *Erysiphe fischeri* (Ben-Kalio & Clarke 1979), is not clear until the dynamics of seed production in the species is known. The effect of a foliar disease may be to reduce root growth or otherwise affect water uptake (Ayres & Paul 1986), which may not be very apparent until perhaps the plant is stressed, e.g. by a dry summer, whereupon it wilts and dies. A reduced vertical growth or leaf surface area, e.g. when *Dichanthium annulatum* is infected by *Sphacelotheca annulata* (Mall & Tugnawat 1973), may not seem very important until the plant is in competition with another species and succumbs because of reduced efficiency.

Thus it is not easy to appreciate the true role a pathogen plays in the population dynamics of a plant species. The best evidence often comes from disturbing the ecological equilibrium and some of the classic cases cited above are good examples of this. One of the best known examples of biological control is exactly similar in that the population density of form A of the European species *Chondrilla juncea*, introduced into Australia in the absence of its specific pathogens, increased to a level much higher than normal. The deliberate introduction of a strain of the rust *Puccinia chondrillina* in 1971 from Europe caused an epidemic (Cullen *et al.* 1973; Hasan 1974*a*), which has gradually reduced the density to approximately one hundredth of its previous value (Cullen 1988) i.e. the normal level in Europe (Wapshere 1971; Wapshere *et al.* 1974). Further, its effect is now not so obvious, and casual observers and some farmers have begun to doubt how it could be effective. These cases should not be thought of as exceptional reactions of host and pathogen, but rather as results of extreme disturbance of what is itself a normal course of events.

*The potential for control*

Given that actual or potential controlling effects of pathogens are not uncommon, it is their recognition and translation into effective action for the control of plants, when these are considered to be weeds, that is the challenge. Clearly, if presented with a plant system without the pathogen(s) normally associated with it, the opportunity exists to introduce the pathogen(s) to restore the appropriate equilibrium, with a reduced plant population as the expected result. Alternatively, if the pathogen is already present, or is introduced, but the resulting equilibrium still gives a higher plant population than desired, there is the possibility of displacing the equilibrium to the detriment of the plant e.g. by increasing the inoculum of the pathogen. These alternatives correspond to the two main forms of biological control of weeds: the classical approach, that of introducing exotic organisms, pathogens in this case, and the bioherbicide approach, involving treatment of the plants with artificially high levels of an organism, a mycoherbicide in the case of fungal pathogens.

The two approaches are obviously complementary, but involve different emphases and different sorts of problems. The classical approach is principally concerned with controlling exotic weeds, by finding the pathogens associated with them, or their close relatives, in their country of origin, or elsewhere, and importing them into the country where the weed is a problem so as to recreate a natural balance, both numerically and genetically. The bulk of the research is concerned with finding the pathogens, evaluating them for effectiveness and safety for introduction (a matter of specificity), establishing them and evaluating their effect. The mycoherbicide approach again involves finding a suitable pathogen, but often has endemic weeds as targets and therefore often uses indigenous pathogens. The problems associated with introducing an exotic organism are therefore rare, but production, storage and application problems are considerable. The two major requirements for any pathogen to be used in biological control are the same as for any prophylactic measure. It must be safe and effective, i.e. it damages or kills the weed without presenting any risk to other plant species. Problems arise when it is deficient in either of these requirements or when the demonstration of an adequate level in either proves difficult or impossible. In general, it is obligatory to demonstrate safety, i.e. specificity, before contemplating introduction or mass release, and it is highly desirable, from the point of view of research investment, if effectiveness is also demonstrated at an early stage.

### CLASSICAL BIOLOGICAL CONTROL

A pathogen normally associated with a weed species, and presumably reasonably frequently if it is to be of any promise, should not be too difficult to find if the correct regions are searched. In this, one is guided by a knowledge of the history of the distribution of the weed host. The original area of occurrence of a species, i.e. its evolutionary centre, is logically the area where the greatest variety of organisms will be found that are sufficiently specialized on the weed (Goeden 1971; Harris & Piper 1970; Wapshere 1974). However, if the plant has been present in other areas for a sufficiently long period, it is possible that there has been adaptation and evolution of other pathogen species or strains not present at the origin. Room (1981) has considered this point, but concluded that generally, the native range offers the best prospects. However, this author also admitted the possibility of effectiveness eventually declining with increasing evolutionary time, a possibility considered primarily by Pimentel (1961) in relation to biological control and considered again recently in detail by Hokkanen & Pimentel (1984) and Hokkanen (1985). These authors suggest that the area of origin may not be the best prospect and that new host–parasite associations have in fact been twice as effective in biological control of weeds. The example of chestnut blight, where the pathogen was introduced to a new, though closely related, host, would support this argument, but as pointed out by Moran et al. (1986), the data put forward by Hokkanen & Pimentel (1984) in support of their argument are considerably biased by one programme and although the basic principle should not be rejected, searching for new associations is not generally accepted as a guideline for practical programmes. The significance of the concept of co-evolution to a point of homeostasis is considered again later.

In practice, highly co-evolved and specialized pathogens, e.g. obligate parasites, have been damaging agents. A strain of *Phragmidium violaceum* has been extremely effective against at least one form of *Rubus fruticosus* in Chile (Oehrens & Gonzales 1974). In a similar situation, the use of *P. chondrillina* against *C. juncea* has shown the need for strains of the pathogen extremely specialized for their host. *C. juncea* is an apomict and exists as several distinct genetic clones or forms. Strains of *P. chondrillina* have specialized to the extent that one form will only be attacked by certain strains of *P. chondrillina* (Hasan 1972). To have any effect, a very high level of specialization and co-evolution is necessary. It is not known yet whether strain IT 32, which has been so virulent against form A of the weed did evolve with this form in Europe or whether, perhaps, it co-evolved with a closely related form and would thus constitute a 'new association' (*sensu* Hokkanen 1985), albeit at an extremely specialized level. Recent evidence does suggest that form A of *C. juncea* is very close or identical to the form occurring in the European locality where strain IT 32 was obtained (P. Chaboudez, personal communication).

In terms of Room's (1981) concept of a peak in effectiveness of an agent at some intermediate point in evolutionary time, present experience suggests that this peak is well towards the later end of the evolutionary time scale.

Leaving aside the above issues, judging the effectiveness of a pathogen is often more important and difficult than simply finding a promising species. Assessments of effectiveness in terms of infection type in the laboratory are often used, but they do not always translate to effectiveness under field conditions, as witnessed by the discrepancy between the number of species regarded as promising on the basis of laboratory data and the number of eventually successful effective species. Searching for biological control agents in those regions of the original range of pathogens that are ecologically and climatically similar to the regions where the weed is a problem and examining their effectiveness in the field (Hasan & Wapshere 1973), has given extra insight into the eventual field effectiveness following introduction (Cullen & Groves 1977).

The major problem for classical biological control using pathogens is that of demonstrating satisfactory specificity before introducing a new exotic pathogen. At times it seems that such a radical change from the philosophy of protection against pathogens has been too difficult to accept, and occasionally there have been problems in finding a course of experimentation and approval that might allow a proposal to be considered. Concerns have been expressed about the stability of specificity, and the interpretation and extrapolation of test results, while the complexity of life cycles and ignorance of mechanisms of specificity and their genetic bases have tended to foster a climate of extreme caution. However, guidelines for testing and introduction have now been in use in Australia and the U.S.A. for several years (Charudattan 1982). Watson (1985) has comprehensively reviewed current procedures and problems. In general, the emphasis is on defining the host range as carefully as possible, with extensive testing of species closely related to the host, examination and interpretation of degrees of susceptible and resistant reactions and consideration of alternate hosts and different spore types. Efforts are essentially limited to those groups of fungi with records of well-developed and stable host specificity, including many obligate pathogens. Many potentially useful species are currently not seriously considered because of a lack of knowledge of the mechanisms of host specificity. Biological control is making significant contributions to the level of knowledge in this area (Clement & Watson 1985; Hasan 1974*b*; Mortensen 1985; Politis *et al.* 1984; Watson 1985; Watson & Alkhoury 1981).

A final concern about classical biological control, which is not unique to the use of pathogens, is related to the inherent aim of establishing a new self-perpetuating organism, capable of causing damage throughout the distribution of a weed species. Serious conflicts of interest can arise if the weed is considered desirable in some situations. Cullen & Delfosse (1985) have recently described a classic example of such a case and the legislation it has given rise to in order to resolve such disputes.

## MYCOHERBICIDES

The development of mycoherbicides is the current growth area in the biological control of weeds. With the current increased sensitivity to the effects of chemicals in the environment, the realization that plant resistance to herbicides is already a problem and likely to increase, and the demonstration that successful, commercially viable products can be developed, several major agricultural chemical companies are now investing considerable resources in this development.

The importance of specificity for a mycoherbicide, particularly when developed from an indigenous pathogen, is different from that for an exotic pathogen imported for classical biological control. The pathogen already exists in the environment and would not be considered if it were already known to cause a disease of any crop in the area. However, the amount of inoculum is enormously increased and is applied in the manner of a chemical product. Registration is necessary and, although sufficient specificity still needs to be demonstrated with regard to species likely to be exposed to infection, assurance is also necessary that the large quantity present will not be harmful in any way to other forms of life (Charudattan 1982). However, the fact that the distribution of the pathogen at artificially high densities is under the control of man, allows a little more flexibility than when using an exotic species intended to spread and establish itself in areas where it was unknown before. Thus, it is possible to use particular host specific strains of a pathogen, the host range of which at the species level could be quite broad (Hasan 1987), or pathogens with a relatively broad range, which will not come into contact with susceptible hosts under the conditions of intended use (Watson 1985). The use of mycoherbicides is also less likely to run into the problems of conflict of interest.

The problems of developing mycoherbicides are essentially related to having an effective, marketable product. To some extent, problems of insufficient virulence or sporulation or both of the pathogen for example, can be overcome by increasing the inoculum. However, commercial mass production, maintenance of viability in storage and environmental requirements for infection, can pose severe problems. These are essentially technical and economic, but demand sophisticated research on the biology and epidemiology of the pathogen concerned, and considerable cooperation between the research scientist and industry (Templeton *et al.* 1980).

The commercial and economic nature of the development of mycoherbicides also poses legislative problems, though of a different nature from those in classical biological control. Related to the development of registration requirements for formulation of mycoherbicides is the right of patent of a commercial product, although it is based on a naturally occurring organism. Patents for formulations related to techniques of storage and application already exist for two products, and are justifiable and necessary to encourage commercial development.

Patenting of organisms as such has not been generally recognized as acceptable or possible, but novel uses for them have been patented, at least in the U.S.A., where patenting of novel forms of microorganisms has also been ruled permissible (Templeton *et al.* 1980). It seems that patenting of specially developed strains will certainly occur, but the definition of 'novel' or 'specially developed' is not yet clear for mycoherbicides. To what extent a change in genetic structure from the wild type has to be deliberately induced as against selected, is not yet well defined. The question of secrecy becomes important when considering commercial development in this field, and the state of research on any weed–pathogen interaction may only be known when public knowledge of it is commercially acceptable. Given the assurances of Templeton *et al.* (1980) that patenting can proceed without undue delay in the dissemination of information, it is to be hoped that the publication and availability of mycoherbicide research and application will be encouraged by commercial interest rather than hindered in any way.

### RESISTANCE, VARIABILITY AND COEVOLUTION

Variation in susceptibility to a pathogen or to a particular strain is normal. Apart from the potential for the selection of resistant populations, the presence of a mixture of susceptible and non-susceptible host forms may hinder the development of disease in the population (Burdon & Chilvers 1976, 1977). Burdon & Marshall (1981) took this point further to suggest that outcrossing plant species, which thus possess a more variable genome, would be less suitable targets for biological control by pathogens or insects, and demonstrated the existence of a positive correlation between inbreeding and level of success of classical biological control programmes. This suggestion has not been generally accepted by entomologists, who find most insect agents slightly less finely tuned to their hosts and more capable of coping with a broader range of genetic variation within the host. It might be considered more applicable to pathogens. It does not however, take into account the evolutionary potential of the agent, and pathogens in particular, turn over their generations several times faster than the plant. The equilibrium between the host and pathogen in the original environment may be complex, as suggested by Harlan (1976), involving differing susceptibilities on the part of the plant to different strains of a pathogen and the presence of more than one strain of the pathogen, but there is no reason why a similar balance should not be obtained in the new environment, i.e. the equilibrium is both ecological and genetic, and the basic principle of classical biological control should still operate. If not, one would expect to see far more native outbreeding species escaping any control by pathogens and becoming important new weeds. From a practical point of view, in at least one important project, it is the variation between forms of an apomict, *C. juncea*, that is causing more problems, the extremely specialized strains of the pathogen associated with these 'stable' forms also showing considerable stability and requiring considerable searching.

Thus the tendency is to suppose that the evolution of resistant populations will not be a major problem in classical control, particularly if efforts are made to broaden the genetic base of the pathogen population when imported, e.g. by using a selection of several strains of *Phragmidium violacaeum* for control of *Rubus fruticosus* (Bruzzese & Hasan 1986). However, in the case of mycoherbicides, the operative strain is that produced and applied by man and, if unchanged, will exert considerable directed selection pressure on the weed to favour the production of one or more resistant forms. Commercial use of mycoherbicides will therefore have to consider the use of mixtures of strains or be prepared to change strains as required. In fact many of the pathogen–host interactions, which from a practical point of view are likely to be used in mycoherbicide programmes, i.e. non-obligate pathogens, seem to involve variable pathogen populations that can produce a range of new virulence types. They should thus be able to overcome the variation in resistance of the host population rapidly, and where this is characterized by partial resistance genes, the increased inoculum load would also help overcome this potential problem (J. J. Burdon & R. H. Groves, personal communication). Obligate pathogens, showing perhaps less variation, are in any case, unlikely to be used in mycoherbicide programmes, at least at present, because of the difficulties of mass production.

Reference has already been made to the possibility of decreased virulence of a pathogen in a highly co-evolved host–pathogen relation and the consequences this could have for the sources and choice of biological control agents. Although the recommendation of Hokkanen & Pimentel (1984) that priority should be given to seeking new parasite–host associations is not accepted, the potential inherent in the suggestion probably merits further attention. However, this line of reasoning has been taken further, to the extent of suggesting that the use of obligate pathogens in any form of biological control is unlikely to be successful. Harper (1977) has described such pathogens as 'trapped in the co-evolutionary rut of host specialization and cause little damage to the host', and objections were raised to the utility of introducing P. chondrillina for control of C. juncea on these grounds. Co-evolution to favour decreased virulence might be possible in some circumstances, e.g. where group selection does not need to be invoked, but the relation between host and pathogen populations is still a dynamic equilibrium. An increase in density of the host will produce a numerical response by the pathogen such as to increase its rate of infection and therefore the damage inflicted. This is one of the basic conditions for starting an epidemic and is readily observed in monocultures. Although the level of the population equilibrium may be influenced by the history of co-evolution of the system, control is still being exerted by the pathogen. If that host population density at equilibrium is acceptable as a level of control in a new environment, where the host plant has increased to a much higher density in the absence of its obligate, co-evolved pathogen, there is every possibility that biological control would be successful. The effectiveness of introducing P. chondrillina into Australia should not be seen as exceptional but to be expected. Such an outcome has been achieved several times in insect parasite systems.

## Current status

It is appropriate to summarize what has been achieved in practical terms before considering, finally, the current direction of development and prospects.

### Classical programmes

The introduction of P. chondrillina has already been cited as an illustration of several points raised in this discussion. The outstanding success of the introduction of strain IT32 against form A of C. juncea has been adequately reported and quantified, and the significance of the status of the other two forms has been described (Cullen 1978, 1985). The successful introduction of P. violacaeum to Chile has also been reported (Oehrens & Gonzales 1974), and the introduction of Cercosporella sp. into Hawaii has been successful in controlling Ageratina riparia (Trujillo 1985). Currently, there are programmes in various stages of development on Uromyces heliotropii for control of *Heliotropium europaeum* (Hasan 1985), *Puccinia jaceae* for *Centaurea diffusa* and *Puccinia carduorum* for *Carduus nutans*.

## Mycoherbicides

Two products are currently registered for commercial use, in the U.S.A.: *Colletotrichum gloeosporioides* f. sp. *aeschynomene* for control of *Aeschynomene virginica*, and *Phytophthora palmivora* for control of *Morrenia odorata* (TeBeest & Templeton 1985). A third pathogen, *Cercospora rodmanii*, is also a candidate for use and is likely to be registered soon for the control of *Eichornia crassipes* (Charudattan 1986). In addition, Hasan (1987) reports 35 other projects in both areas currently in course of investigation.

## POTENTIAL AND PROSPECTS

Apart from a steady increase in the number of pathogens put into practical use and a refining of techniques, particularly in the commercial production of mycoherbicides, what else can be expected?

A field that has been slow to develop has been integrated control or weed management, where biological control techniques are integrated with other systems, including use of chemicals, to produce the level of control desired. There is a relatively long history of development in this field for insect control, but for weeds it is still in its infancy. Although of interest, the reasons are not relevant here, being mainly historical. The fact is that integrated control is long overdue for development and its basic requirements are at last beginning to be realized by biological control workers, weed scientists and by the agrochemical industry. The interaction between herbicide effects and pathogens seems a fertile area for research. It has been found for instance, that the destructive action of the fungus *Cochliobolus lunatus* on *Echinochloa crus-galli*, normally quite limited, is increased considerably when used with 10% of the normal dose of a chemical herbicide (Scheepens & van Zon 1982).

Weed management implies the ability to manage the whole weed environment, i.e. the local agroecosystem and therefore a knowledge of the ecology of the weed, the ecology of the biological control agents, the interaction of these and the weed with the agricultural system, and the level of control desired. The necessary ecological knowledge has often been lacking in weed control programmes, but quantitative, population-orientated approaches are becoming more common so that management of weed populations incorporating the use of pathogens and other methods now seems to be an achievable aim.

Finally, it is virtually certain that the expanding field of biotechnology and genetic engineering will be called on to improve the pathogens. Induction and screening of mutants for finding more virulent strains of pathogens is routine procedure in plant breeding for resistance and studies on the genetics of host–pathogen relations (McIntosh & Watson 1982; Simons 1979) but as yet untried in any serious manner in the use of pathogens for weed control. For insect control, it is now possible to use transformation techniques to construct new strains of entomopathogens without the need for sexual reproduction (Faull 1986). For weed pathogens, the identification of key features for improvement by genetic engineering is still difficult except possibly for resistance to fungicides that can be incorporated into integrated crop protection schemes. A comprehensive knowledge of the genetics of resistance–virulence will be necessary.

There is currently no shortage of projects or interest, and an impression that the potential is enormous. Despite some acceleration in the pace of technical development with increasing investment from private industry, progress towards effective control will continue to be slow and steady, because of the time involved in host specificity testing and, in the case of mycoherbicides, the development of economic production and storage techniques. The potential will therefore only be slowly realized, but there is every confidence that pathogens will become a commonplace component of weed management systems.

REFERENCES

Ayres, P. G. & Paul, N. D. 1986 Foliar pathogens alter the water relations of their hosts with consequences for both host and pathogen. In *Water, fungi and plants* (ed. P. G. Ayres & L. Boddy) (*British Mycological Society Symposium no. 11*), pp. 267–285. Cambridge University Press.

Ben-Kalio, V. D. & Clarke, D. D. 1979 Studies on tolerance in wild plants: effects of *Erysiphe fischeri* on the growth and development of *Senecio vulgaris*. *Physiol. Pl. Path.* **14**, 203–211.

Bruzzese, E. & Hasan, S. 1986 The collection and selection in Europe of isolates of *Phragmidium violaceum* (Uredinales) pathogenic to species of European blackberry naturalised in Australia. *Ann. appl. Biol.* **108**, 527–533.

Burdon, J. J. & Chilvers, G. A. 1976 Epidemiology of *Pythium*-induced damping-off in mixed seedling stands. *Ann. appl. Biol.* **82**, 233–240.

Burdon, J. J. & Chilvers, G. A. 1977 Controlled environment experiments in epidemic rates of barley mildew in different mixtures of barley and wheat. *Oecologia* **28**, 141–146.

Burdon, J. J. & Marshall, D. R. 1981 Biological control and the reproductive mode of weeds. *J. appl. Ecol.* **18**, 649–658.

Burdon, J. J. & Shattock, R. C. 1980 Disease in plant communities. In *Applied biology* (ed. T. H. Coaker), vol. 5, pp. 145–219. London: Academic Press.

Charudattan, R. 1982 Regulation of microbial weed control agents. In *Biological control of weeds with plant pathogens* (ed. R. Charudattan & H. L. Walker), pp. 175–188. New York: J. Wiley.

Charudattan, R. 1986 Integrated control of water hyacinth (*Eichhornia crassipes*) with a pathogen, insects and herbicides. *Weed Sci.* **34** (suppl. 1), 26–30.

Clement, M. & Watson, A. K. 1985 Biological control of spotted knapweed (*Centaurea maculosa*) – host range of *Puccinia centaureae*. In *Proceedings of the VIth International Symposium on the Biological Control of Weeds, Vancouver, Canada, 1984* (ed. E. S. Delfosse), p. 423. Agriculture Canada.

Cullen, J. M. 1978 Evaluating the success of the program for the biological control of *Chondrilla juncea* L. In *Proceedings of the IVth International Symposium on the Biological Control Weeds, Gainesville, Florida, 1976* (ed. T. E. Freeman), pp. 117–121. Institute of Food and Agricultural Science, University of Florida.

Cullen, J. M. 1985 Bringing the cost benefit analysis of biological control of *Chondrilla juncea* up to date. In *Proceedings of the VIth International Symposium on the Biological Control of Weeds, Vancouver, Canada, 1984* (ed. E. S. Delfosse), pp. 145–152. Agriculture Canada.

Cullen, J. M. 1988 *Chondrilla juncea* L. Skeleton weed. In *The biological control of weeds: a practical and ecological appraisal* (ed. M. J. Crawley & V. C. Moran). (In the press.)

Cullen, J. M. & Delfosse, E. S. 1985 *Echium plantagineum*: catalyst for conflict and change in Australia. In *Proceedings of the VIth International Symposium on the Biological Control of Weeds, Vancouver, Canada, 1984* (ed. E. S. Delfosse), pp. 249–292. Agriculture Canada.

Cullen, J. M. & Groves, R. H. 1977 The population biology of *Chondrilla juncea* L. in Australia. *Proc. ecol. Soc. Aust.* **10**, 121–134.

Cullen, J. M., Kable, P. F. & Catt, M. 1973 Epidemic spread of a rust imported for biological control. *Nature, Lond.* **224**, 462–464.

Faull, J. L. 1986 Fungi and their role in crop protection. In *Biotechnology and crop improvement and protection* pp. 141–150. British Crop Protection Council Monograph no. 34.

Goeden, R. D. 1971 Insect ecology of silver leaf nightshade. *Weed Sci.* **19**, 45–51.

Harlan, J. R. 1976 Diseases as a factor in plant evolution. *A. Rev. Phytopath.* **14**, 31–51.

Harper, J. L. 1977 *Population biology of plants*, pp. 483–496. London: Academic Press.

Harris, P. & Piper, G. L. 1970 Ragweed (*Ambrosia* spp.; Compositae), its North American insects and the possibilities for its biological control. *CIBC tech. Bull.* **13**, 117–140.

Hasan, S. 1972 Specificity and host specialisation of *Puccinia chondrillina*. *Ann. appl. Biol.* **72**, 257–263.

Hasan, S. 1974a First introduction of a rust fungus into Australia for the biological control of skeleton weed. *Phytopathology* **64**, 253–254.

Hasan, S. 1974 *b* Host specialisation of a powdery mildew, *Erysiphe cichoracearum* from *Chondrilla juncea*. *Aust. J. agric. Res.* **25**, 459–465.

Hasan, S. 1985 Prospects for biological control of *Heliotropium europaeum* by fungal pathogens. In *Proceedings of the VIth International Symposium on the Biological Control of Weeds, Vancouver, Canada, 1984* (ed. E. S. Delfosse), pp. 617–623. Agriculture Canada.

Hasan, S. 1988 Biocontrol of weeds with microbes. In *Biocontrol of plant diseases*, vol. 1 (ed. K. G. Mukerji & K. L. Karg). Boca Raton, Florida: CRC Press. (In the press.)

Hasan, S. & Wapshere, A. J. 1973 The biology of *Puccinia chondrillina* a potential biological control agent of skeleton weed. *Ann. appl. Biol.* **74**, 325–332.

Hokkanen, H. M. T. 1985 Success in classical biological control. In *CRC critical reviews in plant sciences*, vol. 3, pp. 35–72. Boca Raton, Florida: CRC Press.

Hokkanen, H. M. T. & Pimentel, D. 1984 New approach for selecting biological control agents. *Can. Ent.* **116**, 1109–1121.

McIntosh, R. A. & Watson, I. A. 1982 Genetics of host-pathogen interactions in rusts. In *The rust fungi* (ed. K. J. Scott & A. K. Chakrabarthy), pp. 121–150. London: Academic Press.

Mall, L. P. & Tugnawat, R. K. 1973 Ecopathological investigations (1). Influence of plant pathogenic fungus on production of *Dichanthium annulatum* (Forsk.) Stapf. *Flora* **162**, 437–441.

Moran, V. C., Neser, S. & Hoffman, J. H. 1986 The potential of insect herbivores for the biological control of invasive plants in South Africa. In *The ecology and management of biological invasions in southern Africa*. (ed. I. A. W. Macdonald, F. J. Kruger & A. A. Ferrar), pp. 261–268. Cape Town: Oxford University Press.

Mortensen, K. 1985 A proposal for a standardised scale of attack and its application to biocontrol agents of weeds in laboratory screening tests. In *Proceedings of the VIth International Symposium on the Biological Control of Weeds, Vancouver, Canada, 1984* (ed. E. S. Delfosse), pp. 643–650. Agriculture Canada.

Oehrens, E. B. & Gonzales, S. M. 1974 Introduction de *Phragmidium violaceum* (Schulz) Winter como factor de control biologico de zarzamora (*Rubus constrictus* Lef. et M. y *R. ulmifolius* Schott.). *Agro Sur* **2**, 30–33.

Pimentel, D. 1961 Animal population regulation by the genetic feedback mechanism. *Am. Nat.* **95**, 65–79.

Politis, D. J., Watson, A. K. & Bruckart, W. L. 1984 Susceptibility of musk thistle and related composites *Puccinia carduorum*. *Phytopathology* **74**, 687–691.

Room, P. M. 1981 Biogeography, apparency and exploration for biological control agents in exotic ranges of weeds. In *Proceedings of the VIth International Symposium on the Biological Control of Weeds, Brisbane, Australia, 1980* (ed. E. S. Delfosse), pp. 113–124. C.S.I.R.O. Melbourne.

Scheepens, P. C. & van Zon, H. C. J. 1982 Microbial herbicides. In *Microbial and viral pesticides* (ed. E. Kurstak), pp. 623–641. New York: Marcel Dekker.

Simons, M. D. 1979 Modification of host–parasite interactions through artificial mutagenesis. *Rev. Phytopathol.* **17**, 75–96.

TeBeest, D. O. & Templeton, G. E. 1985 Mycoherbicide: progress in the biological control of weeds. *Pl. Dis.* **69**, 6–10.

Templeton, G. E., Smith, R. J. & Klomparens, W. 1980 Commercialisation of fungi and bacteria for biological control. *Biocontrol News Inf.* **1**, 291–294.

Trujillo, E. E. 1985 Biological control of Hamakua pa-makani with *Cercosporella* sp. in Hawaii. In *Proceedings of the VIth International Symposium on the Biological Control of Weeds, Vancouver, Canada, 1984* (ed. E. S. Delfosse), pp. 661–671. Agriculture Canada.

Wapshere, A. J. 1971 The effect of human intervention on the distribution and abundance of *Chondrillina juncea* L. In *Proceedings of the Advanced Study Institute on the dynamics and numbers of populations, Oosterbeck, 1970*, pp. 469–477. (ed. P. J. den Boer & G. R. Gradwell). Wageningen: Centre for Agricultural Publishing and Documention.

Wapshere, A. J. 1974 Host specificity of phytophagous organisms and the evolutionary centres of plant geneva or sub-genera. *Entomophaga* **19**, 301–309.

Wapshere, A. J., Hasan, S., Wahba, W. K. & Caresche, L. 1974 The ecology of *Chondrilla juncea* in the western Mediterranean. *J. appl. Ecol.* **11**, 783–800.

Watson, A. K. 1985 Host specificity of plant pathogens in biological weed control. In *Proceedings of the VIth International Symposium on the Biological Control of Weeds, Vancouver, Canada, 1984* (ed. E. S. Delfosse), pp. 577–586. Agriculture Canada.

Watson, A. K. & Alkhoury, I. 1981 Response of safflower cultivars to *Puccinia jaceae* collected from diffuse knapweed in eastern Europe. In *Proceedings of the VIth International Symposium on the Biological Control of Weeds, Brisbane, Australia, 1980*. (ed. E. S. Delfosse), pp. 301–305. Melbourne: C.S.I.R.O.

*Discussion*

W. D. HAMILTON, F.R.S. (*Department of Zoology, University of Oxford, U.K.*). Dr Hasan indicated that his main examples of weeds controlled by fungi, skeleton weed and *Rubus*, were apomicts. Although conceding the evidence of apomixis most of the time, I have always found it surprising that plants claimed to be long-established apomicts still have large showy flowers and are still very attractive to insects. I have wondered whether occasional successful crosses may not be quite important to them, and indeed the very success of his control programme might suggest why it should be important from their point of view as hosts. I wanted to ask whether his work threw any light on how completely apomicitic your plants are. For example, did any unexpected and resistant strains appear that might be the result of sexual recombination?

S. HASAN. *Chondrilla juncea* was accidentally introduced into Australia towards 1910 and, since then, it has gradually spread in the southeastern parts, infesting mainly the cereal crops. Studies on the reproduction of the weed have shown that it is an apomicitic triploid ($3n = 15$) and there is no exchange of genetic material in seed formation. Later on, it was demonstrated that in Australia, *C. juncea* occurs in three distinct morphological forms (narrow-, intermediate- and broad-leaved). These three clones have been further confirmed by the modern techniques of electrophoresis.

A strain of the rust fungus *Puccinia chondrillina* was found to be aggressive against the most common narrow leaf form and was released in the field in Australia in 1971. Shortly after the rust became well established and widespread, progressively reducing populations of the weed. The pathogen has continued its destructive action and skeleton weed is no longer a problem. However, during the past 15 years the introduced strain of the rust has attacked only the narrow-leaf form whereas the intermediate and broad leaf forms have remained unaffected and have been increasing in some places. More strains of the rust virulent to these other forms are being discovered in Europe and studies on the efficacy as biological control agents are currently underway.

These results show again how distinct and stable are the three skeleton weed clones. Also, so far, there is no evidence of change in the pathogenicity of the rust or of the presence of other forms of the weed in Australia. However, Burdon *et al.* (1980) have raised doubts about obligate apomyxis in the three Australian forms and suggest the possible formation of new variants through occasional sexual recombination, autosegregation and or random mutation. Thus, studies are currently underway, using electrophoretic techniques, on clonal variation in skeleton weed in Europe and Australia and on the possible existence of a genetic pool close to the weed's centre of distribution giving rise to new forms.

*Reference*

Burdon, J. J., Marshall, D. R. & Groves, R. H. 1980 Isozyme variation in *Chandrilla juncea* L. in Australia. *Aust. J. Bot.* **28**, 193–198.

A. E. AKINGBOHUNGBE (*Department of Plant Science, University of Ife, Nigeria*). (1) I noted that some well-established crop pathogens such as *Phytophthora palmivora* have been mentioned as part of D. Hasan's agents released in control programmes. What steps are taken to ensure that these do not re-establish on other crops?

(2) Is there any possibility of utilizing toxins of known plant pathogens for herbicide formulations?

S. Hasan. (1) The particular isolate of *P. palmivora* from milkweed vine (*Morrenia odorata*) was tested for specificity against 58 plant species from 12 families. A few plants other than milkweed vine were found to be infected, but only with a very high dose of the fungus. Although *P. palmivora* was pathogenic to several citrus rootstocks in pre-emergence tests, no pathogenicity of the isolate from milkweed vine could be demonstrated in the field. Also, isolates from roots of citrus trees treated with *P. palmivora* in the field did not reveal infection by this pathogen.

(2) It may be possible to use host-selective toxins produced by plant pathogens in biological control of weeds. However, their action will be short term, limited to each application, whereas mycoherbicide formulations based on mycelia or spores of pathogens may continue to infect the host, and thus have a prolonged effect in the field.

J. W. Deacon (*Department of Microbiology, Edinburgh University, U.K.*). Are there any programmes to investigate the potential use of mycoherbicides against parasitic higher plants such as *Striga* and *Orobanche* spp.?

S. Hasan. Attempts are being made to control parasitic weeds with plant pathogens. Thus, among fungal pathogens of *Orobanche* spp. (broomrape), *Fusarium oxysporum* var. *orthoceras* destroys 70% of the seed. It has been formulated for field use in the U.S.S.R. as 'Product F', which remains effective for 80 d, and has been applied to infested water melon and tobacco with encouraging results. Also in the U.S.S.R., *Alternaria cuscutacidae* is reported to have been successfully used against dodder (*Cuscuta* spp.).

Considerable interest has been shown in the use of plant pathogens for biological control of dwarf mistletoe, *Arceuthobium* spp. in the U.S.A. Among several pathogens, the anthracnose fungus *Glomerella cingulata* has been shown to be most effective.

There has not yet been any practical application of biological control to witchweeds (*Striga* spp.).

*Phil. Trans. R. Soc. Lond.* B **318**, 225–248 (1988)

*Printed in Great Britain*

# Pathogens for the control of insects: where next?

By C. C. Payne

*Institute of Horticultural Research, Worthing Road, Littlehampton, West Sussex BN17 6LP, U.K.*

Insect populations succumb to a variety of infections caused by pathogenic microorganisms (bacteria, fungi, Protozoa) and viruses. The narrow host-range of many of these agents makes them natural candidates for use within integrated pest management systems. Some, such as *Bacillus thuringiensis* and several baculoviruses, may be applied to crops at regular intervals as microbial pesticides, achieving short-term control of a pest population. Longer-term suppression of insect populations requires some degree of persistence of the pathogen in the target host population. Examples of sustained, natural, insect population regulation by microorganisms are rare; regulation demands stable ecosystems and a capacity for the pathogen to spread.

We cannot ignore the fact that many of the microbial pathogens available today fail to meet the expectations of an agricultural industry used to the rapid and broad-spectrum pest knockdown achieved by many chemical pesticides. Despite the many advantages to be gained in selective pest management from the use of naturally occurring strains of insect pathogens, much recent attention has focused on the improvement of strains by genetic manipulation. Significant advances have already been made in the manipulation of bacterial and viral pathogens to increase virulence and modify host range. The environmental persistence of the insect-pathogenic toxin of *B. thuringiensis* has also been extended by inserting the toxin gene into other bacterial hosts and plants. Exciting future opportunities for biological control may be created by such strategies. However, to make responsible use of these manipulated organisms we must understand more about their long-term impact on insect populations and the environment. Such information should come not only from detailed ecological studies of the host–pathogen interaction but also from laboratory and field studies of the frequency and consequences of genetic exchange between modified strains and naturally occurring microorganisms.

## 1. Introduction

The basic concept of using microorganisms to control insect pests is long-standing with many, largely unsuccessful, attempts in the nineteenth century to exploit fungal diseases for the control of economically important pests (reviewed in Miller *et al.* (1984)). It is now known that a wide range of naturally occurring pathogens of insects (e.g. bacteria, viruses, fungi and Protozoa) can be used as highly selective pest control agents. The development of resistance by certain key pests to chemical pesticides and the increasing production costs for new compounds are encouraging greater interest and investment in such biological control agents. In addition, increased awareness of the adverse environmental consequences of using certain toxic chemical pesticides is further enhancing the desire to control pests with agents that have no damaging effects on non-target species.

Despite these pressures, microbial pest control agents at present form a very small part (less than 1%) of total pesticide sales (Jutsum, this symposium). It is my aim in this paper to examine the reasons for this and to consider the future use of insect pathogens by methods that could increase their contribution to new integrated pest management systems. To achieve this aim, it is necessary first to consider the properties of pathogens that are currently available.

## 2. The current status of insect pathogens as biocontrol agents

### (a) Bacteria

Although about 100 insect-pathogenic species of bacteria have been identified, only certain *Bacillus* spp. have shown clear potential as insect-specific pest control agents (Lüthy 1986a). Of these, *B. thuringiensis* (*B.t.*), *B. sphaericus* and *B. popilliae* have received most attention. *B.t.* is the only microbial pest control agent that has been commercialized world-wide on a large scale. It is an aerobic, spore-forming bacterium, easy to grow on many media, including those composed of cheap waste products of the fish- and food-processing industry (Lüthy 1986a). At sporulation, the bacterium produces both a spore and a large proteinaceous crystal. When the protein crystal is ingested by certain insects, it dissolves in the gut juices and is degraded by proteases to release toxic polypeptides. In the simplest situation, the protein crystal (δ-endotoxin) consists of protoxin molecules with a relative molecular mass ($M_r$) of about 130000, which are degraded in the insect gut to a protein toxin with an $M_r$ of about 60000. Studies with one strain of *B.t.* var. *kurstaki*, active against Lepidoptera, have suggested that the toxin binds to glycoproteins in the plasma membrane of larval gut epithelial cells, generating small pores in the membrane and destroying regulation of ion exchange (Eller *et al.* 1986). Simultaneously, the muscles of gut and mouthparts are paralysed, feeding stops, and death occurs 30 min to 3 days after ingestion (Burges 1986a).

Many strains of *B.t.* have now been isolated and classified within more than 20 different varieties by serological techniques. On the basis of their potency for insects, Ellar *et al.* (1986) have grouped these varieties into at least five pathotypes: (*a*) lepidopteran-specific (e.g. var. *thuringiensis*); (*b*) dipteran-specific (e.g. var. *israelensis*); (*c*) coleopteran-specific (e.g. var. *tenebrionis*); (*d*) those active against both Lepidoptera and Diptera (e.g. var. *aizawai*); (*e*) those with no toxicity recorded in insects (e.g. var. *dakota*). Within each of these pathotypes there are marked differences in both specificity and potency.

Recent intensive research on the molecular biology and genetics of *B.t.* toxins is providing insights into the reasons behind the specificity differences. It has been confirmed that the crystal protoxins are single gene products and that the genes are located in many *B.t.* strains on plasmids (Kronstad *et al.* 1982). From the DNA sequence of the protoxin gene from the HD1-Dipel strain of *B.t.* var. *kurstaki* the amino acid sequence has been deduced (Schnepf *et al.* 1985). Comparison of this gene with other cloned protoxin genes from vars. *kurstaki*, *thuringiensis* (= *berliner*), *sotto* and *alesti* has revealed considerable similarities between the deduced structures of the protoxin molecules. In the total of approximately 1170 amino acids, *ca.* 280 at the N-terminus and *ca.* 400–600 at the C-terminus are highly conserved (Ellar *et al.* 1966; Lüthy 1986b; Adang *et al.* 1987). The region between these conserved areas, particularly between residues 340 and 617, shows considerable variability in amino acid sequence (Adang *et al.* 1987). The insecticidal activity of the toxin itself (*ca.* 60000 $M_r$) is located towards the N-terminus and includes most of the conserved N-terminal region and much of the variable region (Lüthy 1986b; Adang *et al.* 1987).

Although the relation between toxin structure and biological specificity needs further scrutiny, variation in potency between different strains could be partly accounted for by differences in the variable region of the toxin. In addition, some *B.t.* strains have been shown to contain more than one distinct toxin gene (three in *kurstaki* HD-1) (Adang *et al.* 1987) with up to five recorded in some strains (Carlton 1986). Although insecticidal activity in some insect species may require more than one toxin, some toxins may have dual specificity (Haider *et al.* 1987). These exciting studies go some way towards understanding the wide variations in *B.t.* specificity and potency, and provide the basis for future *B.t.* strain improvement and genetic engineering (see §4).

Despite the existence of many *B.t.* strains, at present very few varieties are commercially available (table 1). *B.t.* var. *kurstaki* HD-1 has been extensively used to control larvae of pest Lepidoptera as it has a relatively broad activity spectrum (Lüthy 1986a). It has now been used widely against lepidopterous pests of horticulture, agriculture and forestry (Burges 1986a). *B.t.* var. *israelensis* (Goldberg & Margalit 1977) was recognized as having great potency for larvae of biting blackflies and many species of mosquitoes. Urged on by the need to develop alternative methods to control pesticide-resistant blackfly vectors of onchocerciasis in West Africa, this strain was commercialized within six years of its discovery and has made a major contribution to blackfly and mosquito control (Burges & Pillai 1986). Recently, the potential spectrum of activity of *B.t.* has been increased by the discovery of isolates active against beetles (Krieg *et al.* 1983; Herrnstadt *et al.* 1986).

TABLE 1. PRINCIPAL BACTERIAL PEST CONTROL AGENTS

| species | target pests | commercial products |
|---|---|---|
| *Bacillus thuringiensis* var. *kurstaki* | caterpillars (Lepidoptera) | e.g. Dipel (Abbott), Bactospeine (Philips Duphar), Thuricide (Zoecon), world-wide use. |
| *B.t.* var *aizawai* | waxmoth (*Galleria mellonella*) | e.g. Certan (Zoecon), U.S.A. |
| *B.t.* var. *israelensis* | mosquitoes and blackflies | e.g. Vectobac (Abbott), Bactimos (Philips Duphar), Teknar (Zoecon), world-wide use |
| *B.t.* var. *tenebrionis* / *B.t.* var. *san diego* | beetles | in development |
| *Bacillus sphaericus* | mosquitoes | in development |
| *Bacillus popilliae* | Japanese beetle (*Popillia japonica*) | e.g. Doom (Fairfax Biological Laboratory), Milky Spore (Reuter Labs), U.S.A. |

Although *B.t.* is known to cause natural epizootics in enclosed environments (e.g. granaries), it is otherwise not a highly infectious natural pathogen as it generally fails to spread. This means that it must be used as a microbial pesticide, with regular applications needed for adequate pest control. Because it has no contact action and must be ingested to be effective, it should be applied to sites (and at ambient temperatures) where larvae are feeding. In most susceptible species, ingestion of the toxin crystal alone seems sufficient to ensure death. However, efficacy in some insects (e.g. the wax moth, *Galleria mellonella*) is dependent on the presence of at least some *B.t.* spores in the ingested material (Li *et al.* 1987); most commercial products of *B.t.* contain a mixture of spores and crystals. Like other microbial agents applied in the field, the bacterial spore is inactivated quite rapidly by the ultraviolet (uv) component of sunlight. Although active crystal toxin will persist on foliage for longer than spores, its half-life may be only about 8 days (Kirschbaum 1985).

Although *B.t. israelensis* is very active against larvae of the Diptera *Anopheles*, *Culex*, *Aedes* and *Simulium*, another bacterium, *Bacillus sphaericus*, is more active against *Culex* and some *Anopheles* spp. *B. sphaericus* is an aerobic, spore-forming bacterium common world-wide in soil and aquatic environments. Like *B.t.*, some *B. sphaericus* strains produce a crystalline protein toxin (*ca.* 40000 $M_r$) from a putative protoxin precursor of 125000 $M_r$ (Baumann *et al.* 1986). After a mosquito larva ingests the toxin, its gut epithelium distends and the gut is paralysed, followed by cell lysis and larval death (World Health Organization (WHO) 1985). Unlike *B.t.*, some strains of *B. sphaericus* are able to grow saprophytically in heavily-polluted water, providing opportunities for the maintenance or increase of inoculum in the absence of the insect host (WHO 1985).

In contrast to *B.t.* and *B. sphaericus*, *Bacillus popilliae* (isolated from the Japanese beetle *Popillia japonica*) does not produce toxins. It also spreads naturally, and persists even in low density host populations. Spores applied to pastures in the U.S.A. during the 1930s promoted disease in the Japanese beetle population that was still present 25–30 years later. After larvae ingest bacterial spores the progress of the disease is slow, leading eventually to large cadavers packed with spores that are very persistent in the soil. The bacterium is an obligate pathogen and it has not proved possible to produce spores adequately *in vitro*. Two small companies in the U.S.A. produce and market bacterial spores grown in larvae (Klein 1981, 1986).

### (b) Viruses

More than 1600 virus isolates have been recorded causing disease in about 1100 species of insects and mites (Martignoni & Iwai 1986). These viruses can be grouped into several categories on the basis of their morphological and biochemical properties (Payne & Kelly 1981). Among these groups, only baculoviruses have been given extensive consideration as microbial control agents. They share no obvious biochemical properties with viruses of vertebrates, plants or microorganisms, and present isolates are restricted in their host range to a small number of insect orders (principally Lepidoptera and Hymenoptera) and a few crustaceans and mites. Many individual isolates are genus- or species-specific and are often highly virulent. Being obligate intracellular parasites they can be produced only in larvae or insect cells in culture.

Baculoviruses are large, rod-shaped, enveloped, DNA-containing viruses. They are currently classified into three subgroups on the basis of morphological properties. In two groups, granulosis (GV) and nuclear polyhedrosis (NPV) viruses, virus particles are packed within large proteinaceous occlusion bodies (OB) produced late in infection, whereas viruses in a third group (non-occluded baculoviruses) do not produce these OBs. The OBs are stable and provide the means by which virus infectivity is preserved outside the host. Diseased larvae can release up to $10^{10}$ NPV OBs, or well in excess of $10^{11}$ of the smaller GV OBs, when they die. Under suitable conditions these can promote the rapid spread and maintenance of infection within susceptible insect populations. None the less, the hopes that epizootics leading to long-lasting control can be achieved by a single application of a baculovirus have not proved realistic, except for a few special cases such as the control of the coconut rhinoceros beetle, *Oryctes rhinoceros* (Bedford 1980). In general, adequate pest control has been achieved only when these viruses have been applied repeatedly (Benz 1981).

Virus infection in susceptible insects takes place only after larvae eat food contaminated with virus. In GV and NPV infections, the matrix protein of the OBS dissolves in the insect gut, releasing virus particles that infect and multiply in gut epithelial cells. In Lepidoptera, the infection quickly spreads to other tissues, whereas in Hymenoptera (e.g. sawflies), the infection is confined to the gut. Young larvae are consistently more susceptible to virus infection than older larvae (Payne 1982). None the less, death of an insect as a direct consequence of virus infection is unlikely to occur less than 3–4 days after infection, even with the most virulent of currently available virus strains.

As with all biological control agents, several factors influence the efficacy of a virus applied as a microbial insecticide. The most important of these are the deleterious effects of UV radiation from sunlight and adverse plant-surface effects (Entwistle & Evans 1985). Although many baculoviruses are highly host specific and may seem ideal candidates for selective control, pest problems on a single crop can rarely be solved by the application of one highly selective agent because most crops are attacked simultaneously by several different species of Lepidoptera. There is, therefore, considerable interest in some baculoviruses with a less-selective host range. An NPV from the alfalfa semilooper, *Autographa californica* (ACMNPV) has attracted most research, with a recorded host range of 43 species of Lepidoptera in 11 families, many of which are pest species (Payne 1986). ACMNPV is the most extensively characterized insect virus, and recent research has identified prospects for strain improvement of this and related baculoviruses through genetic manipulation, even though the biological bases of variation in host-range and virulence are not yet understood.

At the time of writing, only two baculoviruses are available as commercial products. These are *Neodiprion sertifer* NPV (for the control of pine sawfly) and *Mamestra brassicae* NPV, which infects the cabbage moth and some key noctuid pests of food and fibre crops. Other baculoviruses have attracted, or continue to attract, research and industrial interest (table 2). These include the baculovirus of *O. rhinoceros* which has been successfully introduced into many countries in the South Pacific region for the long-term suppression of rhinoceros beetle (Bedford 1980). The potential use of viruses for the control of forest pests has received much attention. Here, the high economic thresholds of pest damage that can be tolerated allow greater scope for viruses to exert their control over a longer time period than can be permitted on high value agricultural crops.

### (c) Fungi

There are approximately 100 genera of fungi that contain numerous species pathogenic to insects (Hall & Papierok 1982; Zimmermann 1986). Of these, deuteromycete fungi (table 3) have received most attention as they are among the easiest to produce *in vitro* and several have a broad host range. *Metarhizium anisopliae*, for example, has more than 200 known hosts among Coleoptera, Lepidoptera, Orthoptera and Hemiptera, whereas *Beauveria* spp. have been identified from about 500 host species, principally Lepidoptera and Coleoptera (Hall & Papierok 1982). However, this broad view disguises the fact that individual strains of the same fungal species often have different host ranges or pathogenicities.

The infective propagule in natural deuteromycete infections is the conidiospore. Although a few strains enter the host through the gut or through the respiratory tract, the majority invade insects through the cuticle. Because fungi do not, in general, have to be ingested to be effective, they have potential (unlike *B.t.* or viruses) for the control of sap-feeding arthropods which do not ingest pathogens on the plant surface.

TABLE 2. PRINCIPLE BACULOVIRUS CANDIDATES FOR INSECT PEST CONTROL

| virus | target hosts | crop | status of commercial development |
|---|---|---|---|
| nuclear polyhedrosis viruses | | | |
| Anticarsia gemmatalis NPV (Soybean looper) | A. gemmatalis | soybean | local production, Brazil |
| Autographa californica NPV (Alfalfa semilooper) | Orgyia pseudotsugata Trichoplusia ni | forests cabbage | former commercial trials product, USA. |
| Gilpinia hercyniae NPV (spruce sawfly) | G. hercyniae | forests | |
| Heliothis spp. NPV (cotton bollworm) | Heliothis spp. | cotton, maize, sorghum | former commercial product (Elcar), U.S.A. |
| Lymantria dispar NPV (gypsy moth) | L. dispar | forests | produced by U.S. Forest Service |
| Mamestra brassicae NPV (cabbage moth) | Mamestra, Heliothis and Diparopsis spp. | cotton, cabbage and other vegetables | produced commercially in France (Mamestrin) |
| Neodiprion sertifer NPV (pine sawfly) | N. sertifer | forests | produced commercially in U.K. (Virox) and Finland (Monisarmio virus) |
| Neodiprion lecontei NPV (redheaded pine sawfly) | N. lecontei | forests | produced by Canadian Forest Service |
| Orgyia pseudotsugata NPV (Douglas fir tussock moth) | O. pseudotsugata | forests | produced by U.S. (TM–Biocontrol 1) and Canadian Forest Service (Virtuss) |
| Spodoptera littoralis NPV (cotton leafworm) | S. littoralis | cotton | commercial trials product in France (Spodopterin) |
| Trichoplusia ni NPV (cabbage looper) | T. ni | cabbage | former commercial trials product, U.S.A. |
| granulosis viruses | | | |
| Cydia pomonella GV (codling moth) | C. pomonella | orchards | commercial trials product, U.S.A. (Decyde) |
| Plodia interpunctella GV (Indian meal moth) | P. interpunctella | stored products (grain) | — |
| non-occluded baculoviruses | | | |
| Oryctes rhinoceros virus (coconut rhinoceros beetle) | O. rhinoceros | coconut and oil palm | introduced through Food and Agriculture Organization, United Nation/ South Pacific Commission projects |

Fungi are probably more dependent on appropriate microclimate conditions for their success than any other group of microbial insect pathogens. In particular, the high relative humidity (RH) required for spore germination is often very restricting (Drummond *et al.* 1986). Among deuteromycetes infecting terrestrial insects, the lower limit for spore germination is probably about 92% RH and some may require a film of water to germinate.

Specificity of invasion of the insect by a fungal spore may occur at several levels. The pathogen host range may first be influenced by specificity in the ability of spores to adhere to the cuticle. Germination may be influenced not only by humidity but also by the availability of certain nutrients. Successful penetration of the cuticle by the germinating spore probably occurs from a combination of mechanical and enzymic processes (Charnley 1982). Once past any insect defence mechanisms operating in the haemocoel, hyphal growth continues, often with the production of a yeast-like phase (blastospores) which allows the fungus to spread through the insect haemocoel. The insect is killed (generally after more than 4 days) after substantial hyphal growth or toxin production or both (Charnley 1982). Sporulation occurs with the development of conidia on the surface of the insect. Some local spread of infection can occur from these individuals.

TABLE 3. PRINCIPAL DEUTEROMYCETE FUNGAL CANDIDATES FOR ARTHROPOD PEST CONTROL

| species | main target pests | status of commercial development |
|---|---|---|
| Aschersonia aleyrodis | Trialeurodes vaporariorum (whitefly) | — |
| Beauveria bassiana | Leptinotarsa decemlineata (Colorado beetle) | product in U.S.S.R. (Boverin) |
| Beauveria brongniartii | Melolontha melolontha (cockchafer) | — |
| Culicinomyces clavosporus | mosquitoes | — |
| Hirsutella thompsonii | rust mites | former commercial product (Mycar) |
| Metarhizium anisopliae | beetles, bugs | product in Brazil (Metaquino) |
| Nomuraea rileyi | caterpillars | — |
| Tolypocladium cylindrosporum | mosquitoes | — |
| Verticillium lecanii | aphids, whitefly | products in U.K. (Vertalec; Mycotal) |

Apart from deuteromycete fungi, the Entomophthorales (Zygomycetes) contain by far the most insect-pathogenic isolates. Although the optimal growth temperatures for most Deuteromycetes (20–30 °C) fit them best for use against tropical and subtropical pests, members of the Entomophthorales appear more effective in temperate climates where they often produce extensive, if slow-acting, natural epizootics (Wilding 1981; Wilding *et al.* 1986). Unfortunately, most strains have proved difficult to culture and to store for long periods. Consequently, successful field applications have been relatively few (Wilding *et al.* 1986; Zimmermann 1986).

In the western world, only two insect-pathogenic fungal species are currently produced commercially (table 3). These are *Verticillium lecanii* and *M. anisopliae. V. lecanii* was developed to control aphids and whitefly on glasshouse crops (Hall & Papierok 1982), where the protected environment usually maintains the required humidity and temperature levels for effective spore germination and fungal growth. *M. anisopliae* is used as a microbial pesticide for the control of spittle bugs (e.g. *Mahanarva posticata*) on sugar cane in Brazil (Ferron 1981). Whereas *V. lecanii* products are based on blastospores produced by liquid fermentation, other species are applied as conidiospores grown on cereal grain or bran. It is rare for introduced fungal pathogens to recycle or spread extensively or both, over several seasons at the site of introduction. The most frequent method of use for successful pest control is therefore regular application.

### (d) Protozoa

Most insect-parasitic Protozoa of potential interest for pest control are classified within the Microsporida. They have not been successfully used as fast-acting microbial insecticides, and it is unlikely that they will be used in this manner in the future (Maddox 1986b). Infection in susceptible hosts is initiated by ingestion of spores. Microsporida are obligate parasites that require living cells for their development, and the gut or fat body or both provide the main foci of infection. The disease is often not highly pathogenic, but significantly reduces the rate of development of the insect and lowers its fecundity (Wilson 1982; Maddox 1986a). Natural spread and survival of the protozoan may be assured in many cases by vertical transmission within eggs of the host.

Although viral and fungal epizootics are considered more common, epizootics of microsporidia regularly occur in many insect species. Thus populations of the European corn borer, *Ostrinia nubilalis*, crash when incidence of the protozoan *Nosema pyrausta* in the insects approaches 100% (Maddox 1986a). For microbial control, however, only *Nosema locustae* has received great attention. More than 60 species of grasshopper and cricket are susceptible to this protozoan. Although in nature it is generally uncommon (usually less than 1% of individuals are infected), when spores were applied in a wheat-bran bait, infection levels of up to 40% were obtained (Henry & Oma 1981). In the season after application, infections were also common and the disease spread substantially, suggesting that it has some potential for long-term control. A commercial product (Noloc), based on *N. locustae*, is now manufactured on a small scale in the U.S.A.

### (e) *Nematodes*

It may not appear conventional to consider insect-parasitic nematodes alongside microbial pathogens of insects. However, rhabditid nematodes in the genera *Heterorhabditis* and *Steinernema* (= *Neoaplectana*) are mutualistically associated with insect-pathogenic bacteria in the genus *Xenorhabdus* (reviewed in Poiner (1986)). These large Gram-negative, rod-shaped, facultative anaerobic bacteria are held in a pouch in the intestine of the nematode and have been recorded in nature only associated with these nematodes.

Free-living rhabditid nematode larvae in the third of four larval stages are relatively resistant to desiccation and can survive in damp soil without an insect host for several months. When they encounter, or are attracted to, a susceptible host the nematodes enter through the mouth or anus and pass into the haemocoel by penetrating the gut wall. *Heterorhabditis* spp. may enter directly through the cuticle. Once inside the host, the symbiotic bacteria are released and multiply. The insect host is killed by septicaemia within 48 h of invasion. The nematode feeds and develops on the bacteria and decomposing host tissues, and completes its complex life cycle (Wouts 1984). About 10 days after invasion, hundreds or thousands of infective third-stage larval nematodes are released from the cadaver.

In recent years significant advances have been made in the production and formulation of these nematodes (Bedding 1986; Poinar 1986). Both the bacteria and the nematodes can be grown *in vitro* by using diets of homogenized animal tissues or plant products. Unfortunately, phase variation is a common feature of *Xenorhabdus* spp. The primary phase of the bacterium is the phase naturally occurring in the infective nematode. On occasion, this spontaneously converts to a secondary phase bacterium which reduces the capacity for nematode reproduction (Akhurst 1986b). Despite this problem, the wide, insect host range of these nematodes, their ability to kill the insect host relatively quickly, and the durability of the infective stage, have made them attractive selective control agents. The ideal targets are insect pests that live in soil and other moist and protected environments (Akhurst 1986a). The temperature range of activity for most strains isolated to date is between 10 °C and 32 °C, and low humidity and high solar radiation are limiting factors in their use. Strains of these nematodes are now produced commercially on a small scale in the U.S.A. and The Netherlands. At present, these nematodes and their associated bacteria are the only commercially available biological product for use against insect pests in the soil (Poinar 1986).

### (f) Strategies for using insect pathogens

In general, insect pathogens can be utilized in pest control in two ways. They can be applied at frequent intervals as short-term microbial insecticides, or they can be introduced once (or on a limited number of occasions) in the hope or knowledge that they will spread, persist, and hence exert a long-term controlling influence on an insect pest population. Short-term use is an almost inevitable requirement in agricultural situations where crop rotation, cultivation techniques and crop harvesting dilute the pathogen in the ecosystem and interfere with its survival in the environment. In addition, the high quality standards now demanded of much horticultural and agricultural produce impose low pest thresholds which then demand regular spray treatments, whether with chemical or microbial pesticides. In fact, in such situations, few microbial insecticides can compete with the short-term efficacy and speed of kill of most chemical pesticides. In contrast, more stable ecosystems including forests, plantations and pastures provide opportunities for long-term establishment of a pathogen in an insect population.

Because of the different demands of these two strategies the characteristics of pathogens used as microbial insecticides may be quite distinct from those required of agents that must persist for long periods in the pest population or external environment. Pathogens that have potential as microbial insecticides need to be highly virulent and relatively easy to produce. Examples of those that are commercially available include, *B.t.*, NPVs of *N. sertifer* and *M. brassicae*, the fungi *M. anisopliae* and *V. lecanii*, and the nematodes *Heterorhabditis* spp. and *Steinernema* spp. Pathogens effective in long-term, limited release strategies generally have lower virulence but can survive for long periods in the host population or in the environment (e.g. through the production of resistant stages). Examples include *B. popilliae*, *Oryctes* baculovirus, *G. hercyniae* NPV, the fungus *B. brongniartii* and the Protozoa *N. locustae* and *N. pyrausta*. Both groups of agents have important roles in future integrated pest management programmes. Although limited release strategies are not attractive for commercial development it is nevertheless important that such potential uses for insect pathogens are recognized and supported through government or international agency funding if necessary.

### 3. OVERCOMING CONSTRAINTS IN THE WIDER USE OF MICROBIAL CONTROL AGENTS

The demand for alternatives to chemical pesticides has never been greater. The microbial pest control agents described above are specific, harmless to beneficial organisms, non-polluting and, in some cases, will persist to exert long-term control of a pest population. None the less, among the hundreds of potentially useful insect pathogens, very few have been exploited. Some have been developed to, and beyond the point of, commercialization and then discarded in favour of chemical pesticides (e.g. *Heliothis* NPV). It is important to consider the reasons for the restricted use of pathogens, to identify the constraints and to attempt to find methods to optimize their use.

I believe that there are at least two reasons why exploitation of microbial pathogens has been slow. First, they are not seen as having major potential by commercial companies; market size is often restricted by the inherent target specificity of the microbial agent. Secondly, there is a commonly held view that microbial insecticides are not effective pest control agents. Growers accustomed to the broad spectrum, rapid knockdown and kill of many chemical pesticides find it difficult to accept the slower speed of kill of most microbial pesticides. To improve user acceptance, it is most important that unrealistic claims for the control potential of insect pathogens are not made, and that they are used intelligently, in strategies that exploit their strengths. Unfortunately, this policy has not always been followed, and ignorance of the basic biology of certain pathogens has meant that they have not always been used in the most appropriate manner.

In an attempt to identify future uses for insect pathogens it is necessary to consider in more detail the present constraints on their wider use. Future prospects for the use of genetic manipulation in providing new opportunities for microbial agents are considered in a later section (see §4).

### (a) Market potential

There is no doubt that the limited revenues anticipated from the small potential market size of many insects pathogens provide a major disincentive to their commercial development. Lisansky (1984) considered that greater uptake of microbial pesticides would require a change in market philosophy. Naturally occurring microbial agents are virtually all small-market products, whereas the agrochemical industry generally seeks large-market products to recover its development costs. There are probably very few products based on naturally occurring microorganisms that will be of sufficient value to justify production by major industrial companies (Jutsum, this symposium). Genetic manipulation may, in the longer term, derive microbial strains with altered host range and potency and hence increased potential. Greater financial rewards could be gained by transferring genes that code for toxins from certain insect pathogens into crop plants or other organisms that can deliver the toxin to the pest more effectively than can the original pathogen.

It is likely that the future use of natural pathogen strains will remain in the hands of small companies with low overheads, or international agencies that are largely reliant on government-funded research and development. This balance is unlikely to change in the foreseeable future, as microbial agents are only likely to be adjuncts to, rather than replacements for, chemical pesticides. Developments that could create new market opportunities for the microbial agents include requirements for integrated pest managament programmes brought about by severe pest resistance to chemical pesticides or major 'secondary' pest problems induced by the use of chemicals. Glasshouse and other horticultural crops and, in the longer term, cotton, maize and rice should be worthy of consideration. Environmentally sensitive regions such as forests and public amenity areas where chemical pesticide uses are restricted are also important future markets for insect pathogens.

A further consideration is that microbial pathogens must be able to compete in the market place with other selective pesticides, including growth-regulator type compounds such as diflubenzuron. However, even diflubenzuron has some undesirable effects on non-target species, which are not shared by microbial pathogens (Glen & Phillips 1984). Recent studies in Spain have also indicated that diflubenzuron has extreme persistence on pine needles and reduces populations of non-target Lepidoptera (Soria *et al.* 1986). Apart from selective chemicals, certain pathogens are also likely to compete with each other for the same market.

*Bt – broader host range*
*BcV – infectious*

This is true of *B.t.* and baculoviruses. In general, the commercially available *B.t.* var. *kurstaki* HD-1 strain has a broader spectrum of activity than any baculovirus and should prove more effective in situations where a complex of pest Lepidoptera species needs to be controlled. In contrast, because viruses are infectious agents, only small amounts of the most virulent viruses need to be ingested to be effective. This effect in some situations would tip the balance in favour of a viral insecticide.

### (b) Patentability

Industrial property rights provide one way for companies to protect their investment in a new product. The difficulty of protecting natural strains of insect pathogens has been seen as a disadvantage in their commercial exploitation. None the less, patents have been filed on certain novel naturally occurring microorganisms (e.g. *B.t.* var. *tenebrionis*), as well as on production and formulation processes (e.g. with insect-parasitic nematodes) (Bedding 1986). Genetic manipulation offers potential for the development of novel modified strains of insect pathogens with greater scope for patent protection. However, the extent to which large numbers of new patents will be granted, and the will to defend these patents, remain to be tested.

### (c) Production

Microbial pesticides are generally believed to be more expensive to produce than many chemicals. Costs could well fall as demand increases. Thus public pressure in Canada has promoted the use of *B.t.*, in preference to chemical pesticides, for the control of forest pests. Between 1980 and 1983, the average cost of *B.t.* treatments halved to about \$7 ha$^{-1}$† (Morris *et al.* 1986). In contrast to *B.t.*, viruses must be produced *in vivo*. Depending on the virulence of the virus and the ease with which the insect host can be reared, substantial differences in product cost can arise. Martignoni (1984) lists the 1977 cost of Elcar (*Heliothis* NPV) per hectare dose at \$4.45 (including manufacturing cost plus profit margin) compared with \$42.00 per hectare for TM Biocontrol 1 (NPV of *Orgyia pseudotsugata*; manufacturing cost only). There is little doubt that major savings can be made in *in vivo* production systems through greater automation. Future improvements in virus production could also come from the use of host species that are susceptible to the virus and are easier to rear. As Huber & Miltenburger (1986) point out, it is especially important in such circumstances to authenticate carefully the properties of the pathogen produced. Although large-scale production of insect viruses in cell culture is probably still at least ten years away from achievement, significant advances have been made (Tramper & Vlak 1986), and the exploitation of baculoviruses as gene expression vectors (see §4) provides further motivation to improve insect cell culture systems. At present, major savings in media costs are required. The costs of producing sufficient virus, *in vivo*, to treat 1 ha were cited by Huber & Miltenburger (1986) as \$10–20. The same amount of virus produced by current cell culture techniques would cost \$900. Future savings on media costs and improved yield are also central to the economic mass production of bacterial and fungal pathogens as well as insect-parasitic nematodes. Reduction in manufacturing costs through production improvements is seen as an important component in the future genetic engineering of *B.t.* (Kirschbaum 1985). Research is also underway on the improved production in liquid media of conidia of insect-pathogenic fungi.

Product stability is another important consideration. Most microbial insecticides survive

† 1 hectare = $10^4$ m².

well at temperatures of 4 °C or lower but such low-temperature storage is an additional inconvenience and expense for growers accustomed to maintaining chemical pesticides at ambient temperatures. Nevertheless, failure to formulate these biological products effectively and to store them under appropriate conditions has almost certainly contributed to apparent pest control failures in the past. If it proves difficult to produce formulations that retain infectivity, other than by storing them at low temperatures, then growers must be given other incentives to use the products. Alternatively, the pathogens must be employed in control strategies (e.g. as with *Oryctes* virus) where long-term storage outside the laboratory is not required.

Another aspect of product stability is the avoidance of changes in potency during repeated culture of an insect pathogen. The pathogen must be well-characterized, and reliable quality control procedures should be established to ensure that its properties do not change during production. Genetic changes of insect pathogens during passage have been recorded with viruses (Croizier *et al.* 1985; Smith & Crook 1986*a*) and *Bacillus thuringiensis* (Carlton & Gonzalez 1985; Burges 1986*b*).

### (d) Host-range and virulence

The specificity of many microbial agents is seen as advantageous in preserving beneficial species. None the less, the host range of many naturally occurring strains of insect pathogens often limits the potential market size for their use. Thus it has been known for some time that different lepidopteran pests vary in their response to distinct strains of *B.t.* (Dulmage *et al.* 1981), so that few naturally occurring strains are highly pathogenic for all pest species in the complexes of lepidopteran pests that occur on many crops. Similarly, with fungi, important traits for biological control are found separately in different isolates, as with the whitefly- and aphid-pathogenic strains of *V. lecanii* (Hall 1981). Baculoviruses are more specific than *B.t.* or most fungal strains.

The International Strain Screening Programme of new *B.t.* isolates has shown that substantial improvements in biological activity can be obtained by screening naturally occurring strains (Dulmage *et al.* 1981). Further improvements in potency have also been made through the production of new strains by mutation. Although major advances are also likely to come from genetic manipulation, the enormous gene pool of naturally occurring strains of all insect pathogen groups should not be ignored in the search for agents with optimal host-range and virulence characteristics. The first requirement of a screening survey should be the clear identification of target crops and the different regional pest complexes on these crops.

### (e) Resistance

It has often been implied that insects will not develop resistance to microbial control agents. However, as Briese (1986) points out, 'theoretical studies have indicated that intensively applied control measures, whether they be pathogens or chemical insecticides, will invariably select for resistance'. With viruses there is no direct evidence for resistance developing in the field. Huber (1986) detected no difference in susceptibility to *Cydia pomonella* GV (CPGV) between a susceptible laboratory strain of *C. pomonella* and a population collected from an orchard where CPGV had been applied at least four times every year for the previous nine years. However, in a laboratory selection programme, Briese & Mende (1983) recorded a 140-fold increase in the resistance level of *Phthorimaea operculella* larvae to a GV after six generations of selection.

McGaughey (1985) reported that colonies of *Plodia interpunctella*, obtained from grain storage bins routinely treated with *B.t.* var. *kurstaki*, were less susceptible to *B.t.* than insects from untreated bins. This report would seem to be the only convincing example of the development of resistance of an insect to a microbial pathogen under 'field' conditions. Special circumstances probably prevail in the use of *B.t.* in the stored-grain environment. Under such conditions, the *B.t.* formulation remains stable, and successive generations of *P. interpunctella* can breed in contact with *B.t.* spores and toxin crystals. Consequently, the selection pressure is likely to be much greater than in field-cropping systems. None the less, this example illustrates the need for care in the way in which microbial pathogens are used in future. Control programmes should be managed to slow down the development of resistance and, if resistance develops, remedial action may be required through the selection of more virulent strains of the pathogen and pathogens with different modes of action (Briese 1986).

### (*f*) *Persistence*

Some insect pathogens persist in the host population for long periods, or survive as small inocula of relatively stable forms (e.g. spores, occlusion bodies) in protected niches. However, a large proportion of microbial agents, applied as insecticides to the foliage of crop plants, persist for only short periods mainly because they are inactivated by uv light. Many attempts have been made to improve the persistence of different formulations applied to leaves, by the inclusion of compounds that may protect the pathogen from uv (reviewed in Entwistle & Evans (1985)). To a large degree these attempts have been unsuccessful. Although a concerted effort in formulation improvement is still important, other strategies must be considered. Extended persistence of a microbial insecticide becomes of less concern if a satisfactory monitoring system exists for the pest, so that application of the pathogen can be timed more critically. Among those microorganisms that must be ingested to be effective, uptake of the pathogen could be improved by the development of formulations that attract and stimulate the pest to ingest the pathogens. Better targeting of spray deposits (e.g. to underleaf surfaces partly protected from uv and the position where many pests feed most) could extend persistence. Persistence could also be improved through genetic engineering techniques that package the pathogen or its active component into more stable vectors such as other microorganisms or plants (see §4*a*).

In some circumstances, successful pest control will depend on the pathogen establishing itself in the environment. Thus there are considerable future prospects for the use of bacteria, fungi and nematodes for the long-term control of soil-borne pests if satisfactory colonization of the rhizosphere could be achieved. Zimmermann (1986) reported that both *B. bassiana* and *M. anisopliae* are capable of germinating and growing in sterile but not non-sterile soil, presumably because of microbial competition – antagonism with other components of the soil flora. Similar problems may be encountered in the future use of phyllosphere-colonizing insect pathogenic microorganisms (see §4*a*).

### (*g*) *Registration and safety*

It is not possible in this chapter to dwell on safety aspects such as the effects of microbial agents on non-target organisms; these are considered in several excellent reviews (Burges 1981; Harrap 1982; Rogoff 1982). Current evidence suggests that the responsible use of the pathogens described above does not adversely affect non-target vertebrates, plants and beneficial invertebrates. None the less, it is entirely appropriate that new insect pathogens should be safety-tested before widespread use. With the advent of genetically manipulated microorganisms and *B.t.*-transferred plants risk assessment and management is even more important (see §4*c*).

Lisansky (1984) concluded that recent regulatory improvements in the U.S.A. and the U.K. were likely to make microbial pesticides a more attractive proposition to commercial firms. He estimated then that toxicological testing for a new (naturally occurring) microbial product would cost £40000 compared with £3000000 for a new chemical active ingredient. Even so, such registration costs for small-market products are likely to be a significant part of the total development costs. For some pathogens (e.g. baculoviruses) there are some who advocate the idea of a generic registration for all related products. Other methods of reducing product costs are through the sharing of safety data packages by different companies and Government research and development organizations. Government aid towards the registration of such minor use products is also occurring in the U.S.A. in the form of financial support through the IR-4 scheme.

I have attempted in the above description to identify the major constraints to the more widespread, future use of microbial control agents, and to suggest solutions and opportunities for further research and development. Successful use of microbials is a complex process. The main aim of microbial control programmes is to use the minimum quantity of pathogen sufficient to reduce the pest population below the damage threshold. Although the majority of programmes to date have achieved this on a trial and error basis, approaches to the problems through systems models could provide a strong framework for decision making in the future (Evans 1986). Such an approach, however, will demand access to more quantitative information on host–pathogen interactions than is currently available.

## 4. FUTURE PROSPECTS FOR THE USE OF GENETICALLY MANIPULATED MICROBIAL PEST CONTROL AGENTS

As Dean (1984) wrote in a review of *B.t.* genetics, the prospects for genetic manipulation of pathogens are limited only by the imagination of research workers. However, it is probably most useful to try to examine progress to date in considering what may be achievable within the next ten years. This is not an easy task because much of the research in this area is being done 'behind closed doors' by agrochemical and biotechnology companies. It is clear that some sources see major prospects for genetically manipulated control agents. Estimates of the future U.S. sales of genetically improved biological pesticides show an increase from U.S. $24 M (at 1984 prices) in 1990, to U.S. $455 M in 2025 (Stanford Research Institute International 1984). This contrasts with the present world sales value of existing microbial pesticides which is put at $20 M–40 M (Anon. 1986*b*; Jutsum, this symposium).

In earlier sections, I have identified features of pathogens that may be amenable to improvement through genetic manipulation. These include modifications to virulence, host range, persistence and ease of production. A first requirement is that the pathogen should be amenable to genetic manipulation and, secondly, that it is necessary to understand its mode of action and factors influencing its efficacy. Because basic genetic transformation systems are available at present only for *B.t.* and baculoviruses (among the pathogens described above) I shall restrict detailed discussion to these. However, future scope for genetically modifying the characteristics of insect-pathogenic fungi, *Xenorhabdus* spp. and other bacteria, should not be ignored. Genetic engineering of these agents awaits the development of transformation systems and an improved understanding of their biology, particularly of characteristics that govern virulence and host specificity.

### (a) Genetic improvement of Bacillus thuringiensis

There is currently intense research activity in the genetic manipulation of B.t. It is an ideal target as the protoxins are known to be single-gene products, the primary structure of the proteins in several strains is known, and the protoxins are made in large amounts and are readily assayed. B.t. is also commercially important and shown, from almost 30 years of field use, to be safe. As mentioned above (see §1a) the toxin genes are present on plasmids. This fact has permitted the utilization of a non-recombinant methodology to develop novel strains of B.t. With a conjugation-like process (Gonzalez et al. 1982), plasmids can be exchanged between different parental strains to obtain transconjugants, some of which possess the combined toxic properties of both parents. This technique makes possible the tailoring of B.t. strains for improved toxicity and efficacy against a different range of lepidopteran pests. Thus, the transfer of a plasmid from a B.t. strain with high potency against Heliothis armigera but low activity against Spodoptera littoralis, to a recipient B.t. strain with the converse potencies, produced a transconjugant with high activity against both these major lepidopterous pests of cotton (Jarrett & Burges 1986). Likewise, Klier et al. (1983) constructed a B.t. recombinant which had a new combination of Lepidoptera- and mosquito-active toxins. The first field trials of transconjugant B.t. strains were done in the U.S.A. and the U.K. during 1986.

The cloning and expression of B.t. crystal toxin genes in other organisms was first reported by Schnepf & Whitely (1981), who cloned a B.t. var. kurstaki toxin gene into Escherichia coli. Subsequently, the gene has been cloned into other microorganisms that have potential to act as alternative delivery vectors for the toxin gene. The example that has received most publicity is the cloning by a research team at Monsanto Agricultural Products Co. of a B.t. var. kurstaki toxin gene into Pseudomonas fluorescens, a non-pathogenic rhizosphere-colonizing bacterium (Watrud et al. 1985). The aim of this project was to produce an engineered P. fluorescens that could be applied as a seed-dressing or soil-inoculant and would protect plants from soil-borne lepidopteran pests. P. fluorescens was selected as the delivery vector because it is not pathogenic to humans, was sensitive to clinical antibiotics and sterilants, and had limited potential for genetic exchange and environmental persistence. The toxin gene was inserted into the bacterial chromosome rather than into plasmids (to reduce gene transfer) by direct transposition and homologous recombination by using the transposable element Tn5. To further minimize the potential of horizontal gene transfer to other bacteria, the transposon activity of the transformed bacterium was also eliminated. The engineered bacterium produced the 134 000 $M_r$ B.t. protoxin and the host potency of the engineered bacterium was found to parallel that of the original B.t. strain (Watrud et al. 1985). Restrictions on the environmental release of genetically engineered microorganisms in the U.S.A. have not yet allowed field trials of this transformed P. fluorescens strain.

The concept of using plant microflora as delivery vectors for pesticidal genes is a practical and intellectually satisfying approach to the production of new microbial pesticides. The future introduction of the B.t. crystal toxin genes into leaf epiphytes as well as root colonizers would help alleviate the need for insecticide applications to the crop and effectively increase the persistence of the toxin in the environment. In addition to plant colonizing microorganisms, it is likely that attempts are also being made to transfer the B.t. var. israelensis (dipteran-active) toxin gene into prokaryotes that live in water and are present in the feeding zones of mosquito larvae. Lüthy (1986b) indicated that research of this kind was being carried out with the blue-green alga (Cyanobacteria) *Anabaena*.

In a different approach, Mycogen (a San Diego based biotechnology company) are reported to have also cloned the *B.t.* toxin gene into a *Pseudomonas* sp. with the aim of expressing large quantities of the crystal protein and extending its environmental persistence through a bioencapsulation process that kills all the bacteria (Geiser 1986; Barnes & Lavrik 1986). It is understood that clearance has been granted for field trials of this genetically engineered product on the basis that it is classified as a chemical pesticide, containing no live infectious agents. As Lüthy (1986b) points out, the encapsulated protoxin produced in this manner must be capable of digestion to the toxin molecule by insect gut juices for it to be effective.

A further, well publicized, genetic engineering strategy for the use of *B.t.* toxin has been to clone the gene into crop plants, with the aim of producing plants immune to attack by certain Lepidoptera. This has now been achieved in tobacco through the transfer of the entire *B.t.* protoxin gene, or the sequence that codes for the toxic fragment, by using modified Ti plasmid vectors (Vaeck *et al.* 1987; Adang *et al.* 1988). This approach is not without its problems. By using a highly susceptible test insect (larvae of the tobacco hornworm, *Manduca sexta*) significant mortality was observed on transformed plants but insecticidal activity exhibited by different transformants was variable (Vaeck *et al.* 1986). In other experiments, the crystal-protein gene messenger (m) RNA transcripts expressed in the plant were truncated, possibly through some difference in mRNA processing in the plant compared with that in the bacterium (Adang *et al.* 1988). Even so, the shortened mRNA must have been sufficient to encode the toxin sequence as insecticidal activity was recorded in the transformed plants.

With this elegant approach now being extended to a range of other plant species, compatibility of the toxin with plant components could be critical. Will expression of the toxin in plant cells reduce crop yield or vigour (Kirschbaum 1985)? Will the toxin interact with plant compounds, e.g. tannins that are believed to bind to and/or inactivate the toxin (Lüthy 1986a)? Answers to these questions are awaited with interest. In addition, the potentially high selection pressure that would be imposed on larvae feeding on plants, constitutively expressing an insecticidal molecule, could be seen as a powerful mechanism for the rapid development of resistance in insect populations. Perhaps the insertion of several genes, each coding for a different insecticidal molecule, would be a better long-term strategy? In the meantime, results are eagerly awaited on the first field tests in the U.S.A. of tobacco transformed with *B.t.* toxin (Anon. 1986a).

Apart from these exciting developments in the use of new delivery vectors for *B.t.* toxin genes, significant future progress is likely to be made in the construction of new toxins with differences in virulence and host potency through directed mutagenesis and gene ligation.

### (b) Genetic improvement of baculoviruses

Undoubtedly, improvements in baculovirus pathogenicity can be obtained by strain selection. Studies have also shown that genetic recombination occurs between closely related baculoviruses in mixed infections, providing a means of generating new variants (Croizier & Quiot 1981). Perhaps the most intriguing developments have come from studies on baculovirus genetic engineering which illustrate the possibility of introducing new genes into precise positions in baculovirus genomes. Smith *et al.* (1983) were the first to report that a baculovirus

(ACMNPV) could be used as a vector for the propagation and expression of introduced (passenger) genes. This study made use of the fact that some baculovirus proteins, in particular the matrix protein (polyhedrin) of the occlusion bodies, are produced to high levels during infection. When the gene for this protein was replaced by a gene coding for human β-interferon, the new gene was expressed to a very high level and large quantities of interferon were recovered. Further advances have been made with this system such that recombinant baculoviruses are seen as capable of producing many different protein products (Cochran *et al.* 1986). These studies indicate that baculoviruses can accommodate and express additional DNA sequences, and suggest that new and infectious baculovirus strains could be constructed.

At present, there is no published information on the production of genetically engineered baculoviruses with novel insecticidal properties. None the less, it is likely that the Genetics Institute (Boston, U.S.A.) has a novel recombinant NPV with modified host range and potency which may be field tested within the next two years. In addition, I understand that an NPV of *Spodoptera litura* has been adapted in Japan to grow in the silkworm (to improve production) and then engineered so that the virus infests and kills *S. litura* but does not complete its replicative cycle. In future genetic improvement of NPVs and GVs, it may be necessary to leave the polyhedrin gene intact so that the engineered virus will still produce the occlusion bodies that are important for field stability. Therefore new DNA will have to be inserted into other regions of the viral genome that are not essential for virus replication. The genes that influence virus infectivity and host range have not been identified, and directed phenotypic changes are not yet possible. Genetic control of these properties is likely to prove complex. In the meantime, however, it may be possible to modify a baculovirus so that its speed of kill is increased. The insertion of genes that code for insecticidal toxins (e.g. *B.t.* toxin) or oligonucleotides that may code for insect neuropeptides, could yield such an effect. Problems of how to produce such novel viruses in insects or cell cultures will have to be overcome. One solution could be to produce a conditional lethal mutant (e.g. temperature-sensitive mutant) of the virus which only expresses the toxic gene under specific conditions (e.g. over a defined temperature range).

Finally, viruses themselves may in future be used as gene vectors to transform insects. A complex group of DNA containing, insect viruses (polydnaviruses) are intimately associated with many parasitoids. These could be used to transfer genes that improve the pesticide resistance of a parasitoid, or that modify other components of the parasitoid's behaviour to improve its performance as a biological control agent (Vinson 1986).

### (c) Risk assessment and management

A responsible attitude is required to the environmental release of genetically engineered organisms to satisfy both the regulatory authorities and the public. Not only will there be a need for risk assessment; risk management will also be of prime importance. Containment levels, safety precautions, experimental design and monitoring systems, and risk minimization will need definition based on knowledge of the characteristics of the organism, the risk and type of exposure to non-target organisms, the capability of the organism to survive, multiply and spread, and its interactions with other relevant components of the ecosystem (Heusler 1986). Fortunately, *B.t.* has been in operational use for almost three decades and baculoviruses have also been used extensively in field trials. Both pathogen groups have been subjected to extensive safety tests and there has been no substantiated incident of adverse effects on non-target species.

Thus these agents are ideal model systems with which to obtain data relevant to making decisions about the release of genetically engineered organisms. Information required by the U.S. Environmental Protection Agency of the *B.t.* toxin gene-transformed *P. fluorescens* have included details of taxonomy, toxicology, persistence, host range and genetic stability (Barnes & Lavrik 1986).

What issues are particularly relevant in the release of novel microbial pesticides? Firstly, general safety of genetically engineered microorganisms can be evaluated by the conventional series of safety tests that would normally be applied for a non-engineered strain. There may be public concern that the release of novel strains not subjected to the process of natural selection could themselves become major pest species. This seems extremely unlikely with either *B.t.* or baculoviruses, natural strains of which have been clearly established as having no adverse effect on vertebrates or plants and restricted pathogenicity in invertebrates. Unfortunately, there is no guarantee that microorganisms, once released, can be destroyed. Suggestions have been made that engineered strains should be produced with limited ability to survive in the field. With most naturally occurring insect pathogens that are used as microbial insecticides, this is already the case.

Of equal relevance is the genetic stability of the novel organism and the consequences of any instability. It is known that *B.t.* plasmids carrying the toxin gene can be transferred in the laboratory to some other bacterial species through conjugation (Gonzalez *et al.* 1982). What is not known is how frequently this occurs in nature, nor how relevant such transfers would be. Likewise, with baculoviruses, recombinants can be obtained between closely related virus strains (Croizier & Quiot 1981; Smith & Crook 1986a). It is also known that a number of related but distinct baculovirus genotypes can be isolated from a single infected insect in the wild (Smith & Crook 1986b). The potential therefore exists for the transfer of introduced genes at least within a gene pool of related viruses. With what frequency does this occur; to what extent could the genes be transferred to viruses infecting non-target hosts; what would be the consequences of such transfers? These questions can be answered only by ecological investigation of the frequency and consequences of gene transfer. The production of a baculovirus (ACMNPV) 'marked' with a short section of non-coding DNA, and its release in U.K. trials as virus-infected *Spodoptera exigua* larvae is the first attempt to study the molecular epidemiology of a baculovirus strain (Bishop 1986). Such investigations are central to the future successful exploitation of genetically engineered insect pathogens. However, studies with naturally occurring, endemic pathogen strains and insect species would probably be more instructive; neither ACMNPV nor *S. exigua* can be regarded as species endemic to the U.K.

## 6. Conclusions

The examples cited above illustrate some of the potential uses of microbial pest control agents. Factors constraining their potential were identified and suggestions were made as to how these constraints could be resolved in future. The need to select new pathogen strains, to produce new pathogen strains by genetic engineering and to select more effective use strategies will require additional information on the mode of action of many pathogens and the biology of the host–pathogen relation. Future studies on mode of action will provide data not only of use in selecting the most appropriate strains but also in directing research on future genetic improvement. Because the future registration of genetically engineered strains may be a slow process, based on a case-by-case assessment at the outset, there should still be much potential for the exploitation of the naturally occurring variation amongst endemic insect pathogens. In addition, mode-of-action studies (by providing an understanding of the molecular events that allow pathogens to overcome the natural defences of insects) should lead to the discovery of new active molecules that could form the basis for a new generation of synthetic chemical insecticides (Kirschbaum 1985).

Finally, knowledge of the basic biology of the host–pathogen interaction is essential both for the development of new control strategies (Entwistle 1986) and for the future use of genetically engineered agents. Although I was at first concerned that the extensive initial investment of research funds into the genetic manipulation of pathogens would remove resources from basic biological studies, I am now increasingly heartened that investigations into the requirements for the release of genetically engineered microbial pest control agents will now provide the driving force for the essential biological and ecological studies that are still required.

Although the views expressed in this article are those of the author alone, I would like to thank my colleagues at the Institute of Horticultural Research for their generous sharing of results, helpful discussions and constructive criticism of this paper. I am particularly grateful to Denis Burges, Paul Jarrett, John Ballard, Norman Crook, Ian Smith, Adrian Gillespie and Paul Richardson.

## References

Adang, M. J., Firoozabady, E., Klein, J., DeBoer, D., Sekar, V., Kemp, J. D., Murray, E., Rocheleau, T. A., Rashka, K., Staffeld, G., Stock, C., Sutton, D. & Merlo, D. J. 1988 Expression of a *Bacillus thuringiensis* insecticidal crystal protein gene in tobacco plants. In *Molecular strategies for crop protection* (ed. C. J. Arntzen & C. A. Ryan). A Du Pont–UCLA Symposium. (In the press.)

Adang, M. J., Idler, K. F. & Rocheleau, T. A. 1987 Structural and antigenic relationships between three insecticidal crystal proteins of *Bacillus thuringiensis* subsp. *kurstaki*. In *Biotechnology: Advances in invertebrate pathology and cell culture* (ed. K. Maramorosch). New York. Academic Press. (In the press.)

Akhurst, R. J. 1986*a* Controlling insects in soil with entomopathogenic nematodes. In *Fundamental and applied aspects of invertebrate pathology* (ed. R. A. Samson, J. M. Vlak & D. Peters), pp. 265–267. Wageningen: Foundation of the Fourth International Colloquium of Invertebrate Pathology.

Akhurst, R. J. 1986*b* Recent advances in *Xenorhabdus* research. In *Fundamental and applied aspects of invertebrate pathology* (ed. R. A. Samson, J. M. Vlak & D. Peters), pp. 304–307. Wageningen: Foundation of the Fourth International Colloquium of Invertebrate Pathology.

Anon. 1986*a* Rohm and Haas field tests insect-resistant plants. *Genet. Technol. News* **6** (10), 2–3.

Anon. 1986*b* New developments in biotechnology will have major effect on future of biopesticides. *Eur. chem. News* September 22, pp. 23 and 25.

Barnes, G. & Lavrik, P. 1986 Improvements in the efficacy of microbial control agents. In *Proceedings of the British Crop Protection Conference, Pests and Diseases – 1986*, pp. 669–676. Thornton Heath, Surrey: British Crop Protection Council.

Baumann, P., Broadwell, A. M., Baumann, L., Unterman, B. & Bowditch, R. D. 1986 Chemistry of the *Bacillus sphaericus* toxin. In *Fundamental and applied aspects of invertebrate pathology* (ed. R. A. Samson, J. M. Vlak & D. Peters), pp. 23–25. Wageningen: Foundation of the Fourth International Colloquium of Invertebrate Pathology.

Bedding, R. A. 1986 Mass rearing, storage and transport of entomopathogenic nematodes. In *Fundamental and applied aspects of invertebrate pathology* (ed. R. A. Samson, J. M. Vlak & D. Peters), pp. 308–311. Wageningen: Foundation of the Fourth International Colloquium of Invertebrate Pathology.

Bedford, G. O. 1980 Biology, ecology and control of palm rhinoceros beetles. *A. Rev. Ent.* **25**, 309–339.

Benz, G. 1981 Use of viruses for insect suppression. In *Biological control in crop production* (ed. G. C. Papavizas), pp. 259–272. Totowa: Allenheld Osmun.

Bishop, D. H. L. 1986 UK release of genetically marked virus. *Nature, Lond.* **323**, 496.

Briese, D. T. 1986 Host resistance to microbial control agents. In *Biological plant and health protection* (ed. J. M. Franz) (*Fortschr. Zool.* **32**, 233–256).

Briese, D. T. & Mende, H. A. 1983 Selection for increased resistance to a granulosis virus in the potato moth, *Phthorimaea operculella* (Zeller). *Bull. ent. Res.* **73**, 1–9.

Burges, H. D. (ed.) 1981 *Microbial control of pests and plant diseases 1970–1980*. London: Academic Press.

Burges, H. D. 1986*a* Impact of *Bacillus thuringiensis* on pest control with emphasis on genetic manipulation. *MIRCEN J. appl. Microbiol. Biotechnol.* **2**, 101–120.

Burges, H. D. 1986*b* Standardization in relation to registration of bioinsecticides. In *Fundamental and applied aspects of invertebrate pathology* (ed. R. A. Samson, J. M. Vlak & D. Peters), pp. 669–672. Wageningen: Foundation of the Fourth International Colloquium of Invertebrate Pathology.

Burges, H. D. & Pillai, J. S. 1986 Microbial bioinsecticides. In *Microbial technology in the developing world* (ed. E. J. DaSilva, Y. Domergues, E.-J. Nyns & C. Ratledge), pp. 121–150. Oxford University Press.

Carlton, B. C. 1986 Genetic improvement of bacterial insect pathogens. In *Fundamental and applied aspects of invertebrate pathology* (ed. R. A. Samson, J. M. Vlak & D. Peters), pp. 365–368. Wageningen: Foundation of the Fourth International Colloquium of Invertebrate Pathology.

Carlton, B. C. & Gonzalez, J. M. Jr. 1985 The genetics and molecular biology of *Bacillus thuringiensis*. In *The molecular biology of the Bacilli* (ed. D. Dubnau), vol. 2, pp. 211–248. New York: Academic Press.

Charnley, A. K. 1982 Physiological aspects of destructive pathogenesis in insects by fungi: a speculative review. In *Invertebrate-microbial interactions* (ed. J. M. Anderson, A. D. M. Rayner & D. W. H. Walton), pp. 229–270. Cambridge University Press.

Cochran, M. A., Ericson, B. L., Knell, J. D. & Smith, G. E. 1986 Use of recombinant baculoviruses for the production of subunit vaccines. In *Fundamental and applied aspects of invertebrate pathology* (ed. R. A. Samson, J. M. Vlak & D. Peters), pp. 383–386. Wageningen: Foundation of the Fourth International Colloquium of Invertebrate Pathology.

Croizier, G. & Quiot, J. M. 1981 Obtention and analysis of two genetic recombinants of baculoviruses of Lepidoptera, *Autographa californica* Speyer and *Galleria mellonella* L. *Ann. Virol.* **132**, 3–18.

Croizier, G., Croizier, L., Biache, G. & Chaufaux, J. 1985 Évolution de la composition génétique et du pouvoir infectieux du baculovirus de *Mamestra brassicae* L. au cours de 25 multiplications successives sur les larves de la noctuelle du chou. *Entomophaga* **30**, 365–374.

Dean, D. H. 1984 Biochemical genetics of the bacterial insect control agent *Bacillus thuringiensis*; basic principles and prospects for genetic engineering. *Biotechnol. genet. Engg Revs* **2**, 341–363.

Drummond, J., Hussey, N. W. & Heale, J. B. 1986 The effect of humidity on the pathogenicity of *Verticillium lecanii* towards the glasshouse whitefly *Trialeurodes vaporariorum*. In *Fundamental and applied aspects of invertebrate pathology* (ed. R. A. Samson, J. M. Vlak & D. Peters), p. 248. Wageningen: Foundation of the Fourth International Colloquium of Invertebrate Pathology.

Dulmage, H. D. & Co-operators. 1981 Insecticidal activity of isolates of *Bacillus thuringiensis* and their potential for pest control. In *Microbial control of pests and plant diseases 1970–1980* (ed. H. D. Burges), pp. 193–222. London: Academic Press.

Ellar, D. J., Knowles, B. H., Drobniewski, F. A. & Haider, M. Z. 1986 The insecticidal specificity and toxicity of *Bacillus thuringiensis* δ-endotoxins may be determined respectively by an initial binding to membrane-specific receptors followed by a common mechanism of cytolysis. In *Fundamental and applied aspects of invertebrate pathology* (ed. R. A. Samson, J. M. Vlak & D. Peters), pp. 7–10. Wageningen: Foundation of the Fourth International Colloquium of Invertebrate Pathology.

Entwistle, P. F. 1986 Epizootiology and strategies of microbial control. In *Biological plant and health protection* (ed. J. M. Franz) (*Fortschr. Zool.* **32**, 257–278).

Entwistle, P. F. & Evans, H. F. 1985 Viral control. In *Comprehensive insect physiology biochemistry and pharmacology* (ed. G. A. Kerkut & L. I. Gilbert), vol. 13, pp. 347–412. Oxford: Pergamon Press.

Evans, H. F. 1986 Parameter estimation as a basis for developing systems models for microbial control of pests. In *Fundamental and applied aspects of invertebrate pathology* (ed. R. A. Samson, J. M. Vlak & D. Peters), pp. 586–589. Wageningen: Foundation of the Fourth International Colloquium of Invertebrate Pathology.

Ferron, P. 1981 Pest control by the fungi *Beauveria* and *Metarhizium*. In *Microbial control of pests and plant diseases 1970–1980* (ed. H. D. Burges), pp. 465–482. London: Academic Press.

Geiser, M. 1986 The impact of molecular biology on the biotechnological development of *B. thuringiensis* endotoxin as bioinsecticide. In *Fundamental and applied aspects of invertebrate pathology* (ed. R. A. Samson, J. M. Vlak & D. Peters), pp. 599–601. Wageningen: Foundation of the Fourth International Colloquium of Invertebrate Pathology.

Glen, D. M. & Phillips, M. 1984 Integrating control of earwigs. *Grower* **101**, 35–37.

Goldberg, L. J. & Margalit, J. 1977 A bacterial spore demonstrating rapid larvicidal activity against *Anopheles sergentii, Uranothaenia unguiculata, Culex univittatus, Aedes aegypti* and *Culex pipiens*. *Mosq. News* **40**, 67–70.

Gonzalez, J. M. Jr., Brown, B. J. & Carlton, B. C. 1982 Transfer of *Bacillus thuringiensis* plasmids coding for δ-endotoxin among strains of *B. thuringiensis* and *B. cereus*. *Proc. natn. Acad. Sci. U.S.A.* **79**, 6951–6955.

Haider, M. Z., Ward, E. S. & Ellar, D. J. 1987 Cloning and heterologous expression of an insecticidal delta-endotoxin gene from *Bacillus thuringiensis* var. *aizawai* IC1 toxic to both Lepidoptera and Diptera. *Gene* **52**, 285–290.

# PATHOGENIC CONTROL OF INSECTS 245

Hall, R. A. 1981 The fungus *Verticillium lecanii* as a microbial insecticide against aphids and scales. In *Microbial control of pests and plant diseases 1970–1980* (ed. H. D. Burges), pp. 483–498. London: Academic Press.

Hall, R. A. & Papierok, B. 1982 Fungi as biological control agents of arthropods of agricultural and medical importance. *Parasitology* **84**, 205–240.

Harrap, K. A. 1982 Assessment of the human and ecological hazards of microbial insecticides. *Parasitology* **84**, 269–296.

Henry, J. E. & Oma, E. A. 1981 Pest control by *Nosema locustae*, a pathogen of grasshoppers and crickets. In *Microbial control of pests and plant diseases 1970–1980* (ed. H. D. Burges), pp. 573–586. London: Academic Press.

Herrnstadt, C., Soares, G. G., Wilcox, E. R. & Edwards, D. L. 1986 A new strain of *Bacillus thuringiensis* with activity against coleopteran insects. *Biotechnology* **4**, 305–308.

Heusler, K. 1986 Biotechnology: regulating for the unknown. In *Proceedings of the British Crop Protection Conference, Pests and Diseases – 1986*, pp. 677–682. Thornton Heath, Surrey: British Crop Protection Council.

Huber, J. 1986 Use of baculoviruses in pest management programs. In *The biology of baculoviruses. Vol. II. Practical application for insect control* (ed. R. R. Granados & B. A. Federici), pp. 181–202. Boca Raton, Florida: CRC Press.

Huber, J. & Miltenburger, H. G. 1986 Production of pathogens. In *Biological plant and health protection* (ed. J. M. Franz) (*Fortschr. Zool.* **32**, 167–181).

Jarrett, P. & Burges, H. D. 1986 *Bacillus thuringiensis*: tailoring the strain to fit the pest complex on the crop. In *Biotechnology and crop improvement and protection* (ed. P. R. Day), pp. 259–264. (*BCPC Mong. No. 34.*) Thornton Heath, Surrey: British Crop Protection Council.

Kirschbaum, J. B. 1985 Potential implication of genetic engineering and other biotechnologies to insect control. *A. Rev. Ent.* **30**, 51–70.

Klein, M. G. 1981 Advances in the use of *Bacillus popilliae* for pest control. In *Microbial control of pests and plant diseases 1970–1980* (ed. H. D. Burges), pp. 183–192. London: Academic Press.

Klein, M. G. 1986 *Bacillus popilliae* – prospects and problems. In *Fundamental and applied aspects of invertebrate pathology* (ed. R. A. Samson, J. M. Vlak & D. Peters), pp. 534–537. Wageningen: Foundation of the Fourth International Colloquium of Invertebrate Pathology.

Klier, A., Bourgouin, C. & Rapoport, G. 1983 Mating between *Bacillus subtilis* and *Bacillus thuringiensis* and transfer of cloned crystal genes. *Molec. gen. Genet.* **191**, 257–262.

Krieg, A., Huger, A., Langenbruch, G. A. & Schnetter, W. 1983 *Bacillus thuringiensis* var. *tenebrionis*: ein neuer, genüber larven von Coleopteren wirksomer pathotyp. *Z. angew. Ent.* **96**, 500–508.

Kronstad, J. W., Schnepf, H. E. & Whiteley, H. R. 1983 Diversity of locations for *Bacillus thuringiensis* crystal protein genes. *J. Bact.* **154**, 419–428.

Li, R. S., Jarrett, P. & Burges, H. D. 1987 Importance of spores, crystals and delta endotoxins in the pathogenicity of different varieties of *Bacillus thuringiensis* in *Galleria mellonella* and *Pieris brassicae*. *J. invert. Path.* **50**.

Lisansky, S. G. 1984 Biological alternatives to chemical pesticides. *Wld Biotechnol. Rep.* **1**, 455–466. Pinner: Online Publications.

Lüthy, P. 1986*a* Insect pathogenic bacteria as pest control agents. In *Biological plant and health protection* (ed. J. M. Franz) (*Fortschr. Zool.* **32**, 201–206).

Lüthy, P. 1986*b* Genetics and aspects of genetic manipulation of *Bacillus thuringiensis*. In *Symposium in memoriam Dr Ernst Berliner anlässlich des 75 Jahrestages der Erstbeschreibung von Bacillus thuringiensis* (ed. A. Krieg & A. M. Huger), pp. 97–110. Berlin: Kommissionsverlag Paul Parey.

Maddox, J. V. 1986*a* Current status on the use of microsporidia as biocontrol agents. In *Fundamental and applied aspects of invertebrate pathology* (ed. R. A. Samson, J. M. Vlak & D. Peters), pp. 518–521. Wageningen: Foundation of the Fourth International Colloquium of Invertebrate Pathology.

Maddox, J. V. 1986*b* Possibilities for manipulating epizootics caused by protozoa: a representative case-history of *Nosema pyrausta*. In *Fundamental and applied aspects of invertebrate pathology* (ed. R. A. Samson, J. M. Vlak & D. Peters), pp. 563–566. Wageningen: Foundation of the Fourth International Colloquium of Invertebrate Pathology.

Martignoni, M. E. 1984 Baculovirus: an attractive biological alternative. In *Chemical and biological controls in forestry* (ed. W. Y. Garner & J. Harvey, Jr.), pp. 55–67. (*ACS Symp. Ser. no. 238.*) American Chemical Society.

Martignoni, M. E. & Iwai, P. J. 1986 *A catalog of viral diseases of insects, mites and ticks*, 4th edn, revised. (*General Technical Report PNW-195*). Pacific Northwest Research Station, United States Department of Agriculture.

McGaughey, W. H. 1985 Insect resistance to the biological insecticide *Bacillus thuringiensis*. *Science, Wash.* **229**, 193–195.

Miller, L. K., Lingg, A. J., Bulla, L. A. Jr. 1984 Bacterial, viral and fungal insecticides. In *Biotechnology and biological frontiers* (ed. P. H. Abelson), pp. 214–229. American Society for the Advancement of Science.

Morris, O. N., Cunningham, J. C., Finney-Crawley, J. R., Jaques, R. P. & Kinoshita, G. 1986 Microbial insecticides in Canada: their registration and use in agriculture, forestry and public and animal health. A Report prepared by the Special Committee of the Science Policy Committee, Entomological Society of Canada. *Bull. ent. Soc. Can.* **18** (2) (suppl.), 1–43.

Payne, C. C. 1982 Insect viruses as control agents. *Parasitology* **84**, 35–77.

Payne, C. C. 1986 Insect pathogenic viruses as pest control agents. In *Biological plant and health protection* (ed. J. M. Franz) (*Fortschr. Zool.* **32**, 183–200).

Payne, C. C. & Kelly, D. C. 1981 Identification of insect and mite viruses. In *Microbial control of pests and plant diseases 1970–1980* (ed. H. D. Burges), pp. 61–91. London: Academic Press.

Poinar, G. O. Jr. 1986 Entomophagous nematodes. In *Biological plant and health protection* (ed. J. M. Franz) (*Fortschr. Zool.* **32**, 95–121).

Rogoff, M. H. 1982 Regulatory safety data requirements for registration of microbial pesticides. In *Microbial and viral pesticides* (ed. E. Kurstak), pp. 645–679.

Schnepf, H. E. & Whiteley, H. R. 1981 Cloning and expression of the *Bacillus thuringiensis* crystal protein gene in *Escherichia coli*. *Proc. natn. Acad. Sci. U.S.A.* **78**, 2893–2897.

Schnepf, H. E., Wong, H. C. & Whiteley, H. R. 1985 The amino acid sequences of a crystal protein from *Bacillus thuringiensis* deduced from the DNA base sequence. *J. biol. Chem.* **260**, 6264–6272.

Smith, G. E., Summers, M. D. & Fraser, M. J. 1983 Production of human beta interferon in insect cells infected with a baculovirus expression vector. *Molec. cell. Biol.* **3**, 2156–2165.

Smith, I. R. L. & Crook, N. E. 1986a Latent granulosis virus sequences in *Pieris brassicae*. In *Fundamental and applied aspects of invertebrate pathology* (ed. R. A. Samson, J. M. Vlak & D. Peters), p. 109. Wageningen: Foundation of the Fourth International Colloquium of Invertebrate Pathology.

Smith, I. R. L. & Crook, N. E. 1986b *In vivo* isolation of several distinct genotypes from wild-type granulosis virus. In *Fundamental and applied aspects of invertebrate pathology* (ed. R. A. Samson, J. M. Vlak & D. Peters), p. 115. Wageningen: Foundation of the Fourth International Colloquium of Invertebrate Pathology.

Soria, S., Abos, F. & Martin, E. 1986 Influencia de los tratamientos con diflubenzuron ODC 45% sobre pinares en las poblaciones de *Graellsia isabelae* (Graells) (Lep. Syssphingidae) y resena de su biologia. *Bol. San. Veg. Plagas* **12**, 29–50.

Stanford Research Institute International 1984 *Agricultural biotechnology – its potential impacts on: producers of agricultural chemicals, fertilizers and seeds; genetic engineering companies.* Biotechnology Program – 1984. Menlo Park, California: SRI International.

Tramper, J. & Vlak, J. M. 1986 Some engineering and economic aspects of continuous cultivation of insect cells for the production of baculoviruses. In *Biochemical engineering IV* (ed. H. C. Lim & K. Venkatasubramanian), pp. 279–288. New York: The New York Academy of Sciences.

Vaeck, M., Reynaerts, A., Höfte, H., Jansens, S., De Beuckeleer, M., Dean, C., Zabeau, M., Van Montagu, M. & Leemans, J. 1987 Transgenic plants protected from insect attack. *Nature, Lond.* **328**, 33–37.

Vinson, S. B. 1986 The role of behavioural chemicals for biological control. In *Biological plant and health protection* (ed. J. M. Franz) (*Fortschr. Zool.* **32**, 75–87).

Watrud, L. S., Perlak, F. J., Tran, M.-T., Kusano, K., Mayer, E. J., Miller-Wideman, M. A., Obukowicz, M. G., Nelson, D. R., Kreitinger, J. P. & Kaufman, R. J. 1985 Cloning of the *Bacillus thuringiensis* subsp. *kurstaki* delta-endotoxin gene into *Pseudomonas fluorescens*: molecular biology and ecology of an engineered microbial pesticide. In *Engineered organisms in the environment: scientific issues* (ed. H. O. Halvorsen, D. Palmer & M. Rogul), pp. 40–46. New York: American Society for Microbiology.

WHO 1985 Informal consultation on the development of *Bacillus sphaericus* as a microbial larvicide. *TDR/BCV/SPHAERICUS/85.3*. Geneva: World Health Organization.

Wilding, N. 1981 Pest control by Entomophthorales. In *Microbial control of pests and plant diseases 1970–1980* (ed. H. D. Burges), pp. 539–554. London: Academic Press.

Wilding, N., Latteur, G. & Dedryver, C. A. 1986 Evaluation of Entomophthorales for aphid control: laboratory and field data. In *Fundamental and applied aspects of invertebrate pathology* (ed. R. A. Samson, J. M. Vlak & D. Peters), pp. 159–162. Wageningen: Foundation of the Fourth International Colloquium of Invertebrate Pathology.

Wilson, G. G. 1982 Protozoans for insect control. In *Microbial and viral pesticides* (ed. E. Kurstak), pp. 587–600. New York: Marcel Dekker.

Wouts, W. M. 1984 Nematode parasites of Lepidopterans. In *Plant and insect nematodes* (ed. W. R. Nickle), pp. 655–696. New York: Marcel Dekker.

Zimmermann, G. 1986 Insect pathogenic fungi as pest control agents. In *Biological plant and health protection* (ed. J. M. Franz) (*Fortschr. Zool.* **32**, 217–232).

## Discussion

M. Hafez (*Entomology Department, Cairo University, Egypt*). What does Dr Payne think about the efficacy of the polyhedrosis virus of *Spodoptera littoralis* under adverse physical conditions such as excessive heat? Secondly, what about the value of combining this virus with a pheromone against this pest?

C. C. PAYNE. I doubt that the temperatures encountered on cotton in Egypt would be sufficient to inactivate the virus but I will ask K. Jones to comment on the first part of the question. I know of no experiments combining the use of virus with an attractant pheromone against *Spodoptera littoralis*. However, some work in the U.S.A. by L. Falcon suggested that virus held in a powdered form in specially constructed light traps could be spread through the insect population by moths attracted to these traps. As viruses have to be ingested to be effective there may also be considerable merit in producing formulations of viruses that attract and stimulate larvae to feed on them.

K. JONES (*Tropical Development and Research Institute, Salisbury, U.K.*). The NPV of *S. littoralis* is extremely virulent against the target for control, that is, first-instar larvae. The $LD_{50}$ against this stage is about one polyhedral inclusion body per larva.

Turning to the persistence of the virus in the field, the effect of field temperatures is insignificant. The temperature on the crop rarely exceeds 40 °C, and such temperatures in the field do not inactivate the virus over the required period for control (*ca.* 2 weeks). A more significant problem is the effect of sunlight: exposure to the ultraviolet region of sunlight rapidly inactivates the virus. However, the site in which the target is located on the undersurface of the leaves provides considerable shade. Thus the virus in this region persists for longer than many studies, in which virus deposits have been exposed to direct sunlight, would suggest. Several uv protectants are in the process of being evaluated and the results of this work should lead to the development of a more persistent formulation.

I. HARPAZ (*Department of Entomology, Hebrew University of Jerusalem, Israel*). Will Dr Payne comment on prospects for activating latent baculovirus infections which are quite prevalent among field populations of lepidopterous pest species?

C. C. PAYNE. Research recently conducted at the Institute of Horticultural Research, Littlehampton, U.K., by I. Smith and N. Crook strongly supports the idea that latent baculovirus infections occur in certain insects, and that these can be activated by certain stresses including 'infection' by another baculovirus. In a series of experiments with a laboratory culture of *Pieris brassicae*, larvae were fed with a very high dose of a granulosis virus (GV) which was believed to have little or no infectivity for this insect species. A few of the larvae died of a GV infection. Virus was purified separately from each infected larva and then characterized by restriction endonuclease analysis of the DNA. Different genotypes (more than 20) were identified from these larvae, which were distinct from the inoculum virus and from each other. This and other experiments have led us to believe that the DNA of the inoculum virus (non-infective, or of low infectivity for *P. brassicae*) is recombining with latent viral DNA sequences contained in the insect population to produce new virus genotypes, some of which have higher virulence for *P. brassicae*. If this explanation is correct (the large number of genotypes obtained tends to rule out contamination or selection from an inoculum of mixed genotypes), then it suggests that recombination between baculovirus DNAs can be a frequent event, at least in laboratory tests. Thus if genetically engineered baculoviruses are to be used in future, foreign genes inserted into the baculovirus DNA could become distributed within a gene pool of related viruses. The potential significance of this should be borne in mind in any risk assessment studies on the release into the environment of genetically engineered baculoviruses.

A. E. AKINGBOHUNGBE (*Department of Plant Science, University of Ife, Nigeria*). Is there any possibility of integrating chemical insecticide use with microbial insecticide? Has there been any work done on compatibility of synergistic interactions?

C. C. PAYNE. It is often feasible to combine the use of chemical pesticides and microbial insecticides and this would be the aim in an integrated pest and disease management system. Thus the granulosis virus of *C. pomonella* can be tank-mixed with orchard fungicides without adverse effects. However, it would clearly be unwise to integrate fungicides with fungal pathogens of insects, without first testing the compatibility of the two. Synergism between certain microbial and chemical insecticides has been reported, for example, research groups in France have demonstrated that mixtures of some baculoviruses with low doses of synthetic pyrethroids increase larval mortality due to virus.

R. R. M. PATERSON (*C.A.B. International Mycological Institute, Kew, U.K.*). In my opinion, a new approach has to be taken with fungal pathogens, which involves more work on the toxins produced by these organisms (and other fungi), to discover selective mycopesticides: would Dr Payne go along with that?

C. C. PAYNE. There is already some interest in toxins and other secondary metabolites produced by fungal pathogens of insects (e.g. the destruxins of *Metarhizium anisopliae*). Such interest is not only restricted to their potential as pesticides but also their prospective value as biologically active molecules in the chemical and pharmaceutical industry. If one is to make use of such compounds directly as pesticides, careful toxicological testing will be required to ensure that they are selective and harmless to non-target species.

S. M. K. HAG AHMED (*Wye College, University of London, U.K.*). The first law of control should be to safeguard humans. It seems the use of pathogens may pose a threat to the image of biological control relative to chemical control. It does not seem to be 100% certain that even specific pathogenic microorganisms could not become human pathogens. How can this dilemma be overcome?

C. C. PAYNE. In using microorganisms as biological control agents one must be sure that they are specific and do not have adverse effects on non-target species. I would like to reassure the questioner that representatives of the agents that I have described in my talk have been shown to be safe to use, through programmes of toxicological and infectivity testing and practical field use. *Bacillus thuringiensis*, for example, has been used commercially for almost 30 years with no substantiated adverse effects on the environment. It is nevertheless important to ensure that appropriate quality control criteria are imposed on microbial agents, both to ensure the identity of the agents themselves and to confirm that no adventitious pathogens of non-target organisms are present in the final formulation.

*Phil. Trans. R. Soc. Lond.* B **318**, 249–264 (1988)

*Printed in Great Britain*

# Biocontrol of soil-borne plant pathogens with introduced inocula

By J. W. Deacon

*Microbiology Department, School of Agriculture, University of Edinburgh, West Mains Road,
Edinburgh EH9 3JG, U.K.*

Despite more than 60 years of research on biocontrol of plant pathogens, introduced inocula of only two control agents are used widely and successfully against soil-borne or root-infecting pathogens in current commercial practice. Several others are undergoing exploratory commercial development or are used on a limited or local commercial scale. This review adopts a critical approach to the strategies for control of soil-borne pathogens with applied antagonists, and identifies some areas in which rapid developments could occur. In most instances it will be necessary to combine the use of microbial inocula with management practices designed to minimize disease losses. Also, in most instances, biocontrol strategies should be targeted against small pathogen populations, to prevent or delay the build up of disease, rather than to control existing high levels of pathogens. Natural, rapid senescence of cereal root cortices, which is influenced by both genetic and environmental factors, offers prospects for developing the use of weak parasites for control of take-all disease, caused by *Gaeumannomyces graminis* var. *tritici*. Recent studies on biocontrol of take-all by the fungus *Microdochium bolleyi* are presented, and special emphasis is given to the strategies most likely to be of value for take-all control.

## INTRODUCTION

Soil is an intensely competitive environment for pathogens. As early as 1931, Sanford & Broadfoot showed that a wide range of common soil fungi and bacteria could, individually, control the take-all disease of wheat when introduced with the pathogen *Gaeumannomyces graminis* var. *tritici*, into previously sterilized soil. Similar demonstrations have since been made for many diseases, and now are regarded as commonplace. Gerlagh (1968) described this phenomenon as 'general antagonism' and contrasted it with 'specific antagonism' which occurs in only some soils, affects specific diseases or types of disease, and occurs in addition to general antagonism. Examples of specific antagonism, now often termed 'suppressiveness', include take-all decline, discussed by Hornby (1979), and the failure of some cyst nematodes to increase in continuous cropping systems (Kerry 1981). Such naturally occurring biocontrol mechanisms operate in normal agricultural practice and have been exploited purposefully or by default for many centuries. More recently, our understanding of them has enabled biocontrol to be managed by manipulation of the crop, the environment or other factors (Cook, this symposium), and this must be seen as a direct product of the years of research into biocontrol. It is reflected in many books and reviews that have appeared over the years (Baker & Snyder 1965; Toussoun *et al.* 1970; Baker & Cook 1974; Bruehl 1975; Schippers & Gams 1979; Papavizas 1981; Cook & Baker 1983; Parker *et al.* 1985).

In contrast to biocontrol by disease management, however, the direct, purposeful application of organisms to achieve control of soil-borne pathogens has met with only limited success. One of the main reasons for this is that the very complexity of the soil environment and the antagonisms that are exploited so successfully in disease management mediate also against introduced control agents. Table 1 lists some of the few biocontrol agents that have been used commercially, are said to be undergoing commercial development, or for which research results seem to be directly translatable into normal agricultural practice. It is difficult to appraise the

TABLE 1. EXAMPLES OF BIOCONTROL AGENTS USED COMMERCIALLY OR IN NEAR-COMMERCIAL CONDITIONS AGAINST SOIL-BORNE OR ROOT-INFECTING PATHOGENS

| control agent | disease | crop | reference |
|---|---|---|---|
| Phlebia gigantea | Heterobasidion root rot | pine | Rishbeth (1975) |
| Agrobacterium radiobacter var. radiobacter | crown gall | rose, others | Kerr (1980) |
| Trichoderma harzianum | white rot | onion | Abd-El Moity (1983) |
| Bacillus subtilis | stem rot | carnation | Aldrich & Baker (1970) |
| Sporidesmium sclerotivorum | lettuce drop | lettuce | Adams & Ayers (1982) |
| Gaeumannomyces graminis (hypovirulent) | take all | wheat | Lemaire et al. (1977) |
| Talaromyces flavus | Verticillium wilt | aubergine | Marois et al. (1982) |
| Pythium oligandrum | damping-off | sugar beet | Veslý (1979) |

degree of commercial interest in most of these agents, but to date only two of them have been adopted widely and with obvious success: the use of Phlebia (Peniophora) gigantea to control Heterobasidion annosum root rot of pines, and the use of Agrobacterium radiobacter var. radiobacter for control of crown gall (A. radiobacter var. tumefaciens). These methods were first reported in 1963 and 1972, respectively, and are discussed by Rishbeth (this symposium). The fact that no major advance in commercial exploitation of this biocontrol strategy has occurred over the past 15 years gives cause for serious concern and justifies (indeed, necessitates) a critical appraisal of the approaches that have been adopted to date.

In this paper I shall address the prospects for biocontrol of soil-borne pathogens by means of introduced antagonists, with particular emphasis on take-all disease of cereals. I shall avoid undue overlap with topics covered by other contributors to this symposium. My purpose is not to assess the academic advances of the past decades, except insofar as they relate directly to the application of biocontrol; rather, there is a more urgent need to consider the prospects for commercial realization of biocontrol with introduced antagonists and the strategies that we should adopt in future work.

PHASES OF THE PATHOGEN CYCLE AMENABLE TO BIOCONTROL

Figure 1 shows four main stages in a generalized cycle of the activities of a soil-borne pathogen. Each stage represents a potential target for biocontrol, and together the stages provide a conceptual framework within which to assess the prospects for development of commercial biocontrol strategies.

*Soil-borne inoculum*

Soil-borne pathogens survive in the absence of hosts either as dormant propagules or as active populations. The dormant propagules include spores, sclerotia and resting mycelia of

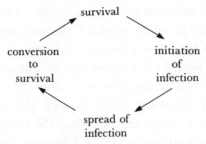

FIGURE 1. Phases in the pathogen cycle that are amenable to biocontrol.

fungi, cysts of some nematodes, and seeds of parasitic higher plants. The active populations may subsist on roots and residues of non-host plants or as declining populations in host residues that were colonized in the parasitic phase; very few important pathogens can increase their populations in the absence of an appropriate host by competitive colonization of soil organic matter.

The logistical problems of targeting biocontrol agents at this phase of the pathogen cycle are considerable, because of the volume of soil that may need to be treated and the non-uniform distribution of pathogen inoculum in soil, reflecting foci of disease in previous crops. Only one of the examples in table 1 is targeted primarily at this phase: the experimental use of *Sporidesmium sclerotivorum* to control soil-borne sclerotia of *Sclerotinia minor*.

*S. sclerotivorum* grows as a parasite on sclerotia but not on mycelia of its hosts, apparently destroying them by inducing autolysis of the central sclerotial tissues and by using the autolytic products to support its own growth and sporulation. Its spores germinate in response to substances released by sclerotia, and it can form radiating hyphae to infect sclerotia up to 1 cm away from those already infected in soil. Adams & Ayers (1982) found that a single application of *S. sclerotivorum* to field plots, dispersed thoroughly at a rate of 100 spores per gram of soil in the plough layer, resulted in 40–55% control of lettuce drop caused by *S. minor* in three successive lettuce crops grown over the next two seasons; with 1000 spores per gram, control was increased to 63–83%, but with 10 spores per g of soil, the degree of control was only 23–28%. In this trial the inoculum density of the pathogen was 16–24 sclerotia per 100 g of soil, which is not unusual in some commercial fields (Adams *et al.* 1984). The results are thus encouraging and have led both to patenting of *S. sclerotivorum* as a biocontrol agent, and to the production of experimental commercial inocula on a vermiculite-based nutrient medium. From laboratory studies, Adams *et al.* (1984) suggested that the lowest application rate of the commercial product at which control of diseases caused by *S. minor* could be expected is about 22 kg per hectare†, equivalent to 5 spores per gram of soil. But this assessment apparently was based on soil samples supplemented with 600 sclerotia per gram, and the degree of control was much smaller at sclerotial densities equivalent to those usually found in the field. Also, and perhaps most importantly, the spores of the control agent were thoroughly mixed into the soil in a way that would be impractical on a commercial scale. So the rate of 22 kg inoculum per hectare is perhaps the theoretical lower limit, and the field experiments suggest that at least twenty times this amount may be needed to achieve 50% disease control by incorporation into soil.

Even if biocontrol agents could be applied economically to the mass of soil in commercial fields to destroy much of the inoculum, they might not bring about significant disease control

† 1 hectare = $10^4$ m².

if the inoculum is present well in excess of amounts needed to cause economic crop losses. A recent example illustrating this problem involved the use of artificial stimulants to trigger germination of the sclerotia of *Sclerotium cepivorum* (white rot of onion), causing them to die in the absence of an appropriate host. In field plots heavily infested with sclerotia, the stimulant diallyl disulphide (a constituent of artificial onion flavouring) reduced sclerotial numbers by up to 40% but had no effect on disease levels because the remaining sclerotia (50–60 per kilogram of soil) were sufficient to cause severe disease (Merriman 1983). Even *S. sclerotivorum* is not so effective against lettuce drop caused by *Sclerotinia sclerotiorum* as against the similar disease caused by *S. minor*. The main reason is that sclerotia of *S. sclerotiorum* germinate to produce air-borne ascospores, so any surviving sclerotia produce a considerable number of infective propagules, whereas sclerotia of *S. minor* germinate to produce mycelia capable of only localized infection in normal field conditions.

There is, nevertheless, much scope for 'introductions' of control agents such as *S. sclerotivorum* in sites where they do not occur, to achieve a degree of 'natural' disease control that may be sufficient in itself or may facilitate other control methods. This approach has been used repeatedly by entomologists but seldom by plant pathologists, who have tended to assume (despite evidence to the contrary for pathogenic species) that most microorganisms occur wherever ecological conditions suit them. In nature, *S. sclerotivorum* grows only as a sclerotial parasite of *Sclerotinia* spp., *Sclerotium cepivorum* and *Botrytis* spp. It may not be generally distributed, although it occurs quite widely in the U.S.A. The sclerotial mycoparasite *Coniothyrium minitans* might similarly be used for introductions; it too is an effective biocontrol agent in field conditions, being able to parasitize both the sclerotia and mycelia of its hosts (references in Cook & Baker (1983)). Parasites of the thick-walled resting spores of other pathogens such as *Pythium*, *Phytophthora* and *Aphanomyces* spp. have been known but largely neglected for some decades; they are attracting attention once again as potential biocontrol agents (Ayers & Lumsden 1977; Sneh *et al.* 1977; Wynn & Epton 1979; Humble & Lockwood 1981). Several of these control agents are host-dependent; so they would need to be introduced where the population levels of their hosts (the pathogens) are uniformly high, but they could subsequently help to maintain lower pathogen populations.

A further possibility for control of soil-borne inoculum is to combine the use of antagonists with soil treatments such as organic amendment or partial sterilization with heat or fumigants. This has attracted much experimental attention and has been reviewed by Papavizas (1981) among others. The antagonists most suited to this approach are mentioned in a later section, but to date the method has not been used widely, if at all, in commercial practice.

### Initiation of infection

For most root-infecting pathogens, soil inoculum is triggered into activity by a nearby root. In a few instances the effect is host-specific, as for *Sclerotium cepivorum* on *Allium* spp. (Coley-Smith & King 1970), some cyst nematodes (Clarke & Perry 1977) and some parasitic higher plants (Musselman 1980). In most instances, however, the effect is not host-specific. Other soil-borne pathogens are induced to develop infective stages not by the host but by seasonal factors such as low temperatures, which stimulate sporulation by the eyespot fungus (*Pseudocercosporella herpotrichoides*) of cereal stem bases.

Initiation of infection is an especially vulnerable stage for a pathogen, which has committed all or part of its inoculum resources for infection and finds itself in a zone of intense microbial activity supported by host-derived nutrients in the rhizosphere or spermosphere. Targeting of biocontrol against this stage is particularly attractive if the control agent can be applied to seeds or other planting material or can be introduced with the seed in drill rows. Relatively small amounts of inoculum are then required if the control agent can proliferate on plant-derived nutrients. In fact, all of the commercially successful examples of biocontrol with introduced antagonists are of this type. Spores of *Phlebia gigantea* are applied to freshly exposed surfaces of pine stumps during forest thinning or felling operations, to protect the stumps against colonization by *Heterobasidion annosum* (Rishbeth 1975). Strain K84 of *Agrobacterium radiobacter* var. *radiobacter* is applied to roses and other horticultural crops during transplanting from nurseries to field sites, to protect wounds against invasion by *A. radiobacter* var. *tumefaciens* (Kerr 1980). Commercial control of white rot of onion (*Sclerotium cepivorum*) was achieved on 230 ha in Egypt by adding to drill rows (at 425 kg per hectare) barley grain colonized by *Trichoderma harzianum* (Abd-El Moity 1983). Carnation cuttings are dipped in inoculum of *Bacillus subtilis* (Aldrich & Baker 1970) or other bacteria to protect the exposed wounds from invasion by *Fusarium* spp., a method used on a limited scale in the Colorado glasshouse industry.

The success of the two most widely used biocontrol agents, *P. gigantea* and *A. radiobacter* var. *radiobacter*, depends in large part on the fact that they gain prior occupancy of the infection court and also that their populations exceed those of the pathogens. Control of the initiation of infection, therefore, might often be most effective against relatively small pathogen populations.

We should consider applying microbial inocula to all transplanted crops, not only because root wounds could be protected, as above, but also because a considerable volume of root material is exposed for inoculation at this time, and in many instances the plants will be transferred from pathogen-free nurseries to potentially contaminated field sites. Marois *et al.* (1982) obtained impressive control of *Verticillium dahliae* wilt of aubergine in field experiments, by inoculating potting composts or field planting holes with spores of *Talaromyces flavus*. It was stated that the inoculum from one two week old colony on potato-dextrose agar is enough to treat 100 plants and that the methods can be implemented readily in present production systems; based on this report the method is included in table 1. The technology for inoculation of bare-rooted plants is easily developed, particularly now that a range of suitable gels is available. This year some three million one year old Sitka-spruce seedlings will be inoculated with ectomycorrhizal fungi, with a gel-based procedure, during transplanting of the seedlings to 'lining-out' beds in a commercial forest nursery; the total cost of this procedure is currently £2 per 1000 seedlings (F. M. Fox & J. W. Deacon, unpublished data) but could be reduced considerably. For larger plants such as orchard crops it may be more convenient to place biocontrol inocula or even disease-suppressive soil into planting holes. Indeed, the papaya replant problem caused by *Phytophthora parasitica* in Hawaii has been overcome simply by filling planting holes with pathogen-free soil (Ko 1982). Replant problems of orchard crops such as apple (Sewell 1981) might be amenable to similar control strategies. It is remarkable that the potential for applying microbial inocula to roots of transplanted crops has been exploited so little; this could become one of the main areas of commercial development in the coming years.

Ironically, numerous biocontrol agents have been applied experimentally to seeds or other planting material, to give short-term protection against seed rots and seedling diseases, for which there is, in general, adequate, cheap and environmentally safe fungicidal control at present. In several cases the biocontrol agents were as effective as conventional fungicide treatments, though somewhat less predictable. This topic was first reviewed by Wood & Tveit (1955) and more recently by Kommedahl & Windels (1981). There has, however, been little commercial uptake of this biocontrol strategy. Al-Hamdani *et al.* (1983) reported that commercial seed-coating with *Pythium oligandrum* for protection against damping off would be more expensive than conventional chemical treatment. The economics might be transformed if biocontrol agents can be shown consistently to control disease and also to enhance plant growth in the absence of pathogens. Such growth enhancement is reported for fluorescent pseudomonads (see Schippers, this symposium), some bacilli (Merriman *et al.* 1974), and most recently for *Trichoderma harzianum* (Chang *et al.* 1986). Irrespective of this, national, state and self-regulatory bodies might consider encouraging the use of biocontrol strategies when these are proved to be as effective or nearly as effective as current chemical control methods. Is there a case to be made for positive discrimination in agricultural legislation?

### Spread of infection

Biocontrol in this and in the previous phase of the pathogen cycle might operate through induced host resistance. This is the suggested mechanism whereby some vascular wilt fusaria that are not pathogenic to particular hosts protect those hosts against pathogenic strains (Wymore & Baker 1982; Ogawa & Komada 1985). It is implicated in the protection of carnation cuttings against stem rot (*Fusarium avenaceum*) when they are pre-dipped in suspensions of *Bacillus subtilis* or other non-pathogens (Baker *et al.* 1978). Biocontrol of take-all of wheat by prior inoculation with *Phialophora graminicola* may operate in part by induced endodermal and stelar lignification (Speakman & Lewis 1978), although this could not be confirmed in the case of grasses and maize (Speakman *et al.* 1978). Immersion of potato tuber seed pieces in suspensions of non-pathogenic pseudomonads gave some protection of the plants when they were challenged 3–4 weeks later by stem or root inoculation with a highly pathogenic strain of *Pseudomonas solanacearum* (Kempe & Sequeira 1983). Induced systemic resistance also has been demonstrated experimentally for pathogens of shoots (Kuć 1982). Interest in the practical application of these phenomena is heightened by evidence that the systemic fungicides metalaxyl and especially fosetyl-Al may act at least partly by induction of host-resistance (Guest 1984; Ward 1984; but see Cohen & Coffey 1986).

Control of the spread of infection can operate also by direct antagonism in the root zone, because many root pathogens produce only limited lesions (for example, *Pythium* and *Phytophthora* spp. in individual root tips) and thus undergo several cycles of infection on a single host, whereas other pathogens characteristically spread along the root surface. Lesions caused by necrotrophic pathogens are invariably colonized by secondary invaders, which exploit the food base that could otherwise be used by pathogens for spread of infection. Some types of fluorescent pseudomonad, for example, show a predilection for lesions caused by the take-all fungus on cereal roots. The ratio of their numbers on diseased compared with healthy roots greatly exceeds that for other soil bacteria (Weller 1983), a fact that implicates fluorescent pseudomonads in take-all decline (Cook & Rovira 1976; Rovira & Wildermuth 1981).

Despite all these examples, we still lack a commercial biocontrol agent that can be applied economically to any of a wide range of field crops such as cereals, legumes, potatoes or crucifers, and that will limit the spread of any of their root diseases. The practical difficulties centre around the ability of biocontrol agents to colonize roots from inocula applied to seeds or other planting material. Roots release substantial amounts of nutrients that support microbial growth, but on any one root region the microbial population increases to a maximum at which its energy requirements match the rate of nutrient supply (Newman 1985). So a biocontrol agent applied to seeds, for example, would need to keep pace with the rate of root growth, unless it can utilize nutrients unavailable to other microbes, increase the rate of nutrient release, or antagonize the existing population and progressively replace it. In general, a microorganism is excluded from a root region once this has been colonized by others.

Much remains to be learned about the dynamics of colonization of plant roots. *Rhizobium* spp. and *Agrobacterium* spp. are very effective colonizers of roots, including those of non-hosts such as grasses (Schroth *et al.* 1979). Fluorescent pseudomonads also are good rhizosphere colonizers (Schippers, this symposium). Several other organisms have been detected on roots at some distance from their sites of application: for example, the biocontrol agents *Talaromyces flavus* (Fravel *et al.* 1985), *Penicillium oxalicum* (Windels & Kommedahl 1982) and *Enterobacter cloacae* (Chao *et al.* 1986). But *Trichoderma* spp., despite their often highly antagonistic properties, are relatively poor root colonizers (Papavizas 1985). Chao *et al.* (1986) recently demonstrated the importance of percolating water in carrying spores or bacterial cells down roots. This may help to explain the poor performance of *Trichoderma* spp., which require light for sporulation and thus may be able to spread only as hyphae along roots.

### Cereal roots, with special reference to take-all

The work of Holden (1975, 1976) opened new avenues for the study of root colonization, especially for cereals and grasses. By means of nuclear and cytoplasmic stains, the root cortex can be shown to senesce early in the lives of these plants, even in the absence of pathogens or other microorganisms and long before the roots show evidence of cortical browning or sloughing. It is not unusual for several cortical cell layers to be anucleate and evidently incapable of defence in only 6–10 day old regions of wheat roots in glasshouse conditions. Data on the rates of natural cortical senescence in various glasshouse and field conditions, and differences between species and cultivars in this respect, are given in Henry & Deacon (1981), Deacon & Henry (1981), Deacon & Lewis (1982), Deacon & Mitchell (1985) and Kirk & Deacon (1986).

Cortical senescence seems to provide a major source of nutrients for rhizosphere bacteria (Van Vuurde & Schippers 1980; Deacon & Lewis 1982). Equally important, it enables weakly parasitic fungi to invade the cortex as resistance of the cells declines. Some of these weak parasites might contribute to disease complexes, but others are known to control major root pathogens. *Phialophora graminicola* is one such example, a non-pathogenic parasite that depends on root cortical senescence (Holden 1976; Deacon 1980; Deacon & Lewis 1986). Natural populations of this fungus in British grasslands are thought to delay the establishment of severe take-all in subsequent cereal crops (Deacon 1973; Slope *et al.* 1978), and also to restrict the occurrence of take-all patch disease of sports turf (Deacon 1974). In field trials in Australia, inoculum of weak parasites closely related to *P. graminicola*, namely *Gaeumannomyces graminis* var. *graminis* and a *Phialophora* sp., gave significant control of take-all of wheat (Wong & Southwell 1980). Take-all patch of turf grass was similarly controlled by these fungi in glasshouse trials (Wong & Siviour 1979). Hypovirulent isolates of the take-all fungus itself have been shown to control take-all of wheat in field trials in France (Lemaire *et al.* 1977). Fungal

viruses were suggested to be involved in this case (discussed by Buck, this symposium) but the
similar behaviour of all these control agents on roots suggests a common biocontrol mechanism
based on exclusion of the pathogen from senescing cortical tissues (Deacon & Henry 1980;
Kirk 1984) and perhaps accompanied by induced endodermal resistance (Speakman & Lewis
1978).

From the above, it is seen that we have some understanding of the ecology of the cereal root
zone, as well as field demonstrations of the effectiveness of biocontrol inocula and evidence for
a role of some weak parasites in natural control of take-all. So how close are we to achieving
a commercially viable biocontrol strategy for this disease? There are still two major limitations.
Firstly, although significant disease control has been obtained in field trials, in most instances
it has been insufficient to give economically worthwhile grain yields; this is true not only for
control by weak parasites but also for control by fluorescent pseudomonads and *Bacillus* spp.,
as summarized in table 2. The reason seems clear: our efforts have been directed towards

TABLE 2. REPORTED YIELD RESPONSES OF WHEAT TO BIOCONTROL AGENTS IN FIELD SITES
NATURALLY OR ARTIFICIALLY INFESTED WITH THE TAKE-ALL FUNGUS, *GAEUMANNOMYCES
GRAMINIS* VAR. *TRITICI*

| biocontrol agent (source of data) | grain yield as the percentage of yield in healthy (uninfested) sites | |
| --- | --- | --- |
| | no treatment | with biocontrol agent |
| *G. graminis* var. *graminis* (Wong & Southwell 1980) | 92 | 100 |
| | 68 | 80 |
| | 68 | 82 |
| | 68 | 80 |
| | 67 | 89 |
| | 55 | 70 |
| | 53 | 61 |
| | 32 | 45 |
| *Pseudomonas fluorescens* (Weller & Cook 1983) | 88 | 90–93 |
| | 16 | 19–40 |
| *Bacillus pumilus* (Capper & Campbell 1986) | 13† | 29† |

† Calculated from the presented data as the percentage of mean grain yield (4.99 t ha$^{-1}$) for healthy crops on
the farm.

control of the disease at or near its maximum levels, whereas the weak parasites, at least, give
best control at much lower inoculum levels of the pathogen (Wong & Southwell 1980; Lemaire
*et al.* 1977) when the take-all fungus itself may depend on senescing root cortical tissues as a
food base for infection (Deacon & Henry 1980; Kirk 1984). It may be more appropriate,
therefore, to use biocontrol agents to delay the development of severe disease in a sequence of
cereals, as *P. graminicola* seems to do naturally after grass crops. The second limitation is that
all the field demonstrations of control by weak parasites have involved inocula of biocontrol
agents produced on solid substrates, usually sterilized oat grains. Cheap liquid fermentation
methods will be needed, preferably for production of spore inocula that can be applied to
seeds.

With this last point in mind, Kirk & Deacon (1987*a, b*) investigated other weak parasites
of cereal and grass roots, especially those that readily produce spores in culture. The fungus

*Microdochium bolleyi* was found to colonize senescing root cortices, with no detrimental effect on its hosts, and in glasshouse conditions it gave as good control of take-all as did *P. graminicola* at equivalent inoculum levels. *M. bolleyi* has been implicated in control of other pathogens of cereal roots and stem bases, such as *Pythium graminicola*, *Fusarium* spp. and *Pseudocercosporella herpotrichoides*, and is known to be a common inhabitant of these parts of plants in field conditions. So *M. bolleyi* would be attractive for use in biocontrol if naturally occurring levels of its population could be augmented sufficiently. It differs from *P. graminicola* and similar fungi in this respect, because the populations of these decline progressively in cereal monocultures, a point that may help to explain their temporary but not lasting ability to control the development of take-all disease.

*M. bolleyi* produces abundant spores by a budding process in liquid culture. In preliminary studies (J. W. Deacon, unpublished data) after spores have been applied to wheat seeds in water or carboxymethylcellulose gels, *M. bolleyi* was found to colonize both the seed coat and the root cortex when the seeds were sown in soil. Viable counts of up to $1.5 \times 10^5$ spores per seed were detected on seeds after brief immersion in water- or gel-based spore suspensions containing $1.8 \times 10^6$ spores per millilitre, and in the best treatments viable counts of $2.7 \times 10^4$ per seed were obtained after the seeds had been air-dried overnight by exposure on a laminar-flow bench. In addition, spores of *M. bolleyi* applied to seeds, without drying, significantly reduced the spread of take-all lesions up roots from an inoculum layer positioned 2 cm below seeding level in pots of soil in a glasshouse (J. W. Deacon, unpublished data). *M. bolleyi* thus joins the increasing list of potentially usable biocontrol agents for take-all. It has yet to be tested in field conditions, but it has the attributes required of a potentially commercial control agent and its development for this can be based on an understanding of its ability to colonize roots in soil.

Before leaving this subject, I will attempt to identify strategies for biocontrol of the spread of infection. Take-all will again be used to illustrate the sorts of factors that need to be considered. First, the overwhelming weight of evidence suggests that economically feasible biocontrol strategies should not be directed against massive disease levels, as illustrated for take-all in table 2 and mentioned earlier for control of the initiation of infection by *Phlebia gigantea* and *Agrobacterium radiobacter* var. *radiobacter*. Cross-protection involving induced host resistance also is usually most effective against relatively low inoculum levels of pathogens. Indeed, the only case in which biocontrol might logically be directed against high pathogen levels is when the control agent depends on, or is favoured by, the pathogen. Secondly, it is probably unrealistic to expect that an applied antagonist could colonize and dominate all or even most of the root system. So we should attempt to identify key protectable sites. In the case of take-all, which spreads along roots by mycelial growth, such key sites are the proximal regions of roots, close to the stem base, and also the basal stem tissues themselves. If the pathogen can be excluded from these regions, then it must infect each root separately rather than grow from one to all others near their points of origin. Fortunately, this key region for the pathogen is also the region most easily protectable with seed-applied inocula. On the other hand, there are circumstances in which biocontrol of take-all might be unachievable by any practical method. An example is when relatively few roots penetrate deeply into soil, because of impedance, and when there is little rainfall during the later part of the growing season, so the crop depends increasingly on water stored in the lower part of the soil profile. Then only the few roots that have penetrated deeply would need to sustain local vascular lesions at some point along their lengths for the crop to fail. The crater disease of wheat in South Africa occurs in conditions such as these, where dramatic crop losses are associated with only localized root lesions caused by *Rhizoctonia solani* (Deacon & Scott 1985). A third and vital part of a biocontrol strategy involves manipulation of the crop or its environment, either to promote growth and activity of the control agent or to minimize pathogen activities and their effects on the crop. The opportunities here are many and varied (Cook, this symposium) but one example will suffice. Of the many factors now known to affect the rate of cortical senescence in cereal roots, the availability of nitrogen seems to be of over-riding importance. I. M. M. Gillespie (personal communication) has shown that the rate of senescence in both attached seedling roots and excised root pieces is greatly increased if nitrogen is present at sub-optimal levels, whereas phosphorus and potassium supply have much lesser effects. Because several biocontrol agents that decrease take-all exploit and even depend on naturally senescing root cortices, it might be possible to manipulate the rate of senescence to aid their establishment from inocula applied to seeds or in the drill rows.

### Conversion to the survival phase

The importance of this relatively short phase in the pathogen cycle is illustrated by the finding of Christias & Lockwood (1973) that 39–52 % of mycelial carbon content can be remobilized and converted into newly formed sclerotia within 4 days when mycelial mats are subjected to stress conditions, as in soil. Pathogens that survive by slow saprophytic growth also depend on efficient conversion to the survival phase; in most instances they lack the competitive saprophytic ability necessary to colonize organic substrates in soil and so can persist only by exploiting host residues that they colonized as parasites or shortly after the host died. Such 'residue possession' (Bruehl 1975) is typical of the take-all fungus, the eyespot fungus and *Cephalosporium gramineum* (leaf stripe) of cereals, as also of *Armillaria mellea* in tree roots.

Any factor that reduces pathogenic activity in the living host will reduce the amount of inoculum available for infection of subsequent crops. For example, the take-all fungus survives less well in the rather ephemeral dead roots than in the more massive stem base tissues of cereals, so biocontrol agents that restrict or prevent invasion of the crown at the end of the growing season will have a corresponding effect on pathogen survival. The low level of damage by cereal cyst nematode (*Heterodera avenae*) in some continuous cereal cropping systems is associated with a low population of eggs in the soil. This is due in part to the activities of egg-parasitic fungi such as *Verticillium chlamydosporium*, but in largest part to parasitism of the female cyst nematodes by the zoosporic fungus *Nematophthora gynophila* (Kerry 1981). Unfortunately, *N. gynophila* has not been grown in axenic culture, so it cannot easily be produced as a biocontrol agent, but it might be a good candidate for introductions.

There may well be scope for applying biocontrol agents to crop residues before these are incorporated into soil, the objective being to limit substrate possession by pathogens. This phenomenon probably contributes to the success of *Phlebia gigantea* in controlling *Heterobasidion annosum* in pine plantations; *P. gigantea* not only restricts colonization of the stump surface from air-borne spores of the pathogen but also can prevent colonization of the stump tissues by the pathogen from infected roots (Rishbeth 1975). In general, applications of biocontrol agents to crop residues may be preferable to direct soil-application (as discussed earlier), even when the control agents are targeted primarily at the survival phase.

Several organisms seem to be good candidates for inoculation of crop residues but at present are among the ranks of the unemployed or, at least, under-employed. They include *Trichoderma* spp., *Gliocladium virens*, *G. roseum*, *Talaromyces flavus* (*Penicillium vermiculatum*), *Pythium oligandrum*, *P. acanthicum* and *P. periplocum*. These fungi share the interesting and rather unusual property of being able to overgrow colonies of other fungi in culture, often parasitizing or otherwise antagonizing their 'hosts'. They can be selectively isolated merely by placing soil organic matter on agar plates precolonized by susceptible fungi (Deacon & Henry 1978; Jager *et al.* 1979; Foley & Deacon 1985) or by burying hyphal mats of these in soil (Liu & Baker 1980). In many instances they have been recorded as secondary invaders of diseased plant tissues. Of all these fungi, *Trichoderma* spp. merit special comment because they have been implicated in numerous examples of natural biocontrol and have been shown repeatedly to control soil-borne pathogens in experimental conditions (reviewed by Papavizas (1985)). Commercial preparations based on *T. viride* and *T. polysporum* (Ricard 1981) are now available for control of silver leaf disease of fruit trees and for disease of mushrooms caused by *Verticillium malthousei* but have yet to find a major commercial role against diseases of crop plants caused by soil-borne pathogens.

## CONCLUSION

The scope for biocontrol of soil-borne pathogens with directly applied antagonists is considerable. But so it has been for at least the past decade because, despite substantial advances in our knowledge, little has changed that alters our ability to put the knowledge into practice. I think we must concede, therefore, that our approaches have been wrong, and that we have failed (or have not tried) to adopt appropriate strategies. The most apposite definition of strategy that I can find is in the Oxford Pocket Dictionary: 'The art of war, especially the part of it concerned with the conduct of campaigns, choice of operations to be attempted, and getting of forces into favourable positions for attempting them.' Every aspect of this definition applies directly to our subject. In terms of the 'choice of operations to be attempted' one is forced reluctantly to ask if the work of the past 30 years on biocontrol of seed and seedling diseases has been strategic. It has led to some advances in basic knowledge, of which the recent work by Nelson *et al.* (1986) is among the most exciting. But we seem to be no closer to applying biocontrol against seedling diseases than when Wood & Tveit (1955) first reviewed this topic. We could do so, and perhaps we should, but still there is no pressing need for it in the agricultural industry. Similarly, despite a wealth of research on massive augmentation of soil with biocontrol agents (reviewed by Papavizas (1984)), there are few, if any, instances in which the economic and practical feasibility of this has been tested on a large scale.

On the other hand, there are now many practical opportunities to be exploited. Disease control by classical introductions remains to be explored in many cases, and new technologies offer exciting prospects for inoculation of transplanted crops and containerized plants, and for biocontrol in glasshouse and nursery situations in general. The prospects for obtaining season-long protection against root- and stem-base pathogens of common field crops seem more distant, unless use can be made of induced resistance. There will be no short cuts in these respects (Garrett 1965), so it is important to ensure that we are travelling along the right paths. To date, we have attempted to control the initiation and spread of infection in field sites heavily infested with the target pathogens, but this approach must now seriously be questioned because the evidence suggests that it is wrong. The corollary is that we should start to apply control agents before a problem develops, a recommendation that will require considerable confidence on the grower's part but will commend itself to the producer of commercial inocula. We need also precisely to define our objectives, whether they be to delay disease long enough for the crop to come through to maturity, to protect specific regions of the host, or even to reduce disease in one crop such that less pathogen inoculum is available for the next. And perhaps most importantly, we should not regard biocontrol necessarily as an alternative to other control strategies, even chemical control. Instead, our attempts to develop biocontrol methods should incorporate any other factors that can minimize disease or its effects on yield. For example, yield losses in the peak take-all years of a cereal sequence seem to be minimized in late-sown crops in southern Britain (Yarham 1986), whereas early sowing is desirable in the absence of take-all. If biocontrol for field crops is to become a practical reality, then we may have to offer growers a strategy, a package of simple and economic measures, not just a packet of inoculum. Further research must reflect this need if the pace of commercialization of biocontrol is to be increased.

## References

Abd-El Moity, T. H. 1983 Biological control of white rot of onion in the field. In *Proceedings of the Second International Workshop on Allium white rot.* Beltsville, U.S.A.: ARS–USDA Soilborne Diseases Laboratory.

Adams, P. B. & Ayers, W. A. 1982 Biological control of *Sclerotinia* lettuce drop in the field by *Sporidesmium sclerotivorum. Phytopathology* **72**, 485–488.

Adams, P. B., Marois, J. J. & Ayers, W. A. 1984 Population dynamics of the mycoparasite, *Sporidesmium sclerotivorum*, and its host, *Sclerotinia minor*, in soil. *Soil Biol. Biochem.* **16**, 627–633.

Aldrich, J. & Baker, R. 1970 Biological control of *Fusarium roseum* f.sp. *dianthi* by *Bacillus subtilis. Pl. Dis. Reptr.* **54**, 446–448.

Al-Hamdani, A. M., Lutchmeah, R. S. & Cooke, R. C. 1983 Biological control of *Pythium ultimum*-induced damping-off by treating cress seed with the mycoparasite *Pythium oligandrum. Pl. Path.* **32**, 449–454.

Ayers, W. A. & Lumsden, R. D. 1977 Mycoparasitism of oospores of *Pythium* and *Aphanomyces* species by *Hyphochytrium catenoides. Can. J. Microbiol.* **23**, 38–44.

Baker, K. F. & Cook, R. J. 1974 *Biological control of plant pathogens.* (433 pages.) San Francisco: Freeman.

Baker, K. F. & Snyder, W. C. 1965 *Ecology of soil-borne plant pathogens: prelude to biological control.* (571 pages.) London: Murray.

Baker, R. R., Hanchey, P. & Dottarar, S. D. 1978 Protection of carnation against *Fusarium* stem rot by fungi. *Phytopathology* **68**, 1495–1501.

Bruehl, G. W. 1975 *Biology and control of soil-borne plant pathogens.* (216 pages.) St Paul, Minnesota: American Phytopathological Society.

Capper, A. L. & Campbell, R. 1986 The effect of artificially inoculated antagonistic bacteria on the prevalence of take-all disease of wheat in field experiments. *J. appl. Bact.* **60**, 155–160.

Chang, Y.-C., Chang, Y.-C., Baker, R., Kleifield, O. & Chet, I. 1986 Increased growth of plants in the presence of the biological control agent *Trichoderma harzianum. Pl. Dis.* **70**, 145–148.

Chao, W. L., Nelson, E. B., Harman, G. E. & Hoch, H. C. 1986 Colonization of the rhizosphere by biological control agents applied to seeds. *Phytopathology* **76**, 60–65.

Christias, C. & Lockwood, J. L. 1973 Conservation of mycelial constituents in four sclerotium-forming fungi in nutrient-deprived conditions. *Phytopathology* **63**, 602–605.

Clarke, A. J. & Perry, R. N. 1977 Hatching of cyst-nematodes. *Nematologia* **23**, 350–368.

Cohen, Y. & Coffey, M. D. 1986 Systemic fungicides and the control of Oomycetes. *A. Rev. Phytopath.* **24**, 311–338.

Coley-Smith, J. R. & King, J. E. 1970 Response of resting structures of root-infecting fungi to host exudates: an example of specificity. In *Root diseases and soil-borne pathogens* (ed. T. A. Toussoun, R. V. Bega and P. E. Nelson), pp. 130–133. Berkeley: University of California Press.

Cook, R. J. & Baker, K. F. 1983 *The nature and practice of biological control of plant pathogens.* (539 pages.) St Paul, Minnesota: American Phytopathological Society.

Cook, R. J. & Rovira, A. D. 1976 The role of bacteria in the biological control of *Gaeumannomyces graminis* by suppressive soils. *Soil Biol. Biochem.* **8**, 269–273.

Deacon, J. W. 1973 Control of the take-all fungus by grass leys in intensive cereal cropping. *Pl. Path.* **22**, 88–94.

Deacon, J. W. 1974 Factors affecting the *Ophiobolus* patch disease of turf and its control by *Phialophora radicicola*. *Pl. Path.* **22**, 149–155.

Deacon, J. W. 1980 Ectotrophic growth by *Phialophora radicicola* var. *graminicola* and other parasites of cereal and grass roots. *Trans. Br. mycol. Soc.* **75**, 158–160.

Deacon, J. W. & Henry, C. M. 1978 Mycoparasitism by *Pythium oligandrum* and *P. acanthicum. Soil Biol. Biochem.* **10**, 409–415.

Deacon, J. W. & Henry, C. M. 1980 Age of wheat and barley roots and infection by *Gaeumannomyces graminis* var. *tritici. Soil Biol. Biochem.* **12**, 113–118.

Deacon, J. W. & Henry, C. M. 1981 Death of the root cortex of winter wheat in field conditions; effects of break crops and possible implications for the take-all fungus and its biological control agent, *Phialophora radicicola* var. *graminicola. J. agric. Sci., Camb.* **96**, 579–585.

Deacon, J. W. & Lewis, S. J. 1982 Natural senescence of the root cortex of spring wheat in relation to susceptibility to common root rot (*Cochliobolus sativus*) and growth of a free-living nitrogen-fixing bacterium. *Pl. Soil.* **66**, 13–20.

Deacon, J. W. & Lewis, S. J. 1986 Invasion of pieces of sterile wheat root by *Gaeumannomyces graminis* and *Phialophora graminicola. Soil Biol. Biochem.* **18**, 167–172.

Deacon, J. W. & Mitchell, R. T. 1985 Comparison of rates of natural senescence of the root cortex of wheat (with and without mildew infection), barley, oats and rye. *Pl. Soil* **84**, 129–131.

Deacon, J. W. & Scott, P. R. 1985 *Rhizoctonia solani* associated with crater disease (stunting) of wheat in South Africa. *Trans. Br. mycol. Soc.* **85**, 319–327.

Foley, M. F. & Deacon, J. W. 1985 Isolation of *Pythium oligandrum* and other necrotrophic mycoparasites from soil. *Trans. Br. mycol. Soc.* **85**, 631–639.

Fravel, D. R., Marois, J. J., Dunn, M. T. & Papavizas, G. C. 1985 Compatibility of *Talaromyces flavus* with potato seedpiece fungicides. *Soil Biol. Biochem.* **17**, 163–166.

Garrett, S. D. 1965 Toward biological control of soil-borne plant pathogens. In *Ecology of soil-borne plant pathogens: prelude to biological control* (ed. K. F. Baker & W. C. Snyder), pp. 4–17. London: John Murray.

Gerlagh, M. 1968 Introduction of *Ophiobolus graminis* into new polders and its decline. *Neth. J. Pl. Path.* **74** (suppl. 2), 1–97.

Guest, D. I. 1984 Modification of defence responses in tobacco and capsicum following treatment with Fosetyl-Al (Aluminium tris (o-ethyl phosphonate)). *Physiol. Pl. Path.* **25**, 125–134.

Henry, C. M. & Deacon, J. W. 1981 Natural (non-pathogenic) death of the cortex of wheat and barley seminal roots, as evidenced by nuclear staining with acridine orange. *Pl. Soil* **60**, 255–274.

Holden, J. 1975 Use of nuclear staining to assess rates of cell death in cortices of cereal roots. *Soil Biol. Biochem.* **7**, 333–334.

Holden, J. 1976 Infection of wheat seminal roots by varieties of *Phialophora radicicola* and *Gaeumannomyces graminis. Soil Biol. Biochem.* **8**, 109–119.

Hornby, D. 1979 Take-all decline: a theorist's paradise. In *Soil-borne plant pathogens* (ed. B. Schippers & W. Gams), pp. 133–156. London: Academic Press.

Humble, S. J. & Lockwood, J. L. 1981 Hyperparasitism of oospores of *Phytophthora megasperma* var. *sojae. Soil Biol. Biochem.* **13**, 355–360.

Jager, G., Ten Hoopen, A. & Velvis, H. 1979 Hyperparasites of *Rhizoctonia solani* in Dutch potato fields. *Neth. J. Pl. Path.* **85**, 253–268.

Kempe, J. & Sequeira, L. 1983 Biological control of bacterial wilt of potatoes: attempts to induce resistance by treating tubers with bacteria. *Pl. Dis.* **67**, 499–503.

Kerr, A. 1980 Biological control of crown gall through production of agrocin 84. *Pl. Dis.* **64**, 25–30.

Kerry, B. R. 1981 Progress in the use of biological agents for control of nematodes. In *Biological control in crop production* (ed. G. C. Papavizas), pp. 79–90. Totowa, New Jersey: Allanheld, Osmun.

Kirk, J. J. 1984 Ability of *Gaeumannomyces graminis* to benefit from senescence of the cereal root cortex during infection. *Trans. Br. mycol. Soc.* **82**, 107–111.

Kirk, J. J. & Deacon, J. W. 1986 Early senescence of the root cortex of agricultural grasses, and of wheat following root amputation or infection by the take-all fungus. *New Phytol.* **104**, 63–75.

Kirk, J. J. & Deacon, J. W. 1987a Invasion of naturally senescing root cortices of wheat and grass seedlings by *Microdochium bolleyi. Pl. Soil* **98**, 231–237.

Kirk, J. J. & Deacon, J. W. 1987b Control of the take-all fungus by *Microdochium bolleyi*, and interactions involving *M. bolleyi, Phialophora graminicola* and *Periconia macrospinosa* on cereal roots. *Pl. Soil* **98**, 239–246.

Ko, W. H. 1982 Biological control of *Phytophthora* root rot of papaya with virgin soil. *Pl. Dis.* **66**, 446–448.

Kommedahl, T. & Windels, C. E. 1981 Introduction of microbial antagonists to specific courts of infection: seeds, seedlings and wounds. In *Biological control in crop production* (ed. G. C. Papavizas), pp. 227–248. Totowa, New Jersey: Allanheld, Osmun.

Kuć, J. 1982 Induced immunity to plant disease. *BioScience* **32**, 854–860.

Lemaire, J. M., Doussinault, G., Tivoli, B., Jouan, B., Perraton, B., Dosba, F., Carpentier, F. & Sosseau, C. 1977 In *Lutte contre les maladies et les ravageurs des céréales*, pp. 21–32. Paris: Institut Technique des Céréales et des Fourrages.

Liu, S. D. & Baker, R. 1980 Mechanism of biological control in soil suppressive to *Rhizoctonia solani*. *Phytopathology* **70**, 404–412.

Marois, J. J., Johnston, S. A., Dunn, M. T. & Papavizas, G. C. 1982 Biological control of *Verticillium* wilt of eggplant in the field. *Pl. Dis.* **66**, 1166–1168.

Merriman, P. R. 1983 Effects of diallyl disulphide and iprodione on sclerotia of *Sclerotium cepivorum* and incidence of white rot in dry bulb onions. *Proceedings of the second international workshop on Allium white rot*. Beltsville, U.S.A.: ARS–USDA Soilborne Diseases Laboratory.

Merriman, P. R., Price, R. D., Kollmorgen, F., Piggott, T. & Ridge, E. H. 1974 Effect of seed inoculation with *Bacillus subtilis* and *Streptomyces griseus* on the growth of cereals and carrots. *Aust. J. agric. Res.* **25**, 219–226.

Musselman, L. J. 1980 The biology of *Striga*, *Orobanche*, and other root-parasitic weeds. *A. Rev. Phytopath.* **18**, 463–489.

Nelson, E. B., Chao, W.-L., Norton, J. M., Nash, G. T. & Harman, G. E. 1986 Attachment of *Enterobacter cloacae* to hyphae of *Pythium ultimum*: possible role in the biological control of *Pythium* preemergence damping-off. *Phytopathology* **76**, 327–335.

Newman, E. I. 1985 The rhizosphere: carbon sources and microbial populations. In *Ecological interactions in soil* (ed. A. H. Fitter), pp. 107–121. Oxford: Blackwell.

Ogawa, K. & Komada, H. 1985 Biological control of *Fusarium* wilt of sweet potato with cross-protection by nonpathogenic *Fusarium oxysporum*. In *Ecology and management of soilborne plant pathogens* (ed. C. A. Parker, A. D. Rovira, K. J. Moore, P. T. W. Wong & J. F. Kollmorgen), pp. 121–123. St Paul, Minnesota: American Phytopathological Society.

Papavizas, G. C. 1981 *Biological control in crop production*. Totowa, New Jersey: Allanheld, Osmun.

Papavizas, G. C. 1984 Soilborne plant pathogens: new opportunities for biological control. In *Proceedings of the 1984 British Crop Protection Conference – Pests and Diseases*, vol. 1, pp. 371–378. Croydon: BCPC Publications.

Papavizas, G. C. 1985 *Trichoderma* and *Gliocladium*: biology, ecology, and potential for biocontrol. *A. Rev. Phytopath.* **23**, 23–54.

Parker, C. A., Rovira, A. D., Moore, K. J., Wong, P. T. W. & Kollmorgen, J. F. (eds) 1985 *Ecology and management of soilborne plant pathogens*. (358 pages.) St Paul, Minnesota: American Phytopathological Society.

Ricard, J. L. 1981 Commercialization of a *Trichoderma*-based mycofungicide: some problems and solutions. *Commonwealth Institute of Biological Control/Biocontrol News Information* **2**, 95–98.

Rishbeth, J. 1975 Stump inoculation: a biological control of *Fomes annosus*. In *Biology and control of soil-borne plant pathogens* (ed. G. W. Bruehl), pp. 158–162. St Paul, Minnesota: American Phytopathological Society.

Rovira, A. D. & Wildermuth, G. B. 1981 The nature and mechanisms of suppression. In *Biology and control of take-all* (ed. M. J. C. Asher & P. J. Shipton), pp. 385–415. London: Academic Press.

Sanford, G. B. & Broadfoot, W. C. 1931 Studies of the effects of other soil-inhabiting micro-organisms on the virulence of *Ophiobolus graminis*. *Sci. Agric.* **11**, 512–528.

Schippers, B. & Gams, W. 1979 *Soil-borne plant pathogens*. (686 pages.) London: Academic Press.

Schroth, M. N., Thomson, S. V. & Weinhold, A. R. 1979 Behaviour of plant pathogenic bacteria in rhizosphere and non-rhizosphere soils. In *Ecology of root pathogens* (ed. S. V. Krupa & Y. R. Dommergues), pp. 105–156. Amsterdam: Elsevier.

Sewell, G. W. F. 1981 Effects of *Pythium* species on the growth of apple and their possible causal role in apple replant disease. *Ann. appl. Biol.* **97**, 31–42.

Slope, D. B., Salt, G. A., Broom, E. W. & Gutteridge, R. J. 1978 Occurrence of *Phialophora radicicola* var. *graminicola* and *Gaeumannomyces graminis* var. *tritici* on roots of wheat in field crops. *Ann. appl. Biol.* **88**, 239–246.

Sneh, B., Humble, S. J. & Lockwood, J. L. 1977 Parasitism of oospores of *Phytophthora megasperma* var. *sojae*, *P. cactorum*, *Pythium* sp., and *Aphanomyces euteiches* in soil by Oomycetes, Chytridiomycetes, Hyphomycetes, actinomycetes, and bacteria. *Phytopathology* **67**, 622–628.

Speakman, J. B., Garrod, B. & Lewis, B. G. 1978 Responses of grass and maize roots to invasion by *Gaeumannomyces graminis* and *Phialophora radicicola*. *Trans. Br. mycol. Soc.* **70**, 325–328.

Speakman, J. B. & Lewis, B. G. 1978 Limitation of *Gaeumannomyces graminis* by wheat root responses to *Phialophora radicicola*. *New Phytol.* **80**, 373–380.

Toussoun, T. A., Bega, R. V. & Nelson, P. H. 1970 *Root diseases and soil-borne pathogens*. (252 pages.) Berkeley: University of California Press.

Van Vuurde, J. W. L. & Schippers, B. 1980 Bacterial colonization of seminal wheat roots. *Soil Biol. Biochem.* **12**, 559–565.

Veselý, D. 1979 Use of *Pythium oligandrum* to protect emerging sugar beet. In *Soil-borne plant pathogens* (ed. B. Schippers & W. Gams), pp. 593–595. London: Academic Press.

Ward, E. W. B. 1984 Suppression of metalaxyl activity by glyphosate: evidence that host defence mechanisms contribute to metalaxyl inhibition of *Phytophthora megasperma* f.sp. *glycinia* in soybeans. *Physiol. Pl. Path.* **25**, 381–386.

Weller, D. M. 1983 Colonization of wheat roots by a fluorescent pseudomonad suppressive to take-all. *Phytopathology* **73**, 1548–1553.

Weller, D. M. & Cook, R. J. 1983 Suppression of take-all of wheat by seed treatments with fluorescent pseudomonads. *Phytopathology* **73**, 463–469.

Windels, C. E. & Kommedahl, T. 1982 Rhizosphere effects of pea seed treatment with *Penicillium oxalicum*. *Phytopathology* **72**, 190–194.

Wong, P. T. W. & Siviour, T. B. 1979 Control of *Ophiobolus* patch in *Agrostis* turf using avirulent fungi and take-all suppressive soils in pot experiments. *Ann. appl. Biol.* **92**, 191–197.

Wong, P. T. W. & Southwell, R. J. 1980 Field control of take-all by avirulent fungi. *Ann. appl. Biol.* **94**, 41–49.

Wood, R. K. S. & Tveit, M. 1955 Control of plant diseases by use of antagonistic organisms. *Bot. Rev.* **21**, 441–492.

Wymore, L. A. & Baker, R. R. 1982 Factors affecting cross-protection in control of *Fusarium* wilt of tomato. *Pl. Dis.* **66**, 908–910.

Wynn, A. R. & Epton, H. A. S. 1979 Parasitism of oospores of *Phytophthora erythroseptica* in soil. *Trans. Br. mycol. Soc.* **73**, 255–259.

Yarham, D. J. 1986 Change and decay – the sociology of cereal foot rots. In *Proceedings of the 1984 British Crop Protection Conference – Pests and Diseases*, vol. 1, pp. 401–410. Croydon: BCPC Publications.

## Discussion

A. R. ENTWISTLE (*Institute of Horticultural Research, Wellesbourne, U.K.*). There are considerable practical difficulties associated with the screening of organisms for the biological control of soil-borne plant pathogens. These difficulties are often avoided by the use of *in vitro* screening, e.g. by culturing the potential biological agent and the plant pathogen on agar. Organisms with biological control activity *in vitro* may, however, prove to be less promising when tested in field conditions.

Would Dr Deacon advise how biological control agents should be tested against soil-borne plant pathogens?

J. W. DEACON. One of the most fruitful approaches to the selection of biocontrol agents has been to investigate organisms associated with natural reductions in pathogen populations or associated with relatively healthy plants in the midst of diseased ones. This should perhaps be the first line of approach, not least because it will identify control agents likely to be effective in the situations for which we wish to use them. Simple *in vitro* screening methods doubtless have some role to play, even if their results are not always matched by performance in practice. What must be avoided, however, is the mistake so often made in the past: perseverance in research with 'promising' control agents just because they are so promising *in vitro* and despite the sometimes obviously insuperable difficulties attending their use in commercial conditions. Some of the work on soil-augmentation with biocontrol agents such as *Trichoderma* spp. falls into this category: logic dictates that such methods would be impracticable because of the amounts of inoculum required. In short, small field trials in simulated or actual commercial conditions should be done early in the course of development of a biocontrol strategy, and the research should be redirected if the likely costs of inoculum production and application could not reasonably be matched by the benefits likely to accrue.

R. R. M. PATERSON (*C.A.B. International Mycological Institute, Kew, U.K.*). Have the metabolites produced by all the biocontrol fungi been determined, and has it been established if any of the compounds might be responsible for the antagonistic activity?

J. W. DEACON. The modes of action of biocontrol fungi are many and varied, although in several instances I suspect that competition (e.g. for host-derived nutrients or senescing cereal root cortices) is a contributory factor. Among the mechanisms thought to be involved are mycoparasitism (e.g. by *Pythium oligandrum* and *Sporidesmium sclerotivorum*), contact inhibition termed hyphal interference (e.g. by *Phlebia gigantea*) and hyphal lysis (e.g. by *Pythium nunn*).

*Trichoderma* spp. are among the few biocontrol fungi known to produce antifungal agents, but it is unclear if these compounds are responsible for biocontrol in nature. Metabolite production requires access to an available food source, so I suspect that, at best, it is secondary in importance to the attributes that enable a successful biocontrol agent to obtain its nutrients.

J. M. LYNCH (*Glasshouse Crops Research Institute, Littlehampton, U.K.*). I was pleased to hear Dr Deacon's suggestion that the battlefield for the antagonist against the pathogen should be treated at the earliest possible stages of crop growth; unlike biological pest control, disease control should be preventative. However, with pathogens that are borne on crop residues I wonder whether the primary battle should take place on the residue. With colleagues Naresh Magan and Paul Hand, I have found that *Fusarium* can be totally suppressed on stand by a *Trichoderma* spray.

J. W. DEACON. The application of biocontrol agents to crop residues seems to be a profitable area for research and I am pleased to learn of your success with *Trichoderma*. Many types of residue are accessible for inoculation before they are ploughed into the soil, and control agents might be selected for their abilities to utilize and increase their population levels on residues. Disease control then could be effected by (1) interference with conversion of the pathogen to its resting or saprophytic survival phase, (2) antagonism during survival, and (3) interference with the initiation of infection in the next crop (see figure 1).

J. IRVINE (*University College London, U.K.*). In the case of soil-borne problems, where re-infection and inoculum build-up is slow, controlling propagation of a pest may offer little protection in the season of application. Such measures may require government subsidy over a long-term. What are Dr Deacon's views on implementing this kind of strategy?

J. W. DEACON. The type of biocontrol that might attract or even require government subsidy is the classical type introduction of an agent to control an exotic pathogen, as is sometimes practised against insects and weeds. It applies mainly to cases in which control on a single farm would be fruitless because of the threat of re-invasion of the target species from neighbouring areas. We have paid too little attention to the prospects for introductions of control agents against soil-borne pathogens. But, as Mr Irvine says, the rate of re-infestation and inoculum build-up by these pathogens is generally slow, so individual landowners could employ introductions and benefit from them without the need for subsidy.

R. N. STRANGE (*Department of Botany and Microbiology, University College London, U.K.*). I was interested to see Dr Deacon's slides of enuculate cortical cells of wheat. Could he explain why these cells are not rapidly destroyed by the soil microflora?

J. W. DEACON. I cannot explain this, but I should say that we remove our roots very carefully from the soil because we are as much interested in the senescent parts as in the living ones. Even from field plots, we find that one or, usually, two dead cortical cell layers remain attached to cereal roots if these are sampled carefully by collecting soil blocks and washing soil from the roots in the laboratory.

*Phil. Trans. R. Soc. Lond.* B **318**, 265–281 (1988)

*Printed in Great Britain*

# Biological control of air-borne pathogens

By J. Rishbeth, F.R.S.

*Botany School, University of Cambridge, Downing Street, Cambridge CB2 3EA, U.K.*

Some pathogens are partly controlled by microorganisms that occur naturally on aerial surfaces of plants, and many attempts have been made to improve control by applying selected antagonists to such surfaces. Antagonists often compete for nutrients with the pathogen, and antibiotics may be formed that reduce germination of its spores and subsequent growth. Hyphae of fungal pathogens may be killed on contact with the antagonist or by direct penetration. The plant's defences may be stimulated before challenge by a pathogen. Apart from killing the pathogen, an antagonist may reduce its reproductive capacity. The examples given illustrate the operation of these different mechanisms in the control of a wide variety of diseases. For diseases of foliage, flowers or fruit, glasshouse crops offer more attractive possibilities for control than field crops because the population level of antagonists is easier to maintain. In some cases plants can be protected by inoculation before transplanting them to the field. Foliage and canker diseases of forest trees present problems too intractable for successful control, but in orchards the prospects are better; for example, methods are available for combining pruning with application of inoculum. Similarly, in some circumstances tree stumps can be inoculated to prevent colonization by a pathogen. Where biological methods are as effective as chemical ones and comparable in cost, they are to be preferred on environmental grounds. In some cases they can be combined with advantage; for example a lower concentration of fungicide may suffice if applied with an antagonist.

## Introduction

Interest in biological control of pathogens that affect aerial parts of plants developed more slowly than in the case of pathogens affecting roots. This is probably because those of the former type tend to be more readily controlled by chemical methods, which are often very effective. As Baker & Cook (1974) point out, the two types of method are in direct competition. In addition, the ecology of microorganisms present on aerial surfaces, an understanding of which facilitates successful biological control, only became a popular field of investigation comparatively recently. However, when some pathogens developed resistance to fungicides and concern increased about toxic residues in plants, the advantages of biological methods became more evident. Some fungal diseases actually increased in severity as a result of fungicide treatment. Pathologists began to realize that some pathogens are partly controlled by microorganisms occurring naturally on aerial surfaces of plants, and that it is useful to look for ways of increasing this control.

In this account emphasis is laid upon the direct use of microorganisms. As the title implies, the majority of diseases considered affect aerial parts of plants, but there are a few anomalies. Thus air-borne fungi that are controlled by inoculating stumps, such as *Heterobasidion annosum*, are included even though they mainly attack roots. A pathogen regularly transmitted by insects, *Erwinia amylovora*, is mentioned because it is also dispersed by wind. *Agrobacterium radiobacter* var. *tumefaciens*, although soil-borne, is included because the symptoms it causes appear predominantly on stems. The examples that follow have been selected to illustrate the different types of disease that are subject to biological control; methods range from interesting possibilities, which for various reasons may be unsuitable for wide application, to well established procedures employed on a large scale. In many cases the mechanism of control is only partly understood. Inevitably there is some overlap between categories of disease; for example some pathogens that enter stem wounds cause galls or cankers. Many aspects of biological control have been discussed at greater length than is possible here by Blakeman & Fokkema (1982) and Cook & Baker (1983), for example.

## FOLIAGE DISEASES

In recent years considerable attention has been paid to components of the microflora present on the leaf surface, which is a specialized habitat commonly known as the phylloplane. This is often subject to rapid and wide fluctuations of temperature, relative humidity and radiant flux. The nutrient status of water films is usually low but may be increased, especially as leaves grow older, by leakage from their cells and deposition of materials such as honey dew from aphids and pollen. The resident microflora and leaf pathogens compete for nutrients, and the results of such competition and antagonistic reactions between them may largely determine disease severity.

Several cases are known where the existence of natural biological control has been revealed by use of a fungicide. Such an effect was demonstrated experimentally by Fokkema et al. (1975) with rye; they monitored simultaneously colonization of the leaf surface by saprotrophic fungi and leaf infections by Cochliobolus sativus. Spraying leaves with benomyl reduced the population of saprotrophic fungi about tenfold by comparison with water-sprayed controls, and there was a corresponding increase in necrosis when such leaves were inoculated with a strain of C. sativus resistant to benomyl.

Naturally occurring saprotrophic fungi have been used in attempts to control leaf-infecting fungi. An early example is provided by the work of Wood (1951), who inoculated leaves of lettuce plants growing in a frame with selected antagonists and Botrytis cinerea. Subsequent leaf rot by Botrytis was reduced, the most effective fungal antagonists being Penicillium clavariaeforme and a species of Fusarium. Better control was obtained when antagonists were inoculated 3 days before B. cinerea than when they were inoculated simultaneously. Pace & Campbell (1974) made small wounds in leaves of cabbage and Brussels sprout seedlings and inoculated them with suspensions of spores of Epicoccum nigrum ($1.6 \times 10^7$ ml$^{-1}$) or Aureobasidium pullulans ($3.6 \times 10^7$ ml$^{-1}$) and also with spores of the leaf pathogen Alternaria brassicicola ($1.6 \times 10^7$ ml$^{-1}$). Levels of infection were significantly lower ($p < 0.01$) with an antagonist present than with the pathogen alone. If antagonists were introduced into wounds 14 hours before inoculation with A. brassicicola, infection was generally about 50% lower than with simultaneous inoculation. There was evidence that A. pullulans produced an inhibitor.

There have been few reports of field applications. Fokkema et al. (1979) sprayed suspensions of Sporobolomyces roseus and Cryptococcus laurentii var. flavescens, together with nutrients, onto recently expanded wheat leaves and noted a hundredfold increase in their leaf-surface population within a few days. When leaves were subsequently inoculated with Septoria nodorum or Cochliobolus sativus, infection by both pathogens was about 50% less than on leaves sprayed with water. This effect lasted for 3 weeks but later disappeared as the population of inoculated yeasts declined. *Chaetomium globosum* was found to be antagonistic to the apple-scab pathogen, *Venturia inaequalis*, under field conditions (Cullen *et al.* 1984). Suspensions of *C. globosum* ascospores at a concentration of $1$–$2 \times 10^6$ ml$^{-1}$, applied to young apple leaves at intervals of 1–2 weeks, reduced the incidence of scab by more than 20%. Ascospores germinated on scab-infected tissue more freely than on healthy tissue. However, the population of *C. globosum* declined from 314 to 36 propagules per unit area of leaf surface between applications. In the same investigation, *Aureobasidium pullulans* was found to have too low a survival rate after inoculation to exert any useful control. There was evidence that its decline was partly due to desiccation, and other factors such as removal by rain and competition with phylloplane microorganisms probably contributed. The majority of pathogens that are sensitive to antagonism normally grow over the leaf surface to some extent before penetrating it (Blakeman & Fokkema 1982). In many instances such antagonism probably results from competition for nutrients, which restricts surface growth of the pathogen and thus its opportunity to cause infection.

A very different mechanism of control is involved when the host defences are stimulated before challenge by a pathogen. An example of such a method, sometimes referred to as cross-protection (Cook & Baker 1983), is provided by control of tobacco brown spot, caused by *Alternaria alternata*. When a non-pathogenic strain of this species was applied at a concentration of $10^4$ conidia ml$^{-1}$ to tobacco leaves and a pathogenic strain of the same species was inoculated at the same dosage 3 days later, leaf spotting was reduced by 60% in laboratory experiments and 65% under field conditions (Spurr 1977). Similarly, when a cotyledon or the first leaf of a cucumber seedling was inoculated with *Colletotrichum lagenarium*, causing anthracnose, and the plant was again inoculated with the same pathogen 7 days later, the number and size of lesions were reduced (Kuć & Richmond 1977). The extent and persistence of this effect were proportional to the dosage used for the first inoculation. Even more interestingly from a practical viewpoint, appreciable protection of cucumber and watermelon was obtained by applying *C. lagenarium* spores to the first true leaf of seedlings about 7 weeks before transplanting them to the field (Caruso & Kuć 1977). This type of resistance can be induced by microorganisms other than *C. lagenarium* and is therefore not very specific. One of the defence mechanisms has been studied in melons by Esquerré-Tugayé *et al.* 1979), who showed that protection is associated with the appearance in cell walls of glycoproteins rich in hydroxyproline, production of which is triggered by ethylene. In other cases there is evidence that phytoalexins are produced.

By contrast with the fungi considered so far, hyperparasites have a different mode of action because they infect biotrophic pathogens such as powdery mildews and rusts. If used for biological control, hyperparasites must be applied after infection has occurred, rather than before as in the case of saprotrophs. Their potential for control is disputed (Krantz 1981), but some good results have been obtained in the glasshouse. Thus Jarvis & Slingsby (1977) found that infections of cucumber by *Sphaerotheca fuliginea* were significantly reduced by spraying them with a suspension of conidia of *Ampelomyces quisqualis* at a concentration of $10^5$ ml$^{-1}$. This treatment was given at intervals of 7–10 days for about 1 month and was particularly effective when plants were sprayed with water between inoculations. When this was done the yield of cucumbers was increased by 56%. Sundheim (1982) also obtained an increase in yield after spraying infected cucumbers with *A. quisqualis*; this increase was about 60% despite the fact that development of powdery mildew was not retarded. Similar increases of yield were

obtained with the fungicide triforine, and also a combination of the hyperparasite with one
third the normal concentration of triforine. Air-borne dispersal of *A. quisqualis* was indicated by
its parasitism of *S. fuliginea* on unsprayed control plots. Grabski & Mendgen (1985) sprayed
beans with a suspension of spores of *Verticillium lecanii*, a parasite both of rusts and insects,
10 days after they had become infected by *Uromyces appendiculatus* and found that spread of the
rust to adjacent uninoculated plants was reduced by 68 % by comparison with unsprayed
controls.

Hyperparasitism is sometimes exhibited by relatively unspecialized phylloplane fungi. For
example, cucumber powdery mildew has been controlled with *Tilletiopsis minor* (Hijwegen
1986). This fungus restricted growth of *S. fuliginea* when applied to plants growing in a Weiss
climate cabinet or glasshouse at concentrations between $10^6$ and $2 \times 10^8$ propagules ml$^{-1}$;
applications were made 7–9 days after inoculating with the pathogen. The number of
apparently healthy *S. fuliginea* conidiophores bearing conidia was reduced to 1 % of those on
untreated plants. After spraying twice with *T. minor* at an interval of 3 days, no secondary
infections occurred and plants remained free from powdery mildew for 3 weeks. Preventative
spraying 1 day before inoculation with *S. fuliginea* had little effect. A strain of *T. minor* resistant
to the fungicide fenarimol was found that might be useful in a scheme of integrated control.
*Cladosporium* spp. are believed to reduce epidemics of popular rust, caused by *Melampsora
laricipopulina*, in the Canberra district of Australia partly because they are hyperparasitic on this
rust. Sharma & Heather (1983) have demonstrated post-penetrative antagonism by
*Cladosporium tenuissimum* to the rust, which produces fewer uredia; earlier work had shown that
pre-penetration effects also occur.

Newhook (1951) showed that various bacteria gave protection against *Botrytis cinerea* when
they were applied to wounded leaves of lettuce seedlings. He attributed this to production of
antibiotics and increase of pH in lettuce tissue from 6.1 to 7.8–8.4, at which level growth of
*B. cinerea* and activity of any pectinase it produced were minimal. Since then considerable
interest has developed in the use of bacteria for controlling foliage diseases. As in the case of
saprotrophic fungi, bacteria must be applied to plants in time and in sufficient numbers to
antagonize pathogens (Spurr 1981). The search for suitable bacteria may be lengthy: thus
Leben (1964) found that only one of 230 isolates obtained from cucumber leaves was active
against *Colletotrichum lagenarium*. This bacterium, later identified as *Pseudomonas cepacia*, reduced
disease incidence in the glasshouse but not in the field, where fewer than 1 % of cells remained
viable on sprayed leaves after 1 day. After investigation of factors that affect survival of
bacteria and their adherence to leaves, field trials were done on crops of tobacco and peanut
(Spurr 1981). *P. cepacia* was tested, as were *Bacillus cereus mycoides* and *B. thuringiensis*. This last
species had shown activity in earlier bioassays and is of particular interest because it is widely
used against insect pests and readily available in commercial preparations. Aqueous sprays
containing about $10^8$ bacterial propagules ml$^{-1}$ were applied at intervals of 7 or 14 days. A
significant reduction in the number of leaf-spot lesions in tobacco, caused by *Alternaria alternata*,
was obtained with *P. cepacia* and *B. cereus mycoides*, and also with a commercial formulation of
*B. thuringiensis*. Infection by *Mycosphaerella arachidis*, causing leaf-spot on peanut, was also
reduced by these bacteria, but much better control was obtained with benomyl. A noteworthy
feature of this experiment is that significant reductions in disease were obtained over three
successive seasons, which differed in temperature and rainfall.

Work on bean rust, caused by *Uromyces phaseoli*, has shown that a biotroph can also be controlled by bacteria (Baker *et al.* 1983). Under certain conditions in the glasshouse or cold frame, infection by *U. phaseoli* was reduced by *B. subtilis*, *B. cereus mycoides*, *B. thuringiensis* and *Erwinia ananas* pv. *uredovora*. One strain of *B. subtilis* was especially effective, giving 95–98 % reduction in the number of rust pustules when suspensions were sprayed onto plants 2 hours – 5 days before inoculating with *U. phaseoli*. A heat-stable inhibitor was present in culture filtrates of *B. subtilis*. In later field experiments, in which *B. subtilis* was applied three times a week, severity of bean rust was reduced by at least 75 % in two successive years (Baker *et al.* 1985). However, one of the two isolates tested reduced yield greatly; the other did not. In some tests, control by the bacterium was better than the once-weekly application of the fungicide mancozeb. Experiments have also been done with some tropical crops. Purkayastha & Bhattacharyya (1982) found *Bacillus megaterium* to be highly antagonistic towards *Colletotrichum corchori* on jute: spraying leaves with a bacterial suspension 1 day before inoculating with *C. corchori* greatly reduced the number of lesions after 2 days and the spread of lesions after 4 days. The same species was used by Islam & Nandi (1985) in an attempt to control brown spot of rice, caused by *Drechslera oryzae*. In pot experiments infection was prevented by spraying with a relatively low concentration of cells, $10^4$ ml$^{-1}$, 8 hours – more than 15 days before inoculating with the fungus. In field experiments spraying with bacterial suspension at 15 day intervals until the grain was mature reduced disease incidence and improved crop growth and yield.

A remarkable instance of biological control is provided by the use of *Bdellovibrio bacteriovorus* for bacterial blight of soybeans, caused by *Pseudomonas syringae* pv. *glycinea* (Scherff 1973). In a glasshouse experiment, *B. bacteriovorus*, which was isolated from the rhizosphere of soybean roots, inhibited the development of local and systemic lesions when inoculated with the pathogen at ratios of 9:1 or 99:1. The mechanism of control is unusual, for the minute comma-shaped bacterium penetrates the host cell by a very rapid drilling action, and after entering it destroys the contents.

Finally, a method of control that does not involve direct use of microorganisms should be mentioned. Schönbeck & Dehne (1986) describe a method by which resistance to biotrophic leaf pathogens that form haustoria can be induced by applying microbial metabolites. A strain of *Bacillus subtilis* that had no detectable ability to produce antifungal compounds was used. The reduction of powdery mildew on induced-resistant wheat plants was greater in field experiments than in the glasshouse, in marked contrast to results usually obtained with antagonists. In addition, far fewer conidia were produced. Resistance appears to be based on an impairment of fungal nutrition caused by reduced haustorial efficiency. This method may have good potential as an additional means of disease control.

### DISEASES OF FLOWERS AND FRUITS

One line of research in this field developed from the observation that in wind-fall apples *Trichoderma pseudokoningii* often replaces *Botrytis cinerea* in lesions at the top of the fruit. Tronsmo & Raa (1977) found that although *T. pseudokoningii* partly controlled *B. cinerea* infection when they were both sprayed onto flowers, it did not control natural infection because of failure to grow at temperatures below 9 °C. Later it proved possible to control such infection by using cold-tolerant strains: for instance spraying apple blossom in an orchard three times with *T. harzianum* in 1 % malt extract at a concentration of $10^7$ spores ml$^{-1}$ gave a reduction in fruit rot of 41 % and was as effective as fungicides in current use (Tronsmo & Ystaas 1980). In the case of strawberries many fungicide applications may be required to control *B. cinerea* rot; the successful use of *Trichoderma* spp. for spraying during the flowering period (Tronsmo & Dennis 1977) is therefore encouraging, particularly because it was again as effective as using a fungicide. Hyphal interaction and production of non-volatile inhibitors by the antagonists were thought to be important in the control of rot.

Extensive trials in French vineyards have shown that *Trichoderma* sp. also has considerable potential for controlling *B. cinerea* rot of grapes. Dubos *et al.* (1978) applied homogenized cultures of *T. viride* containing $10^8$ spores $ml^{-1}$ to vines from the beginning of flowering until 3 weeks before harvest: the proportion of rotted grapes was reduced from 32 % in controls to 9 %. This method was nearly as effective as using the fungicide dichlofluanid. Treatment before and after flowering probably ensures that much of the senescent floral material is colonized by *T. viride*; this tends to restrict establishment of *Botrytis* and delays the appearance of fruit rot. Inoculum of various *Trichoderma* spp. has been produced in Europe for several years, especially in the form of pellets (Ricard 1981).

In cereals infected by *Claviceps purpurea*, the cause of ergot, several *Fusarium* spp. can colonize ovary tissue containing the parasite. Mower *et al.* (1975) tested a world-wide collection and discovered that certain strains of *F. roseum* were the most virulent hyperparasites of *C. purpurea*. Of these, they discovered that *F. roseum* f.sp. *sambucinum* was a very effective agent of control both in glasshouse and field trials. *F. roseum* spores were sprayed onto field-grown rye, irrigated by sprinkler, in which the disease was at the honey-dew stage. Spores produced on the sphacelial stage were dispersed by insects, thus providing secondary spread. The level of control over ergot was difficult to determine but was probably about 95 %. The isolate used was not pathogenic to cereals, unlike some others, and had the added advantage of breaking down the alkaloid ergotamine into less toxic compounds.

As with foliage diseases, bacteria can sometimes be used for control. *Glomerella camelliae* causes serious damage to an oil-producing tree in southern China, *Camellia oleifera*; one source of loss is the fruits, some 20–50 % of which may drop prematurely. D.-P. Zeng (personal communication) found that when a strain of *Bacillus subtilis* is applied to the wilting flowers the proportion of diseased fruits is reduced: in fifteen field experiments done at six locations, the mean reduction was 59 %. The mode of protection here seems similar to that occurring with *Trichoderma viride* on grapes. Attempts have been made to control fireblight of apples and pears, caused by *Erwinia amylovora*, by using selected bacteria. In this disease the blossom is commonly infected first, and later stages may cause severe dieback of branches. It is usually treated by frequent applications of bactericides such as streptomycin, but populations of *E. amylovora* resistant to this compound are widely present in the western U.S.A., for example. Riggle & Klos (1972) used *E. herbicola*, which is common on leaf surfaces, to inoculate pear blossom 1 day before further inoculation with *E. amylovora*; a suspension containing $10^8$ cells $ml^{-1}$ was applied in each case. The disease was partly controlled both in glasshouse and orchard trials, infection being reduced by up to 50 % in the latter. The antagonistic effect of *E. herbicola* was shown to occur in nectar, and evidence was obtained that the bacterium competes with *E. amylovora* for organic nitrogen and reduces the pH to an inhibitory level.

Stimulation of host resistance has been utilized to protect fruits. D.-P. Zeng (personal communication) discovered that when spores of *Glomerella cingulata*, isolated from poplar, were sprayed onto fruits of *Camellia oleifera*, the fungus penetrated them but caused no symptoms.

When such fruits were subsequently inoculated with a suspension of spores of *Glomerella camelliae*, infection was reduced: in five field experiments done over a 3 year period, the mean reduction was 44%. The species used here is closely related to the pathogen.

Unlike most of the previous examples, a method described by Pusey & Wilson (1984) involves post-harvest treatment. Peaches, nectarines, apricots and plums were wounded, sprayed with bacterial suspension and inoculated 1–2 h later with spores of *Monilia fructicola*. Of the bacteria tested, one strain of *Bacillus subtilis* controlled brown rot on all types of fruit at temperatures ranging from 1–30 °C. Brown rot was partially controlled at bacterial concentrations of $10^6$ and $10^7$ propagules ml$^{-1}$ and completely at $10^8$ propagules ml$^{-1}$. An antifungal metabolite was probably involved in control because a culture filtrate also protected fruit from rot.

## Diseases of woody tissues
### Cankers and galls

Some attention has been given to the role of hyperparasites in controlling rusts that cause tree cankers. Kuhlman & Matthews (1976) made surveys in Florida and found that about 90% of uredial sori of *Cronartium strobilinum* on oak were parasitized by *Sphaerellopsis filum* (*Darluca filum*). Inoculation experiments were done on oak leaves infected by another rust, *C. quercuum* f.sp. *fusiforme*: conidia of *S. filum* were applied at a concentration of $10^6$ ml$^{-1}$, which resulted in 74–90% colonization of telia 1–5 weeks later (Kuhlman *et al.* 1978). *Cladobotryum amazonense* is a newly described hyperparasite of *Crinipellis perniciosa*, which causes witches' broom disease of cocoa; it overgrows the basidiocarps and prevents spore dispersal (Bastos *et al.* 1981). *C. amazonense* produces a heat-stable metabolite which in field applications protected cocoa tissues, particularly pods, from infection by *C. perniciosa*. *Tuberculina virosa* (*T. maxima*) is not a hyperparasite in the strict sense but invades tissues infected by rusts, chiefly those causing cankers or galls on conifers. It degrades the host cells and probably suppresses the rust by destroying the food source vital to its survival (Wicker 1981). The extent to which it exerts natural control seems variable. Kimmey (1969) surveyed stands of white pine in the northwestern U.S.A. and found that 62% of all lethal-type cankers caused by *Cronartium ribicola* were inactivated, and that production of aecia on them was greatly reduced. There was evidence that most of this was due to *T. virosa*. However, Wicker (1981) considers that though the fungus has prolonged the life of infected trees, it has not controlled the disease. These fungi all suppress the formation of inoculum to some extent and, as Cook & Baker (1983) suggest, they may in so doing reduce disease from a potentially epidemic status to a largely endemic one. Little work has been reported on practical application. By contrast, the next disease to be considered provides an example of biological control that is applied very widely.

Crown gall, caused by *Agrobacterium radiobacter* var. *tumefaciens*, affects a wide variety of cultivated plants, especially fruit trees. The bacterium, which is present in the soil and rhizosphere, enters through wounds such as those made during propagation or transplanting. It induces unregulated cell division, leading to the formation of large galls; these are formed in various positions and may reduce yield or kill the plant. During study of agrobacteria in the soil of a stone-fruit nursery in Australia, Kerr (1980) found strains that did not induce galls when inoculated into plants. Experiments with one of these, now known as *A. radiobacter* var. *radiobacter* strain 84, showed that it had a remarkable potential for controlling pathogenic strains. It produces a nucleotide bacteriocin, known as agrocin 84, which selectively inhibits most pathogenic agrobacteria. The bacterium also prevents transfer of the tumour-inducing plasmid from the pathogen to the host and, most importantly, is an effective colonizer of roots.

In the control method devised by Kerr (1980), planting material is dipped in a cell suspension of strain 84 at a concentration of $10^6$–$10^7$ propagules ml$^{-1}$: this gives nearly complete control of the disease in crops such as stone fruits and roses after planting. The treatment is very cheap, costing only a few cents for each tree or shrub. Commercial firms market strain 84 in Australia, New Zealand and the western U.S.A.; it is distributed mainly in the form of cultures on nutrient agar or in a peat formulation, by using techniques developed for *Rhizobium* spp. The practical aspects of using this method and successful applications to host plants in different locations have been reported by Moore (1979); it is the most widely employed method of controlling a plant pathogen by means of an antagonist. Recent examples of its use include application to Colt rootstocks in England (Garrett & Fletcher 1983) and stone fruits in Hungary (Süle 1983). There are some limitations: of the *A. radiobacter* var. *tumefaciens* biotypes recognized so far, 1 and 2 are sensitive to agrocin 84 whereas 3, which occurs on grapevines, is not. In addition, mutants resistant to agrocin 84 sometimes occur, although this has not been a problem in Australia so far.

### Diseases originating from stem wounds

Wound-sealing methods are now believed to have little or no effect in preventing decay (Shigo 1971), and therefore increasing interest is being taken in biological control of pathogens that infect tree wounds. *Chondrostereum purpureum* often causes silver-leaf and branch die-back of fruit and ornamental trees after its basidiospores have entered wounds caused by pruning, for example. In plum tree nurseries Grosclaude (1970) showed that fresh pruning wounds could be completely protected from infection by applying a suspension of *Trichoderma viride* conidia at a concentration of $10^6$ ml$^{-1}$ 2 days before inoculation with *C. purpureum*. Simultaneous inoculation resulted in partial control. Later, pruning shears were designed that could apply a *T. viride* suspension to wounds at the time of pruning (Grosclaude *et al.* 1973). The protective effect of *T. viride* results from its production of antibiotics in the wood vessels and the formation of gum barriers by the host in response to the presence of the fungus (Grosclaude 1974). A curative treatment has been reported by Corke (1978), who inoculated pear trees severely affected by *C. purpureum* with *T. viride* and found that symptoms during the next 3 years were significantly reduced by 61 %, compared with equivalent untreated trees.

*Eutypa armeniacae* causes gummosis and branch die-back of apricots in Australia after infection of pruning wounds by ascospores. Carter (1971) produced evidence that in the past this disease had been aggravated by the use of copper fungicides to control the foliage pathogen *Clasterosporium carpophilum*, because this treatment reduced the population of potential antagonists on the leaf surface. Of several antagonists tested, the best results were given by *Fusarium lateritium*, which reduced the number of infections by *E. armeniacae* through pruning wounds if these were sprayed with a spore suspension 1 day before inoculating with the pathogen. A dosage of $4.4 \times 10^3$ spores ml$^{-1}$ gave effective protection (Carter & Price 1974). *F. lateritium* produces a non-volatile fungitoxin which inhibits germination of *E. armeniacae* ascospores and mycelial growth of the fungus. Later research showed that inoculation gave better results when combined with a fungicide treatment; for example, a wound application containing $10^4$ spores $ml^{-1}$ of *F. lateritium* and 125 µg $ml^{-1}$ of benomyl protected 98 % of shoots against *E. armeniacae* (Carter & Price 1975). *F. lateritium* is much more tolerant of benomyl than *E. armeniacae*. The method provides immediate protection by the fungicide and longer-lasting protection by the anatagonist. A simple pneumatic-powered control device was produced that delivers biocide to wounds made during pruning by a standard pneumatic secateur (Carter & Perrin 1985).

Large, broadleaved trees are often decayed by a variety of wood-rotting hymenomycetes after lopping, particularly in urban areas, or after damage caused by high winds. Pottle & Shigo (1975) made wounds in 45 year old red maples and inoculated them with suspensions of *Trichoderma viride* conidia. When isolations were made after 1 year, *T. viride* was obtained from all inoculated wounds, no hymenomycetes were found and non-hymenomycete fungi were less frequent than in uninoculated wounds. By contrast, hymenomycetes were often isolated from decayed wood associated with uninoculated wounds. Results of later sampling, reported by Pottle *et al.* (1977), showed that *T. viride* had delayed colonization by hymenomycetes for at least 21 months in wounds made during summer. Smith *et al.* (1981) suggested that control by *T. viride* can be partly explained by its replacement of pioneer wound-colonizing fungi, such as *Phialophora melinii*, because these render wood susceptible to decay by reducing the concentration of phenolic compounds that inhibit wood-rotting fungi. More recently, Mercer & Kirk (1984) did similar experiments on 40 year old beech and found that inoculating wounds with *T. viride* significantly reduced colonization by decay fungi over a period of 4 years: the level was only about 15 % of that in controls. Inoculation with *T. viride* resulted in more extensive wood staining than in untreated wounds, and much of the stained area remained sterile during the first year. This may indicate that inoculation with *T. viride* promotes a strong reaction from the tree, thus assisting control of decay fungi.

Lesions on the bark of apple trees caused by *Nectria galligena* are due to infection through leaf scars as well as through pruning wounds. Swinburne (1973) isolated several microorganisms from leaf-scar tissue and found that *Bacillus subtilis* was the most antagonistic to *N. galligena* in culture. When shoots of apples growing in field plots were sprayed after leaf fall with a suspension of *B. subtilis* containing about $10^{10}$ cells $ml^{-1}$, some protection was given against *N. galligena*, which was inoculated 1 day later. The numbers of *B. subtilis* recovered from inoculated leaf scars remained fairly constant until the following spring, when the primary protective layer was shed. In later field trials, reported by Swinburne & Brown (1976), apple shoots that had been manually defoliated were inoculated with *N. galligena* and either sprayed with a suspension of *B. subtilis* or with the fungicide phenylmercuric nitrate; controls were not sprayed. During the following summer some of the shoots were further treated with the fungicide dithianon. The two fungicides alone gave some control over subsequent cankering, but *B. subtilis* was ineffective unless inoculated shoots were treated later with dithianon. However, such shoots had significantly less cankering than uninoculated shoots treated with this fungicide.

Corke & Hunter (1979) applied *B. subtilis* to pruning wounds on apple trees. In one experiment they found that if this was done 1 day before inoculation with *N. galligena* the number of shoots it colonized was reduced by 60 % and the size of lesion that developed by 55 %. By contrast, when *B. subtilis* was inoculated 1 day after *N. galligena*, no lesions were formed. Inoculation of fresh pruning wounds gave as good protection as treatment with benomyl. Inoculation with *B. subtilis* also led to the release during the following year of 96 % fewer conidia of *N. galligena* than uninoculated controls. It was considered much cheaper to reduce inoculum production in this way than by treating with fungicide.

### Diseases originating from stumps

*Heterobasidion annosum* is a wood-rotting fungus that causes serious damage to conifers, mainly through butt-rot and killing. Freshly cut stumps often become colonized by wind-borne basidiospores and infections occur on adjacent trees when the fungus passes to their roots from stump roots in contact with them. Subsequent radial spread may result in the formation of large disease foci. Of several fungi tested as possible antagonists for use on pine stumps, *Peniophora gigantea* gave the best results (Rishbeth 1963). With the largest inoculum of *H. annosum* spores likely to be deposited naturally, a dosage of $10^4$ *P. gigantea* spores gave sufficient control on stumps having a wood diameter of 16 cm. *P. gigantea* competes successfully with *H. annosum* at the cut surface, enters the lateral roots of stumps and usually checks advance of the pathogen in any tissues infected at the time of felling; it also replaces the pathogen to some extent. This latter process is probably due to hyphal interference by *P. gigantea* (Ikediugwu *et al.* 1970). The control method supplements a process that occurs naturally but is too erratic to be reliable.

Inoculum is produced commercially in fluid form and distributed in sachets. Each sachet contains 1 ml suspension in which there are at least $5 \times 10^6$ viable oidia (Greig 1976); these are obtained from cultures of *P. gigantea* growing on malt agar. The contents of a sachet are added to 5 l water and 5 g of dye is added to colour the stumps. At least 100 stumps of 20 cm diameter can be treated with 5 l suspension and the cost, including labour, is from 0.6–1.2 p per stump. In Britain the method is used during thinning of pine plantations over an area of about 62000 ha† (Webb 1973). It has been introduced on a small scale during mechanical harvesting of pines in the southern U.S.A. In an interesting variation of the method, Artman (1972) added oidia of *P. gigantea* to lubrication oil of the chain saw to inoculate the cut. *P. gigantea* is also used fairly extensively in Poland, where only the rate at which inoculum can be produced limits its wider use (Sierota 1981). The method does not adequately protect young pines replanted at sites having extensive root infection at the time of felling. This failure is mainly due to the inability of *P. gigantea* to replace *H. annosum* is very resinous roots. The use of *P. gigantea* for stumps of conifers other than pines has not progressed beyond an experimental stage, although the fungus provides good protection for stumps of Norway spruce (Rishbeth 1970; Kallio & Hallaksela 1979).

Attempts have been made to control other stump-colonizing fungi by means of inoculation. Nelson & Thies (1985) drilled holes in stumps of Douglas fir containing *Phellinus weirii* and introduced inoculum of *Trichoderma viride*. Colonization by this species 1 year later was greatest in the upper, more heavily decayed region of the stump, whereas it was least in the lower region; it had not grown well in sound wood. Stumps of broadleaved trees are sometimes colonized by *Armillaria mellea* and may then become sources of infection for a much wider variety of trees than in the case of *H. annosum*. To enable fungi potentially antagonistic to *A. mellea* to grow, such stumps need to be killed by treating the surface with 40 % aqueous

---

† 1 hectare = $10^4$ m².

ammonium sulphamate directly after cutting. In birch stumps so treated and then inoculated simultaneously with *Coriolus versicolor* and *A. mellea*, the amount of wood occupied by the latter fungus 4 years later was greatly reduced compared with controls inoculated with *A. mellea* alone (Rishbeth 1976, 1979). It was shown that wood-decay fungi differ considerably in their ability to reduce the size of potential food-base available to *A. mellea* in stumps.

## DISCUSSION

The investigations outlined here provide useful information about the conditions necessary for successful biological control. Although most of the methods described are unlikely to be applied on a large scale at present, a few seem sufficiently promising to be employed at once, and it is certainly possible that circumstances will change sufficiently to make others attractive in the future.

There is a fairly strong presumption that the most appropriate microbial antagonists are to be found in or near the natural infection courts of the pathogen, as in the case of *Peniophora gigantea*, isolated from decaying pine stumps. Because *Bacillus thuringiensis* gave some control over infection by *Alternaria alternata* and *Uromyces phaseoli*, it might be useful to test potential antagonists from other sources. However, as Blakeman & Fokkema (1982) point out, microorganisms naturally resident on aerial plant surfaces have become adapted to survive and grow in this habitat, and should therefore be preferred to microorganisms from other habitats which may be equally antagonistic. It is perhaps significant that *Trichoderma* spp., which are only occasionally found in the phyllosphere, have not been used successfully as antagonists on leaf surfaces but are suitable for other purposes such as colonization of withered flowers and some woody tissues. It is interesting that the ubiquitous *Bacillus subtilis* can be used to control such a wide variety of pathogens. Care is needed in the selection of strains, because some otherwise effective antagonists have undesirable side effects, such as reducing crop yield. Field tests are essential for selecting effective strains of some antagonists, such as *Trichoderma* spp. and *P. gigantea*. In addition to providing adequate control, an antagonist must be safe to use. An antagonist that is appropriate for one type of infection court may be unsuitable for another: thus *Trichoderma viride* controls *Chondrostereum purpureum* well in pruning wounds on plum but protects pine stumps relatively poorly from infection by *Heterobasidion annosum*.

The dosage of an antagonist reported as achieving control is often high; in the investigations mentioned here the concentration of propagules ranged from $4 \times 10^3$–$10^{10}$ ml$^{-1}$, with a mean of about $10^6$ ml$^{-1}$. The effect of using different concentrations is not always tested, but the results may be instructive. Thus Doherty & Preece (1978) attempted to control *Puccinia allii* on leek growing in controlled environments by spraying leaves with suspensions of *Bacillus cereus*. A concentration of $2.5 \times 10^7$ bacteria ml$^{-1}$ gave no control, $4.5 \times 10^8$ bacteria ml$^{-1}$ reduced the frequency of rust pustules by 41 %, whereas $6 \times 10^9$ bacteria ml$^{-1}$ reduced it by 93–99 %. Particularly for applications on arable crops, the need for such dosages would involve a massive production of inoculum. For most of the potentially useful antagonists so far considered, this would be difficult but not impossible, as judged by the vast scale on which biological agents are used to control pests of field crops in China. Experience with preparing inoculum of *Bacillus thuringiensis* suggests that this could be done for other potentially useful species of *Bacillus*. Inoculum of various *Trichoderma* species is already produced on a fairly large scale. A wide

J. RISHBETH

range of antagonistic fungi produce asexual spores freely in culture, and even non-sporing fungi could probably be used on a smaller scale, homogenized mycelium serving as inoculum for stumps, for example (Rishbeth 1963).

The timing of protective treatments is clearly important. In experiments the commonest reported period for applying saprotrophic fungi or bacteria is 1–3 days before inoculating with the pathogen, although in one instance a better result was obtained by application soon afterwards. Hyperparasites are often applied 7–10 days after a biotrophic pathogen has become well established; such a delay would be critical if the pathogen had already caused serious damage. As Tronsmo (1986) states, the epidemiology of a disease must be taken into account in order to obtain the maximal effect of the treatment. In certain cases control is more effective when nutrients are added with the antagonist, but in others addition of nutrients might well stimulate growth of the pathogen.

Survival of the antagonist for long enough to control the pathogen is crucial. In this respect less difficulty is likely to arise with relatively protected infection courts such as leaf scars, pruning wounds or stump tissues than with exposed surfaces. Many potential antagonists that seem promising in glasshouse trials fail in subsequent field tests because they are killed by desiccation or exposure to intense sunlight, for instance. Even if an antagonist is shown to reduce infection to an acceptable level under such conditions, frequent applications may be needed to maintain its population at an effective level. Repeated treatment may also be required because tissues susceptible to infection, such as young leaves, are produced over a considerable period; although this also applies to treatment with most fungicides.

The precise circumstances in which air-borne pathogens are best controlled by biological agents is a controversial matter. In the case of diseases that affect foliage, flowers or fruit, glasshouse crops offer more attractive possibilities than field crops because conditions are to some extent controllable and the population level of antagonists is more easily maintained. Procedures such as supplementary spraying with water are more likely to succeed in the glasshouse. Even so, care is needed not to create conditions that favour the pathogen. Inoculation of plants such as cucumbers in the glasshouse with non-pathogenic fungi, to confer protection after transplanting them to the field, is potentially very useful. For most arable crops the problem of antagonist survival seems too formidable in our present state of knowledge to permit application on a really large scale.

In the case of diseases affecting trees, their longevity and the large surface area needing protection create extra difficulties. It seems most unlikely that regular spraying with an antagonist could be used for controlling pathogens such as those causing stem cankers on forest trees. It is not so difficult to envisage biological control of leaf pathogens in orchards, but more effective methods would be needed. However, when the target area for protection is much smaller and the need arises only once, as for instance when a stump is created, the prospect for effective biological control is much better. Similar opportunities arise when orchard trees are pruned, and successful methods are available of combining this operation with introduction of inoculum. Experiments involving larger wounds on trees require many years for adequate assessment, but the preliminary results obtained by inoculation with *Trichoderma viride* are promising.

As mentioned at the outset, biological methods compete directly with chemical ones. In many of the investigations mentioned earlier no comparison was made between the two types of method, but in some the level of control obtained with an antagonist was too low to be of

[ 166 ]

interest to a commercial grower. Nevertheless, such work is valuable in preparing the way for development of more effective methods. Research projects in which biological and chemical methods were compared are particularly useful. Often treatment with a fungicide gave better results than spraying with an antagonist, or fewer fungicide applications were needed to give a similar amount of protection. Sometimes, however, the biological method was as good as the chemical one. On environmental grounds there is good reason for believing that a biological method is preferable if it gives a similar level of control at a comparable cost. In the case of fruits and other edible crops the risk of detrimental effects from metabolites produced by antagonists may well be less than those associated with use of fungicides, but must be taken into account.

Biological and chemical methods are by no means strict alternatives; enough evidence already exists to show that they can sometimes be combined with advantage. In the control of *Eutypa armeniacae*, for example, the two components provide shorter- and longer-term protection. Research with powdery mildew of cucumber indicates that a lower concentration of fungicide may suffice if applied with a suspension of an antagonist. Because sensitivity of an antagonist to a fungicide rules out such a combination, it is encouraging to find awareness in some recent work, for example on *Tilletiopsis minor*, of the potential value of fungicide-resistant strains. However, as Krantz (1981) observes, several biological and technical problems must be solved before hyperparasites can be used in integrated control.

The same need arises throughout the whole field of biological control of air-borne pathogens: thus more research is required to determine the conditions that favour growth and survival of antagonists on plant surfaces, for instance. Studies on the colonization of leaves after inoculation with bacteria and yeasts (Blakeman 1985) provide a useful example. Considerable progress has been made in selecting antagonists for particular purposes. It is tempting to continue testing species such as *Trichoderma viride* and *Bacillus subtilis* in yet further situations, but opportunities abound for finding new antagonists. Within species there is much scope for selecting, and creating by genetic manipulation, new strains capable of more effective antagonism and better survival, for example. Further work on the mechanisms by which control is achieved should assist in the development of better techniques. Continuation of such basic research is undoubtedly necessary, but of at least equal importance are practical aspects, such as the need to test existing methods more fully and to develop new ones. To facilitate sensible choices, adequate comparison with methods of chemical or integrated control is important, as are estimates of cost.

I thank Dr H. J. Hudson for helpful discussion.

### REFERENCES

Artman, J. D. 1972 Further tests in Virginia using chain saw-applied *Peniophora gigantea* in loblolly pine stump inoculation. *Pl. Dis. Reptr* **56**, 958–960.

Baker, C. J., Stavely, J. R., Thomas, C. A., Sasser, M. & MacFall, J. S. 1983 Inhibitory effect of *Bacillus subtilis* on *Uromyces phaseoli* and on development of rust pustules on bean leaves. *Phytopathology* **73**, 1148–1152.

Baker, C. J., Stavely, J. R. & Mock, N. 1985 Biocontrol of bean rust by *Bacillus subtilis* under field conditions. *Pl. Dis.* **69**, 770–772.

Baker, K. F. & Cook, R. J. 1974 *Biological control of plant pathogens*. San Francisco: W. H. Freeman.

Bastos, C. N., Evans, H. C. & Samson, R. A. 1981 A new hyperparasitic fungus, *Cladobotryum amazonense*, with potential for control of fungal pathogens of cocoa. *Trans. Br. mycol. Soc.* **77**, 273–278.

Blakeman, J. P. 1985 Ecological succession of leaf surface microorganisms in relation to biological control. In *Biological control on the phylloplane* (ed. C. E. Windels & S. E. Lindow), pp. 6–30. St Paul, Minnesota: American Phytopathological Society.

Blakeman, J. P. & Fokkema, N. J. 1982 Potential for biological control of plant diseases on the phylloplane. *A. Rev. Phytopath.* **20**, 167–192.

Carter, M. V. 1971 Biological control of *Eutypa armeniacae*. *Aust. J. exp. Agric. Anim. Hus.* **11**, 687–692.

Carter, M. V. & Price, T. V. 1974 Biological control of *Eutypa armeniacae*. II. Studies of the interaction between *E. armeniacae* and *Fusarium lateritium*, and their relative sensitivities to benzimidazole chemicals. *Aust. J. agric. Res.* **25**, 105–119.

Carter, M. V. & Price, T. V. 1975 Biological control of *Eutypa armeniacae*. III. A comparison of chemical, biological and integrated control. *Aust. J. agric. Res.* **26**, 537–543.

Carter, M. V. & Perrin, E. 1985 A pneumatic-powered spraying secateur for use in commercial orchards and vineyards. *Aust. J. exp. Agric.* **25**, 939–942.

Caruso, F. L. & Kuć, J. 1977 Field protection of cucumber, watermelon and muskmelon against *Colletotrichum lagenarium* by *Colletotrichum lagenarium*. *Phytopathology* **67**, 1290–1292.

Cook, R. J. & Baker, K. F. 1983 *The nature and practice of biological control of plant pathogens*. St Paul, Minnesota: American Phytopathological Society.

Corke, A. T. K. 1978 Microbial antagonisms affecting tree diseases. *Ann. appl. Biol.* **89**, 89–93.

Corke, A. T. K. & Hunter, T. 1979 Biocontrol of *Nectria galligena* infection of pruning wounds on apple shoots. *J. hort. Sci.* **54**, 47–55.

Cullen, D., Berbee, F. M. & Andrews, J. H. 1984 *Chaetomium globosum* antagonizes the apple scab pathogen, *Venturia inaequalis*, under field conditions. *Can. J. Bot.* **62**, 1814–1818.

Doherty, M. A. & Preece, T. F. 1978 *Bacillus cereus* prevents germination of uredospores of *Puccinia allii* and the development of rust disease of leek, *Allium porrum*, in controlled environments. *Physiol. Pl. Path.* **12**, 123–132.

Dubos, B., Bulit, J., Bugaret, Y. & Verdu, D. 1978 Possibilités d'utilisation du *Trichoderma viride* Pers. comme moyen biologique de lutte contre la pourriture gris (*Botrytis cinerea* Pers.) et l'excoriose (*Phomopsis viticola* Sacc.) de la vigne. *C. r. hebd. Séanc. Acad. Agric. Fr.* **64**, 1159–1168.

Esquerré-Tugayé, M.-T., Lafitte, C., Mazau, D., Toppan, A. & Touzé, A. 1979 Cell surfaces in plant-microorganism interactions. II. Evidence for the accumulation of hydroxyproline-rich glycoproteins in the cell wall of diseased plants as a defence mechanism. *Pl. Physiol.* **64**, 320–326.

Fokkema, N. J., van de Laar, J. A. J., Nelis-Blomberg, A. L. & Schippers, B. 1975 The buffering capacity of the natural mycoflora of rye leaves to infection by *Cochliobolus sativus*, and its susceptibility to benomyl. *Neth. J. Pl. Path.* **81**, 176–186.

Fokkema, N. J., den Houter, J. G., Kosterman, Y. J. C. & Nelis, A. L. 1979 Manipulation of yeasts on field-grown wheat leaves and their antagonistic effect on *Cochliobolus sativus* and *Septoria nodorum*. *Trans. Br. mycol. Soc.* **72**, 19–29.

Garrett, C. M. E. & Fletcher, D. A. 1983 Crown gall (*Agrobacterium tumefaciens*). *Rep. E. Malling Res. Stn 1982*, 79.

Grabski, G. C. & Mendgen, K. 1985 Einsatz von *V. lecanii* als biologisches Schadlingsbekämpfungsmittel gegen den Bohnenrostpilz *U. appendiculatus* var. *appendiculatus* im Feld und in Gewächschaus. *Phytopath. Z.* **113**, 243–251.

Greig, B. J. W. 1976 Biological control of *Fomes annosus* by *Peniophora gigantea*. *Eur. J. For. Path.* **6**, 65–71.

Grosclaude, C. 1970 Premiers essais de protection biologique des blessures de taille vis-à-vis du *Stereum purpureum* Pers. *Annls. Phytopath.* **2**, 507–516.

Grosclaude, C. 1974 Le pénétration des spores de champignons dans les blessures de taille des arbres fruitiers. Application au cas de la protection biologique vis-à-vis du *Stereum purpureum*. *Revue Zool. Agric. Path. Veg.* **73**, 1–21.

Grosclaude, C., Ricard, J. & Dubos, B. 1973 Inoculation of *Trichoderma viride* spores via pruning shears for biological control of *Stereum purpureum* on plum tree wounds. *Pl. Dis. Reptr* **57**, 25–28.

Hijwegen, T. 1986 Biological control of cucumber powdery mildew by *Tilletiopsis minor*. *Neth. J. Pl. Path.* **92**, 93–95.

Ikediugwu, F. E. O., Dennis, C. & Webster, J. 1970 Hyphal interference by *Peniophora gigantea* against *Heterobasidion annosum*. *Trans. Br. mycol. Soc.* **54**, 307–309.

Islam, K. Z. & Nandi, B. 1985 Control of brown spot of rice by *Bacillus megaterium*. *Z. PflKrankh. PflPath. PflSchutz.* **92**, 241–246.

Jarvis, W. R. & Slingsby, K. 1977 The control of powdery mildew of greenhouse cucumber by water sprays and *Ampelomyces quisqualis*. *Pl. Dis. Reptr* **61**, 728–730.

Kallio, T. & Hallaksela, A.-M. 1979 Biological control of *Heterobasidion annosum* (Fr.) Bref. (*Fomes annosus*) in Finland. *Eur. J. For. Path.* **9**, 298–308.

Kerr, A. 1980 Biological control of crown gall through production of agrocin 84. *Pl. Dis.* **64**, 25–30.

Kimmey, J. W. 1969 Inactivation of lethal-type blister rust cankers on western white pine. *J. For.* **67**, 296–299.

[ 168 ]

Krantz, J. 1981 Hyperparasitism of biotrophic fungi. In *Microbial ecology of the phylloplane* (ed. J. P. Blakeman), pp. 327–352. London: Academic Press.

Kuć, J. & Richmond, S. 1977 Aspects of the protection of cucumber against *Colletotrichum lagenarium* by *Colletotrichum lagenarium*. *Phytopathology* **67**, 533–536.

Kuhlman, E. G. & Matthews, F. R. 1976 Occurrence of *Darluca filum* on *Cronartium strobilinum* and *C. fusiforme* infecting oak. *Phytopathology* **66**, 1195–1197.

Kuhlman, E. G., Matthews, F. R. & Tillerson, H. P. 1978 Efficacy of *Darluca filum* for biological control of *Cronartium fusiforme* and *C. strobilinum*. *Phytopathology* **68**, 507–511.

Leben, C. 1964 Influence of bacteria isolated from healthy cucumber leaves on two leaf diseases of cucumber. *Phytopathology* **54**, 405–408.

Mercer, P. C. & Kirk, S. A. 1984 Biological treatments for the control of decay in tree wounds. II. Field tests. *Ann. appl. Biol.* **104**, 221–229.

Moore, L. W. 1979 Practical use and success of *Agrobacterium radiobacter* strain 84 for crown gall control. In *Soil-borne plant pathogens* (ed. B. Schippers & W. Gams), pp. 553–568. London: Academic Press.

Mower, R. L., Snyder, W. C. & Hancock, J. G. 1975 Biological control of ergot by *Fusarium*. *Phytopathology* **65**, 5–10.

Nelson, E. E. & Thies, W. G. 1985 Colonization of *Phellinus weirii*-infected stumps by *Trichoderma viride*. I. Effect of isolate and inoculum base. *Eur. J. For. Path.* **15**, 425–431.

Newhook, F. J. 1951 Microbiological control of *Botrytis cinerea* Pers. I. The role of pH changes and bacterial antagonism. *Ann. appl. Biol.* **38**, 169–184.

Pace, M. A. & Campbell, R. 1974 The effect of saprophytes on infection of leaves of *Brassica* spp. by *Alternaria brassicicola*. *Trans. Br. mycol. Soc.* **63**, 193–196.

Pottle, H. W. & Shigo, A. L. 1975 Treatment of wounds on *Acer rubrum* with *Trichoderma viride*. *Eur. J. For. Path.* **5**, 274–279.

Pottle, H. W., Shigo, A. L. & Blanchard, R. O. 1977 Biological control of wound hymenomycetes by *Trichoderma harzianum*. *Pl. Dis. Reptr* **61**, 687–690.

Purkayastha, R. P. & Bhattacharyya, B. 1982 Antagonism of microorganisms from jute phyllosphere towards *Colletotrichum corchori*. *Trans. Br. mycol. Soc.* **78**, 509–513.

Pusey, P. L. & Wilson, C. L. 1984 Postharvest biological control of stone fruit brown rot by *Bacillus subtilis*. *Pl. Dis.* **68**, 753–756.

Ricard, J. L. 1981 Commercialization of a *Trichoderma* based mycofungicide: some problems and solutions. *Biocontrol News Inf.* **2**, 95–98.

Riggle, J. H. & Klos, E. J. 1972 Relationship of *Erwinia herbicola* to *Erwinia amylovora*. *Can. J. Bot.* **50**, 1077–1083.

Rishbeth, J. 1963 Stump protection against *Fomes annosus*. III. Inoculation with *Peniophora gigantea*. *Ann. appl. Biol.* **52**, 63–77.

Rishbeth, J. 1970 The possibility of stump inoculation for conifers other than pines. In *Proceedings of the 3rd International Conference on Fomes annosus*. Section 24, pp. 110–120. International Union of Forest Research Organizations. Washington: United States Department of Agriculture Forest Service.

Rishbeth, J. 1976 Chemical treatment and inoculation of hardwood stumps for control of *Armillaria mellea*. *Ann. appl. Biol.* **82**, 57–70.

Rishbeth, J. 1979 Modern aspects of biological control of *Fomes* and *Armillaria*. *Eur. J. For. Path.* **9**, 331–340.

Scherff, R. H. 1973 Control of bacterial blight of soybean by *Bdellovibrio bacteriovorus*. *Phytopathology* **63**, 400–402.

Schönbeck, F. & Dehne, H.-W. 1986 Use of microbial metabolites inducing resistance against plant pathogens. In *Microbiology of the phyllosphere* (ed. N. J. Fokkema & J. Van den Heuvel), pp. 363–375. Cambridge University Press.

Sharma, I. K. & Heather, W. A. 1983 Post-penetration antagonism by *Cladosporium tenuissimum* to uredinial induction by *Melampsora larici-populina*. *Trans. Br. mycol. Soc.* **80**, 373–374.

Shigo, A. L. 1971 Wound dressing research on red maples. *Int. Shade Tree Conf. Proc.* **47**, 97–98.

Sierota, Z. H. 1981 Chances of practical control of *Fomes annosus* (Fr.) Cke. infection using biological methods. In *Root and butt rots in Scotch pine stands* (International Union of Forest Research Organizations Working Party S2.06.01), pp. 62–68. Poznań: Polish Academy of Sciences.

Smith, K. T., Blanchard, R. O. & Shortle, W. C. 1981 Postulated mechanism of biological control of decay fungi in red maple wounds treated with *Trichoderma harzianum*. *Phytopathology* **71**, 496–498.

Spurr, H. W., Jr. 1977 Protective applications of conidia of nonpathogenic *Alternaria* sp. isolates for control of tobacco brown spot disease. *Phytopathology* **67**, 128–132.

Spurr, H. W., Jr. 1981 Experiments on foliar disease control using bacterial antagonists. In *Microbial ecology of the phylloplane* (ed. J. P. Blakeman), pp. 369–381. London: Academic Press.

Süle, S. 1983 Biologiai vedekezes a gyumolcsfak agrobakteriumos gyokergolyvaja ellen. *Novenyvedelem* **19**, 337–340.

Sundheim, L. 1982 Control of cucumber powdery mildew by the hyperparasite *Ampelomyces quisqualis* and fungicides. *Pl. Path.* **31**, 209–214.

[ 169 ]

Swinburne, T. R. 1973 Microflora of apple leaf scars in relation to infection by *Nectria galligena*. *Trans. Br. mycol. Soc.* **60**, 389–403.

Swinburne, T. R. & Brown, A. E. 1976 A comparison of the use of *Bacillus subtilis* with conventional fungicides for the control of apple canker (*Nectria galligena*). *Ann. appl. Biol.* **82**, 365–368.

Tronsmo, A. 1986 Use of *Trichoderma* spp. in biological control of necrotrophic pathogens. In *Microbiology of the phyllosphere* (ed. N. J. Fokkema & J. Van den Heuvel), pp. 348–362. Cambridge University Press.

Tronsmo, A. & Dennis, C. 1977 The use of *Trichoderma* species to control strawberry fruit rots. *Neth. J. Pl. Path.* **83** (suppl. 1), 449–455.

Tronsmo, A. & Raa, J. 1977 Antagonistic action of *Trichoderma pseudokoningii* against the apple pathogen *Botrytis cinerea*. *Phytopath. Z.* **89**, 216–220.

Tronsmo, A. & Ystaas, J. 1980 Biological control of *Botrytis cinerea* on apple. *Pl. Dis.* **64**, 1009.

Webb, P. J. 1973 An alternative to chemical stump protection against *Fomes annosus* on pines in state and private forestry. *Scott. For.* **27**, 24–25.

Wicker, E. F. 1981 Natural control of white pine blister rust by *Tuberculina maxima*. *Phytopathology* **71**, 997–1000.

Wood, R. K. S. 1951 The control of diseases of lettuce by the use of antagonistic organisms. I. The control of *Botrytis cinerea* Pers. *Ann. appl. Biol.* **38**, 203–216.

## Discussion

R. D. LUMSDEN (*United States Department of Agriculture Agricultural Research Service, Beltsville, U.S.A.*). Dr Rishbeth, from your extensive knowledge and experience with the discovery and development of the one major example of successful biological control that we have in our own discipline, what are the factor or factors that you judge to be responsible for the success of *Peniophora gigantea* as a biological control agent against *Heterobasidion annosum*?

J. RISHBETH. *Peniophora gigantea* is one of the few fungi that can colonize the surface of freshly cut pine stumps. It is very competitive, preventing establishment of *Heterobasidion annosum* and often replacing this pathogen if it is already present. *Peniophora* grows extensively in stump roots and rapidly decays the wood, but does not invade living roots. Fortunately it is easy to grow in culture and produces abundant asexual spores which are effective for inoculation.

J. N. GIBBS (*Forest Research Station, Farnham, U.K.*). I wish to emphasize the competitive mode of action of *Peniophora*; its success in practice lies in its ability to grow rapidly into the fresh stump regardless of whether the pathogen (*Heterobasidion*) is present or not.

W. D. HAMILTON, F.R.S. (*Department of Zoology, Oxford University, U.K.*). Is it a possible generalization that the antagonists of air-borne plant pathogens are less air-borne themselves? This might be expected from theory in that species that have poor chances of moving from their present host to another should evolve properties that tend to keep their present host alive. In contrast, species with excellent dispersal may evolve courses of rapid exploitation that result in pathogenesis. Of the antagonists of pathogenic fungi that you mention, I think that the two slightly familiar to me, *Trichoderma viride* and *Peniophora gigantea*, may illustrate poor dispersal. *T. viride*, for example, sporulates under bark and may rely on dispersal by rather loosely associated insects rather than on wind. Do you see such a general contrast between the antagonists and the pathogens?

J. RISHBETH. I doubt whether such a contrast is general, although Professor Hamilton may well be correct about *T. viride*, which I have seldom detected when trapping air-borne spores. On the other hand, spores of *P. gigantea* are at least as common in the air as those of *Heterobasidion annosum* unless conditions are very dry. Of other microorganisms used for biological control, spores of *Bacillus* spp. also occur commonly in the air, whereas ballistospores of *Sporobolomyces* are often extremely abundant in moist air. Hyperparasites such as *Ampelomyces* are probably dispersed fairly effectively in spores of their fungal hosts.

R. J. COOK (*United States Department of Agriculture Agricultural Reseach Service, Washington State University, Pullman, U.S.A.*). In response to the question from Dr Neuenschwander [not printed] of whether or not plant pathologists make use of theory and models of population dynamics in our research on biological control, I think the answer is a qualified no. Modern epidemiology in plant pathology makes considerable use of this approach in describing the increase of a pathogen population or frequency of virulence genes in a pathogen population on a susceptible host crop. This is used to some advantage in biological control systems where the strategy is some kind of gene deployment achieved by a network, sequence, or mixture of plant cultivars designed to control the frequency of a particular race or pathovar of the pathogen. As to a counterpart of the efforts in entomology to describe or model population dynamics of a plant pathogen interacting with its natural enemies, we have done little or nothing along this line. A major reason is that many if not most of our successful biological controls involving introduced or managed populations of antagonists of plant pathogens do not involve the strategy of regulating the pathogen population directly by predatory or hyperparasitic agents. The biological controls of plant pathogens with introduced agents described at this meeting, and in use under study around the world (systems that seem to work best for us), are aimed mostly at defence against the processes of infection, disease development, or reproduction of the pathogen at the end of the disease cycle. Examples exist of hyperparasites or hyperpathogens with ability to lower the inoculum density of a target plant pathogen, but generally these are too inefficient for effective biocontrol. The best use of natural enemies of the inoculum of plant pathogens are those that prevent inoculum from ever forming, e.g. hyperparasites in rust pustules, or those that destroy pathogen propagules of plant parasitic nematodes as they form on the host plant.

*Phil. Trans. R. Soc. Lond.* B **318**, 283–293 (1988)

*Printed in Great Britain*

# Biological control of pathogens with rhizobacteria

By B. Schippers

*Willie Commelin Scholten Phytopathological Laboratory, Department of Plant Pathology, State University of Utrecht, State University of Amsterdam, 3742 CP Baarn, The Netherlands*

Present knowledge on the biological control of soil-borne plant pathogens by rhizosphere inhabiting bacteria, especially fluorescent *Pseudomonas* spp., is discussed. Attention is paid to the use of molecular biological techniques to analyse the mechanism(s) of antagonism (competition for iron, antibiosis) and the population dynamics of the antagonist(s). Special attention is given to the biological control of a new class of pathogen that does not obviously damage the host, except by stunting its growth and yield. The need for more information on mechanisms of root colonization and survival of antagonists to improve their use as biocontrol agents is emphasized.

## 1. Rhizobacteria and pathogens

Bacteria isolated from the rhizosphere and belonging to a wide variety of genera, have the potential to suppress diseases caused by a diversity of soil-borne plant pathogens (table 1). Some of these, especially *Pseudomonas* spp. and *Bacillus* spp., significantly suppress disease and increase yield of crops in field trials.

Most progress in understanding the mechanisms of control and of successes and failures in the field has come from recent studies on the role of fluorescent *Pseudomonas* spp. in promoting plant growth by suppressing deleterious rhizosphere microorganisms (DRM) (Burr & Caesor 1984; Schippers *et al.* 1987 a, b; Suslow 1982), and on their role in soils naturally suppressive to diseases caused by *Fusarium oxysporum* in a variety of crops (Baker *et al.* 1986), by *Gaeumannomyces graminis* in wheat (Weller & Cook 1986a) and by *Thielaviopsis basicola* in tobacco (Ahl *et al.* 1986).

Disease-suppressive soils are attractive model systems for exploring the potentials of rhizosphere microorganisms to control disease because in these soils, the antagonists also function in modern agricultural practices and can give even better results than do pesticides.

Plant growth promotion by rhizobacteria is another attractive model system for research, because it operates with a variety of crops (table 1) by enhancing root function and growth, thereby improving the uptake of nutrients and water from soil.

Experience with *Pseudomonas* spp. as biocontrol agents in these model systems has shown that even within this pre-eminent group of rhizobacteria, interaction with the target organism varies from inhibition of germination and germ tube growth (*F. oxysporum*) in the rhizosphere (Baker *et al.* 1986) to restriction of the pathogenic activity (*G. graminis*) inside infected and necrotic root tissue (Weller & Cook 1986a). In addition, the mechanisms controlling activity of the pathogens are diverse and include competition for $Fe^{3+}$, antibiosis and induction of host resistance. Competition for iron seems to be a major factor in some and to be involved in other mechanisms of biocontrol of diseases caused by microbial plant pathogens.

TABLE 1. RECENT REPORTS ON GENERA OF RHIZOBACTERIA WITH BIOCONTROL POTENTIAL

| bacteria | pathogen | host | reference |
|---|---|---|---|
| *Alcaligenes* | *Fusarium oxysporum* | carnation | Yen & Schroth (1986) |
| *Arthrobacter*† | *Fusarium oxysporum* | carnation | Sneh (1981) |
| *Bacillus*† | *Gaeumannomyces graminis* | wheat | Capper & Campbell (1986) |
| *Bacillus*† | *Phytophthora cactorum* | apple | Gupta & Utkhede (1986) |
| *Bacillus* | *Sclerotium cepivorum* | onion | Utkhede & Rahe (1983) |
| *Enterobacter* | *Phytophthora cactorum* | apple | Gupta & Utkhede (1986) |
| *Hafnia* | *Fusarium oxysporum* | carnation | Sneh *et al.* (1985) |
| *Pseudomonas* | *F. oxysporum* | carnation, flax | Baker *et al.* (1986) |
| *Pseudomonas*† | *Erwinia carotovora* | potato | Xu & Gross (1986) |
| *Pseudomonas*† | *Erwinia carotovora* | potato | Rhodes & Logan (1986) |
| *Pseudomonas*† | *Gaeumannomyces graminis* | wheat | Weller & Cook (1986*a*) |
| *Pseudomonas*† | *Pythium* spp. | wheat | Weller & Cook (1986*b*) |
| *Pseudomonas* | *Pythium* spp. | cotton | Howell & Stipanovic (1979) |
| *Pseudomonas* | *Rhizoctonia solani* | cotton | Howell & Stipanovic (1980) |
| *Pseudomonas* | *Thielaviopsis basicola* | tobacco | Ahl *et al.* (1986) |
| *Pseudomonas*† | deleterious microorganisms | potato | Kloepper *et al.* (1980) |
| *Pseudomonas*† | deleterious microorganisms | potato | Schippers *et al.* (1986) |
| *Pseudomonas* | deleterious microorganisms | beet | Suslow (1982) |
| *Rhizobium* | *Phytophthora megasperma* | soybean | Tu (1978) |
| *Serratia* | *Fusarium oxysporum* | carnation | Sneh *et al.* (1985) |

† Significant control was also obtained in field trials.

## 2. COMPETITION FOR IRON AS A MECHANISM OF DISEASE CONTROL

Iron plays a central role in the energy metabolism of aerobic and semi-anaerobic microorganisms. Its availability in soil for microorganisms and plants drops dramatically with increasing pH above pH6. Microorganisms compete for iron by releasing siderophores (S) which are small proteins with a high binding affinity to $Fe^{3+}$ (Neilands 1981; Leong 1986; Schippers *et al.* 1987*a,b*). The affinity for $Fe^{3+}$ of the many different microbial siderophores varies widely and is *ca.* ten times greater for the catechol-hydroxamate type siderophores of pseudomonads, than for the hydroxamate type siderophores of fungi. Competition for $Fe^{3+}$ can also occur among different strains of *Pseudomonas* spp. It probably depends, for example, on differences in siderophore production, in affinity of their siderophores for $Fe^{3+}$, and also on the specificity of their receptor proteins for their own siderophores. The receptor proteins are located in the outer cell membrane of bacterial cells.

The ability, or inability of microorganisms to use each others $Fe^{3+}$-siderophore complexes seems to be important for their ability to colonize the rhizosphere (Bakker *et al.* 1986*b*). Our plant growth promoting (PGP) *Pseudomonas putida* WCS358 can use siderophores of strains of many other fluorescent *Pseudomonas* spp. isolated from the rhizosphere of potato plants. However, the use of its own siderophore by other strains of *Pseudomonas* spp. is limited. PGP *Pseudomonas fluorescens* WCS374 can use the siderophores of only a few other strains of *Pseudomonas* spp., but its own siderophore can be used by many other strains. Strain WCS358 can use the siderophore of WCS374, but WCS374 cannot use the siderophore of WCS358.

The significance of these differences for the colonization of the rhizosphere was demonstrated in pot experiments. Mutants of WCS358 and WCS374, which had lost their ability to produce siderophores but not their receptors, were obtained by *Tn5* transposon mutagenesis (Marugg *et al.* 1985). When roots that had just emerged from potato sprouts were inoculated before planting with the siderophore-negative mutant (S⁻) of either WCS358 or WCS374 and planted in soil containing the siderophore producing parent strain (S⁺) of either WCS358 or

WCS374, populations of S⁻ mutants on the roots developed differentially (Bakker *et al.* 1986*b*). WCS358 S⁻ was significantly stimulated in the presence of its parent strain and of WCS374, but WCS374 S⁻ only increased in the presence of its parent strain and not in the presence of WCS358 (figure 1). These observations strongly suggest not only that siderophores of

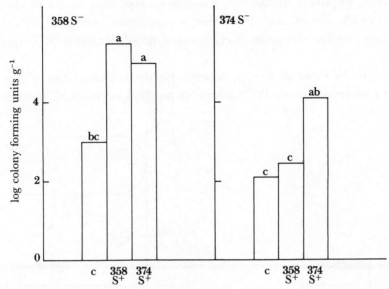

FIGURE 1. The significance of siderophores (S) for root colonization by *Pseudomonas* spp. Root colonization from soil of a transposon *Tn5* mutant of *P. putida* 358 (358 S⁻), which has lost its ability to produce siderophores, is significantly enhanced by the presence on the roots of its siderophore-producing parent strain 358 S⁺, or of *P. fluorescence* 374 S⁺, siderophores of which can be used by 358. Root colonization from soil by *P. fluorescence* 374 S⁻ is only enhanced by its siderophore-producing parent strain 374 S⁺, but not by 358 S⁺, siderophores of which can not be used by 374. Roots were inoculated with *Pseudomonas* strain 358 S⁺ or strain 374 S⁺ before planting in soil inoculated with 358 S⁻ or 374 S⁻. Values with the same letter on top of a bar are not significantly different at $p = 0.01$ based on Student's *t*-test. Control treatment of roots (c).

*Pseudomonas* spp. are being produced in the rhizosphere but also demonstrate the possible impact of siderophore-mediated competition for iron among rhizosphere pseudomonads on their population dynamics in the rhizosphere.

### 3. PLANT GROWTH PROMOTION AND DELETERIOUS RHIZOSPHERE MICROORGANISMS

Siderophores produced by strains of fluorescent *Pseudomonas* play a key role in growth promotion of a variety of crops in pot experiments (Geels & Schippers 1983; Kloepper *et al.* 1980; Leong 1986; Schippers *et al.* 1986; Suslow 1982). Potato tuber treatment with *P. putida* WCS358 improved seed tuber yield by 13%. Its *Tn5* transposon S⁻ mutant, however, had no effect in these field experiments (Bakker *et al.* 1986*a*). This shows that *Pseudomonas* spp. siderophores operate in plant growth promotion and in yield increases in the field.

The growth promotion is attributed to suppression of ill-defined rhizosphere inhabiting microorganisms that impair root function (Kloepper & Schroth 1981; Suslow 1982; Schippers *et al.* 1986, 1987*a*, *b*). In our potato-field experiments they seem to be involved in the progressive decrease in tuber yield with increasing frequency of potato cropping.

We hypothesize that in soils frequently cropped to potato, hydrocyanic acid production by deleterious rhizosphere pseudomonads impairs the energy metabolism of potato root cells thereby decreasing uptake of nutrients from soil. The HCN production of microorganisms probably is then suppressed by the PGP *Pseudomonas* spp. strains (Bakker & Schippers 1988). This hypothesis is supported by the following observations *in vitro*, and in pot experiments (figure 2):

(1) more than 50 % of potato rhizosphere *Pseudomonas* spp. isolates can produce HCN;

(2) potato root cytochrome oxidase respiration is suppressed by less than 5 $\mu$M HCN;

(3) the potato root exudate components glycine and proline enhance HCN production by pseudomonads;

(4) HCN production by *Pseudomonas* spp. depends highly on availability of iron and can be suppressed by PGP *Pseudomonas putida* WCS358 or its purified siderophore pseudobactin 358.

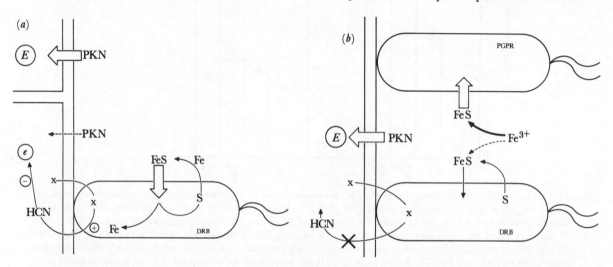

FIGURE 2. Diagram of hypothetical interactions between plant growth promoting rhizobacteria (PGPR), deleterious rhizobacteria (DRB) and the plant root cell. (*a*) Inhibition of potato root cell function by hydrocyanide-producing DRB. The uptake of iron by siderophores of DRB (S) from the soil enhances their HCN production from the root exudate component 'x'. HCN inhibits the energy metabolism (*e*) of the root cell and thus decreases uptake of phosphorus, potassium and nitrogen (PKN). (*b*) Competition for iron by the siderophores of a PGPR inhibits the HCN production by DRB, thereby increasing the available energy (*E*) of the root cell for uptake of PKN.

Microbial HCN production in the rhizosphere is difficult to demonstrate because HCN is rapidly inactivated in soil. It may, however, occur inside healthy root tissue because for many crops, *Pseudomonas* populations have been demonstrated in these microsites (Schippers *et al.* 1987 *a, b*).

Whether the interactions shown in figure 2 function in the field needs further experimental evidence. So far they have attracted little attention. They may, however, have a large impact on crop yields.

## 4. SPONTANEOUS DISEASE SUPPRESSION BY RHIZOBACTERIA

According to Baker *et al.* (1986) the spontaneous suppression of wilt diseases caused by *formae speciales* of *Fusarium oxysporum* in fine sandy loam soils in the Salinas Valley of California, is most likely to be caused by siderophore-mediated competition for iron with certain *Pseudomonas putida* strains. No evidence for the participation of pseudomonads in parasitism, antibiosis, competition for carbon sources or in inducing plant resistance in suppressiveness was obtained. The biocontrol seems to be due particularly to inhibition of chlamydospore germination and of germ-tube growth in the saprophytic phase of the fungus in rhizosphere soil.

Cook and co-workers provided evidence that both siderophore production and production of antibiotic phenazin compounds by certain strains of fluorescent *Pseudomonas* spp. are involved in suppression of take all disease caused by the fungus *G. graminis* in continuous wheat culture in the Pacific Northwest of the U.S.A. Protection is thought to be primarily the result, of interference with the pathogen in its parasitic phase. Antibiotic negative mutants obtained by *Tn5* mutagenesis were significantly less suppressive of disease development than was the parent strain (Cook *et al.* 1988; Weller & Cook 1986 *a*).

Défago *et al.* (1987) selected a *P. fluorescens* strain CHA0 producing siderophores, hydrocyanic acid and several antibiotics, which they consider to be responsible for natural suppression in certain Swiss soils, of black root rot of tobacco caused by the fungus *Thielaviopsis basicola* (Ahl *et al.* 1986). The strain is also highly suppressive of take all in wheat (Défago *et al.* 1987). Its siderophores are not considered to be toxic not because they deplete the environment of $Fe^{3+}$, but because they increase the $Fe^{3+}$ concentration to the point where it becomes toxic to the many fungi tested (Ahl *et al.* 1986). Hydrocyanic acid production by the *P. fluorescens* strain CHA0 is supposed to be produced particularly inside the initially healthy root tissue, and to induce resistance to the pathogen. Mutants obtained by transposon mutagenesis, which had lost their ability to produce hydrocyanic acid, also had lost their ability to suppress disease (G. Défago, personal communication).

These examples demonstrate the rapid increase in our knowledge of biocontrol by rhizosphere pseudomonads, the diversity of the mechanisms and of the sites of disease suppression and the contributions of molecular and cell biological techniques to elucidating these mechanisms.

Interesting information has also recently been obtained on induction of suppression by rhizosphere pseudomonads of seedling diseases in wheat caused by *Pythium* spp. (Weller & Cook 1986 *b*), in cotton by *Pythium* spp. and *Rhizoctonia solani* (Howell & Stipanovic 1979, 1980) and on decreasing infection of potato daughter tubers by *Erwinia carotovora* (Xu & Gross 1986; Rhodes & Logan 1986).

## 5. FIELD TRIALS: SUCCESSES AND FAILURES

Significant control of diseases and consequent increases in plant development and yield have been obtained for a variety of soil-borne pathogens and crops in field trials (table 1). Biocontrol of *Pythium* spp. in wheat with *Pseudomonas* spp. was similar to control with the fungicide metalaxyl (Weller & Cook 1986 *b*). Treatment of potato tubers with *P. putida* WCS358 increased yields of seed tuber of potatoes in short rotations to those of potatoes in long rotations (Bakker *et al.* 1986 *a*).

The major problem, however, is the failure to repeat these results consistently on different soils or in different years in naturally contaminated fields and to make biological control of soil-borne pathogens competitive with chemical control (Capper & Campbell 1986; Geels *et al.* 1986). The factors involved are various and of physical, chemical and biological origin. Insufficient root colonization seems to be a major factor. With spontaneous or natural

288 B. SCHIPPERS

suppression of *Fusarium* wilts and of root rot caused by *Thielaviopsis basicola*, the function and perpetuation of the microbial antagonism seem to depend on soil properties such as the absence (illite) or presence (vermiculite) of particular clay minerals (Stutz *et al.* 1985), iron availability and soil pH (Baker *et al.* 1986). The presence of the pathogen may also be a factor in selectively stimulating and perpetuating the antagonistic *Pseudomonas* populations.

## 6. ROOT COLONIZATION AND SURVIVAL OF RHIZOBACTERIA

Antibiotic resistance labelling of rhizobacteria, either by selection of spontaneous mutants or by transposon mutagenesis, has recently provided much information on their distribution and survival in field soils. When applied to seed or seed tubers, labelled strains of *Pseudomonas* spp. could be reisolated from all parts of potato and wheat plants throughout the summer or winter (Bahme & Schroth 1987; Geels *et al.* 1986; Bakker *et al.* 1986a). Their distribution over the root system, however, is lognormal (Loper *et al.* 1984b, 1985) and parts of roots or even complete roots may not be colonized at all (Bahme & Schroth 1987). Population sizes and distribution were recently shown to be much affected by soil types differing in pore sizes, adsorbing clay particles, organic colloids and water movement, especially along roots (Bahme & Schroth 1987).

Detailed sampling of underground parts of potato plants in the field throughout the season in California and in The Netherlands revealed that population densities of introduced strains of *Pseudomonas* spp. sufficient to protect against pathogens occur primarily on plant roots within ±15 cm from treated seed tubers, depending on soil type (Bahme & Schroth 1987; P. A. H. M. Bakker, A. W. Bakker & B. Schippers, unpublished results). According to Bahme & Schroth (1987), greatest protection therefore is most likely to occur in the crown area against pathogens attacking juvenile tissue, including seed-decaying bacteria, fungi such as *Pythium* spp. and ill-defined deleterious rhizosphere microorganisms. The distribution of antagonistic strains of *Pseudomonas* spp. that develop inside the root tissue, however, may be different and less affected by environmental factors.

Whether strains of *Pseudomonas* spp. that keep pace with growth of roots through soil can be obtained or constructed seems questionable as their generation times are too slow. Differences in abilities to survive in soil and to colonize parts of young roots growing through the soil, however, are worth exploring. Bahme & Schroth (1987) noticed that their *Pseudomonas* strain A1-B persisted in non-rhizosphere soil throughout the season. In our field experiments with fluorescent *Pseudomonas* spp. strain WCS292G, antagonistic to the take-all pathogen of wheat *G. graminis*, improved protection of roots was obtained if the pseudomonads were introduced in the preceding year (J. G. Lamers & B. Schippers, unpublished results).

## 7. GENETIC MANIPULATION

Selective elimination of the production of microbial metabolites such as siderophores, antibiotics or hydrocyanic acid by transposon mutagenesis has enhanced the possibility of understanding mechanisms of antagonism *in vivo*. Similarly, genetic manipulation will be a valuable tool in detecting the traits for microbial survival and root colonizing abilities. This may lead to increased efficacy and consistency of biological control by management of antagonistic rhizobacteria. Analysis of the molecular genetics of siderophore biosynthesis by strains of *Pseudomonas* spp. with potential as biocontrol agents is in progress for three isolates: *P. fluorescens/putida* B10 (Moores *et al.* 1984), *P. syringae* pv. *syringae* JL 2000 (Loper *et al.* 1984*a*) and *P. putida* WCS358 (Marugg *et al.* 1985). These studies may show how to manipulate production of siderophore or siderophore receptors in new, improved strains for use as biocontrol agents.

This approach does, however, raise questions about the risks of introducing microorganisms obtained by recombinant DNA into the environment.

## 8. CONCLUSIONS

Several genera of rhizobacteria have the potential to be used successfully for the biological control of soil-borne plant pathogens. The site of their interactions with the different pathogens and their hosts and the mechanisms of the interactions are diverse even for the genus *Pseudomonas*. The slow development of commercial use of rhizobacteria is due largely to the inconsistency of results in the field. To improve this situation, more fundamental knowledge is needed on the biotic and abiotic factors affecting the population dynamics, survival and antagonistic activity of the rhizobacteria *in situ*, particularly by the use of molecular biological techniques. More research also is needed on the technology of using rhizobacteria, especially in formulating commercial products and manipulation of the environment in which they will be used.

Biological control with rhizobacteria is only one of the many biocontrol mechanisms that operate as part of a complex system in nature. The real challenge is to integrate it with other systems of control such as (induced) resistance, other mechanisms of microbial antagonism and control of the environment.

I thank my co-workers Peter A. H. M. Bakker, Albert W. Bakker and Patrick Geels, whose work I have cited; the Netherlands Technology Foundation (STW) for support of the work and Dr R. Harling for his critical reading of the text.

## REFERENCES

Ahl, P., Voisard, C. & Défago, G. 1986 Iron bound-siderophores, cyanic acid, and antibiotics involved in suppression of *Thielaviopsis basicola* by a *Pseudomonas fluorescens* strain. *J. Phytopath.* **116**, 121–134.
Bahme, J. B. & Schroth, M. N. 1987 Spatial–temporal colonization patterns of a rhizobacterium on underground organs of potato. *Phytopathology* **77**, 1093–1100.
Baker, R., Elad, Y. & Sneh, B. 1986 Physical, biological and host factors in iron competition in soils. In *Iron, siderophores, and plant diseases* (ed. T. R. Swinburne), pp. 77–84. New York: Plenum.
Bakker, A. W. & Schippers, B. 1988 Microbial cyanide production in the rhizosphere in relation to potato yield reduction and *Pseudomonas* spp.-mediated plant growth-stimulation. *Soil Biol. Biochem.* (In the press.)
Bakker, P. A. H. M., Lamers, J. G., Bakker, A. W., Marugg, J. D., Weisbeek, P. J. & Schippers, B. 1986*a* The role of siderophores in potato tuber yield increase by *Pseudomonas putida* in a short rotation of potato. *Neth. J. Pl. Path.* **92**, 249–256.
Bakker, P. A. H. M., Weisbeek, P. J. & Schippers, B. 1986*b* The role of siderophores in plant growth stimulation by fluorescent *Pseudomonas* spp. *Med. Fac. Landbouww. Rijksuniv. Gent* **51**, 1357–1362.
Burr, T. J. & Caesor, A. 1984 Beneficial plant bacteria. *CRC crit Rev. Pl. Sci.* **2**, 1–20.
Capper, A. L. & Campbell, R. 1986 The effect of artificially inoculated antagonistic bacteria on the prevalence of take-all disease of wheat in field experiments. *J. appl. Bacteriol.* **60**, 155–160.

Cook, R. J., Thomashow, L. S. & Weller, D. M. 1988 Fungal–bacterial interactions in the root region, with special reference to antagonism of wheat root-infecting fungi by rhizobacteria. In *Fourth International Symposium on Microbial Ecology, Ljubljana, 1986*. (In the press.)

Défago, G., Berling, C. H., Henggeler, S., Hungerbühler, W., Kern, H., Schleppi, P., Stutz, E. W. & Zürrer, M. 1987 Survie d'un *Pseudomonas fluorescens* dans le sol et protection du blé contre des maladies d'origine fongique. *Schweiz. Landw. Recherche agronom. Suisse* **26**, 155–160.

Geels, F. P. & Schippers, B. 1983 Reduction of yield depressions in high frequency potato cropping soil after seed tuber treatments with antagonistic fluorescent *Pseudomona* spp. *Phytopath. Z.* **108**, 207–214.

Geels, F. P., Lamers, J. G., Hoekstra, O. & Schippers, B. 1986 Potato plant response to seed tuber bacterization in the field in various rotations. *Neth. J. Pl. Path.* **92**, 257–272.

Gupta, V. K. & Utkhede, R. S. 1986 Factors affecting the production of anti-fungal compounds by *Enterobacter aerogenes* and *Bacillus subtilis*, antagonists of *Phytophthore cactorum*. *J. Phytopath.* **117**, 9–16.

Howell, C. R. & Stipanovic, R. D. 1979 Control of *Rhizoctonia solani* on cotton seedlings with *Pseudomonas fluorescens* and with an antibiotic produced by the bacterium. *Phytopathology* **69**, 480–482.

Howell, C. R. & Stipanovic, R. D. 1980 Suppression of *Pythium ultimum*-induced damping-off of cotton seedlings by *Pseudomonas fluorescens* and its antibiotic, pyoluteorin. *Phytopathology* **70**, 712–715.

Kloepper, J. W., Leong, J., Teintze, M., Schroth, M. N. 1980 Enhanced plant growth by siderophores produced by plant growth promoting rhizobacteria. *Nature, Lond.* **286**, 885–886.

Kloepper, J. W. & Schroth, M. N. 1981 Relationship of in vitro antibiosis of PGPR to plant growth and the displacement of root microflora. *Phytopathology* **71**, 1020–1024.

Leong, J. 1986 Siderophores: their biochemistry and possible role in the biocontrol of plant pathogens. *A. Rev. Phytopath.* **24**, 187–209.

Loper, J. E., Haack, C., Schroth, M. N. 1985 Population dynamics of soil pseudomonads in the rhizosphere of potato (*Solanum tuberosum* L.). *Appl. envir. Microbiol.* **49**, 416–427.

Loper, J. E., Orser, C. S., Panopoulos, N. J. & Schroth, M. N. 1984*a* Genetic analysis of fluorescent pigment production in *Pseudomonas syringae* pv. *syringae*. *J. gen. Microbiol.* **130**, 1507–1515.

Loper, J. E., Suslow, T. V. & Schroth, M. N. 1984*b* Lognormal distribution of bacterial populations in the rhizosphere. *Phytopathology* **74**, 1454–1460.

Marugg, J. D., Spanje, M. van, Hoekstra, W. P. M., Schippers, B. & Weisbeek, P. J. 1985 Isolation and analysis of genes involved in siderophore-biosynthesis in the plant growth-stimulating *Pseudomonas putida* strain WCS358. *J. Bacteriol.* **164**, 563–570.

Moores, J. C., Magazin, M., Ditta, G. S., Leong, J. 1984 Cloning of genes involved in the biosynthesis of pseudobactin, a high-affinity iron transport agent of a plant growth-promoting *Pseudomonas* strain. *J. Bacteriol.* **157**, 53–58.

Neilands, J. B. 1981 Microbial iron compounds. *A. Rev. Biochem.* **50**, 715–731.

Rhodes, D. J. & Logan, C. 1986 Effects of fluorescent pseudomonads on the potato blackleg syndrome. *Ann. appl. Biol.* **108**, 511–518.

Schippers, B., Bakker, A. W. & Bakker, P. A. H. M. 1987*a* Interactions of deleterious and beneficial rhizosphere microorganisms and the effect of cropping practices. *A. Rev. Phytopath.* **25**, 339–358.

Schippers, B., Bakker, P. A. H. M., Bakker, A. W., Hofstad, G. A. J. M. van der, Marugg, J. D., Weger, L. A. de, Lamers, J. G., Hoekstra, W. P. M. & Lugtenberg, B. 1986 Molecular aspects of plant growth affecting *Pseudomonas* spp. In *Recognition in microbe-plant symbiotic and pathogenic interactions* (ed. B. Lugtenberg), pp. 395–404. Berlin, Heidelberg and New York: Springer.

Schippers, B., Lugtenberg, B. & Weisbeek, P. J. 1987*b* Plant growth control by fluorescent pseudomonas. In *Innovative approaches to plant disease control* (ed. I. Chet), pp. 19–39. New York and Toronto: John Wiley.

Sneh, B. 1981 Use of rhizosphere chitinolytic bacteria for biological control of *Fusarium oxysporum* f.sp. *dianthi* in carnation. *Phytopath. Z.* **100**, 251–256.

Sneh, B., Agami, O., Baker, R. 1985 Biological control of *Fusarium*-wilt in carnation with *Serratia liquefaciens* and *Hafnia alvi* isolated from rhizosphere of carnation. *Phytopath. Z.* **113**, 271–276.

Stutz, E. W., Défago, G., Hantke, R. & Kern, H. 1985 The effect of parent materials derived from different geological strata on the suppressiveness of soils to black root rot of tobacco. In *Ecology and management of soilborne plant pathogens* (ed. C. A. Parker, A. D. Rovira, K. J. Moore, P. T. W. Wong, & J. F. Kollmorgen), pp. 215–217. St Paul, Minnesota: American Phytopathology Society.

Suslow, T. V. 1982 Role of root-colonizing bacteria in plant growth. In *Phytopathogenic prokaryotes* (ed. M. S. Mount & G. H. Lacy), vol. 1, pp. 187–223. New York and London: Academic Press.

Tu, J. C. 1978 Protection of soybean from severe *Phytophthora* root rot by Rhizobium. *Physiol. Pl. Path.* **12**, 233–240.

Utkhede, R. S. & Rahe, J. E. 1983 Effect of *Bacillus subtilis* on growth and protection of onion against white rot. *Phytopath. Z.* **106**, 199–203.

Weller, D. M. & Cook, R. J. 1986*a* Suppression of root diseases of wheat by fluorescent pseudomonads and mechanisms of action. In *Iron, siderophores and plant diseases* (ed. T. R. Swinburne), pp. 99–107. New York: Plenum.

Weller, D. M. & Cook, R. J. 1986 *b* Increased growth of wheat by seed treatments with fluorescent pseudomonads and implications of *Pythium* control. *Can. J. Plant Path.* **8**, 328–334.
Xu, G. W. & Gross, D. C. 1986 Field evaluation of interactions among fluorescent pseudomonads, *Erwinia carotovora* and potato yields. *Phytopathology* **76**, 423–430.
Yen, G. Y. & Schroth, M. N. 1986 Inhibition of *Fusarium oxysporum* f. sp. *dianthi* by iron competition with an *Alcaligenes* sp. *Phytopathology* **76**, 171–176.

## Discussion

J. M. Lynch (*Glasshouse Crops Research Institute, Littlehampton, U.K.*). Would Professor Schippers please comment on (1) the observation that pseudobactin, the siderophore produced by rhizosphere bacteria, can inhibit the uptake of iron by plants and (2) the relative affinity constants of plant and microbial siderophores?

B. Schippers. (1) Becker *et al.* (1985) showed that addition of pseudobactin to a nutrient solution can inhibit $Fe^{3+}$ assimilation by maize and pea plants. Such a treatment probably leads to a decrease of iron availability over the entire root system because of binding of ferric ions in the nutrient solution by pseudobactin. In soil, pseudobactin will only be produced locally by *Pseudomonas* bacteria in micro-sites. Moreover, other microbial siderophores may enhance $Fe^{3+}$ assimilation by plants. Dicotyledonous plants can react to iron deficiency by releasing protons from the roots. This reaction will create micro-environments with a low pH unfavourable for growth of pseudobactin-producing pseudomonads or pseudobactin production or both. Thus pseudomonads in the rhizosphere do not necessarily interfere with iron acquisition by the plant.

(2) Affinity constants ($\log_{10}Kf$) of microbial siderophores for ferric ion vary from 22.9 (aerobactin) to 52 (enterobactin).

Phytosiderophores such as aminohydroxylcarboxylates (in root washings of graminaceous plants) have a $\log_{10}Kf$ equal to 18. Affinity constants of phytosiderophores seem not to be so high as those of bacterial and fungal siderophores.

### References

Becker, J. O., Messens, E. & Hedges, R. W. 1985 The influence of agrobactin on the uptake of ferric iron by plants. *FEMS microb. Ecol* **31**, 171–175.
Hider, R. C. 1986 The facilitation of iron uptake in bacteria and plants by substituted catechols. In *Iron siderophores and plant diseases* (ed. T. R. Swinburne), pp. 49–60. New York and London: Plenum.
Neilands, J. B. 1981 Microbial iron compounds. *A. Rev. Biochem.* **50**, 715–731.

P. Neuenschwander (*International Institute of Tropical Agriculture, Ibadan, Nigeria*). May I ask a general question as an entomologist to pathologists working in biological control?

Do they do, or can they do, studies in population dynamics? And if so, do they consider such studies relevant?

B. Schippers. Yes, we can do studies in population dynamics. Gilligan (1985) has an introductory chapter and his own chapter on disease progress of soil-borne plant pathogens. He points out that modelling crop disease is a rapidly expanding discipline, but one with a relatively short history compared with the study of insect population dynamics. He nominates work in the 1960s as the beginning of the present mathematical phase (see, for example, Van der Plank 1963).

D. Bouhot & Joannes (1983) have produced a simple deterministic model in population dynamics in soil that is an application of the logistic equation to two competing populations (*Pythium* spp. v. microflora in his bioassay).

For many years there has been much interest in inoculum and infection, which has necessitated knowing about populations of propagules and this can be traced back to Gregory's (1948) multiple infection transformation and beyond. R. Baker's interest in models of root infection go back to the early 1960s (Baker 1965). D. Hornby (1981) tried to quantify inoculum of the take-all fungus.

*References*

Baker, R. 1965 The dynamics of inoculum. In *Ecology of soil-borne plant pathogens*. (ed. K. F. Baker & W. C. Snyder), pp. 395–419. Berkeley: University of California Press.

Bouhot, D. & Joannes, H. 1983 Potential infectieux des sols – concept et modèles. *Bull. OEPP* **13**, 291–295.

Gilligan, C. A. (ed.) 1985 Mathematical modelling of crop diseases. In *Advances in plant pathology*, vol. 3. (245 pages.) London and New York: Academic Press.

Gregory, P. H. 1948 The multiple-infection transformation. *Ann. appl. Biol.* **35**, 412–417.

Hornby, D. 1981 Inoculum. In *Biology and control of take-all* (ed. M. J. C. Asher & P. J. Shipton), pp. 271–293. London: Academic Press.

Scott, P. R. & Bainbridge, A. 1978 *Plant disease epidemiology* (329 pages.) Oxford: Blackwell Scientific Publications.

Van der Plank, 1963 *Plant disease: epidemics and control.* (349 pages.) New York: Academic Press.

Zadoks, J. C. & Schein, R. F. 1977 *Epidemiology and plant disease management.* (427 pages.) Oxford University Press.

J. W. DEACON (*Department of Microbiology, Edinburgh University, U.K.*). If, as Professor Schippers, suggests, some deleterious rhizobacteria produce cyanide, which depends on an adequate supply of iron, and if this benefits these bacteria by making root cells more 'leaky', then I would expect these bacteria to develop effective siderophores and siderophore-uptake mechanisms. In such circumstances it is difficult to see how these deleterious bacteria would be controlled by siderophore-producing beneficial rhizobacteria. In any case, I would expect such control to be only temporary, because it would select for effective siderophore-producers among the deleterious bacteria.

B. SCHIPPERS. Our hypothesis is that by frequent cropping of potato, the production of hydrocyanide by rhizosphere inhabiting pseudomonads increases either by increasing availability of iron for these particular pseudomonads and/or by increasing the availability in soil of precursors of microbial HCN production. The increasing availability of iron for HCN-producing pseudomonads could for example originate in accumulation of *Pseudomonas* spp. $Fe^{3+}$-siderophores, that are recognized and utilized by the HCN-producing pseudomonads. The introduction in the rhizosphere of (plant growth promoting) pseudomonads, the $Fe^{3+}$-siderophores of which cannot be recognized by HCN-producing pseudomonads (such as that of our strain WCS358), then reduces the availability of $Fe^{3+}$. I agree that this may select for deleterious (HCN-producing) bacteria that can use the competitive (WCS358) siderophore, as also stated in Schippers *et al.* (1986) and Schippers *et al.* (1987*a*).

B. C. HEMMING (*Monsanto Life Services Research Center, St Louis, U.S.A.*). Because our *in vitro* experiments have demonstrated that HCN production by fluorescent pseudomonads is medium- or substrate-dependent, what evidence exists for production of HCN *in situ* (i.e. on plants or in soils) by bacterial isolates?

The creation of insertional mutants by Dr Défago, and their evaluation, certainly implicates involvement of HCN in the processes observed. Increased root hair extension and development of epidermal transfer cells has, however, also been shown to occur under plant iron stress.

B. SCHIPPERS. We do not have evidence yet, for HCN production *in situ* by bacterial isolates; however, we recently have demonstrated that growth of potato plants can be decreased significantly by concentrations of HCN below the limits of detection. HCN was produced by bacterial isolates inoculated on sterile squashed potato roots on a mineral nutrients agar plate.

J. A. LUCAS (*Department of Botany, University of Nottingham, U.K.*). I was wondering about this suggested phenomenon of induced resistance in roots. Is it being proposed that these rhizobacteria somehow trigger a host response in root tissues? If so, what mechanisms are envisaged, and how do these bacteria differ from others in the resident rhizosphere microflora that do not induce resistance?

B. SCHIPPERS. Yes, indeed it is hypothesized that specific *Pseudomonas* spp. strains trigger a host response in root tissue. Their HCN production inside the root tissue, by suppressing the cytochrome oxidase respiration pathway and stimulating the alternative respiration pathway, possibly triggers the production of secondary metabolites, toxic to the pathogen.

These bacteria may differ from others in the resident rhizosphere microflora by their strong HCN production and by their ability to develop inside the healthy root tissue.

G. DÉFAGO (*Swiss Federal Institute of Technology, Zürich, Switzerland*). In answer to the question [not printed] about resistance in tobacco to *Thielaviopsis basicola* induced by a selected wild-type strain of *Pseudomonas fluorescens* there are the following points: (1) the wild-type strain produces HCN when colonizing roots; HCN is known to induce in roots an alternative respiratory pathway that is associated with the synthesis of phytoalexins; (2) the strain increases the production of phenolic compounds in the roots; (3) it greatly stimulates the formation of root hairs; and (4) it suppresses disease.

In contrast, an HCN⁻ mutant induced by *Tn5* insertion: (1) did not stimulate formation of root hairs; and (2) did not suppress disease. Also the wild-type strain does suppress disease in soil with vermiculite clay minerals but does not in soil with illite clays. CN bound to vermiculite clays induces root hair formation whereas CN bound to illite clays does not. Finally, a 'rough' mutant that did not suppress disease was confined to root surfaces whereas the effective wild-type strain penetrated and grew inside roots. From these facts it may be concluded that the wild-type strain suppresses disease by growing inside roots and by producing HCN which then alters the physiology of roots in ways that make them resistant to the pathogen.

*Phil. Trans. R. Soc. Lond.* B **318**, 295–317 (1988)

*Printed in Great Britain*

# Control of plant pathogens with viruses and related agents

By K. W. Buck

*Department of Pure and Applied Biology, Imperial College of Science and Technology,
London SW7 2BB, U.K.*

Cytoplasmically transmissible agents causing diseases of plant pathogenic fungi characterized by reductions in pathogenicity, ability to form sexual and asexual spores, spore viability and growth rate, are often associated with the presence of one or more specific segments of virus-like double-stranded RNA (dsRNA). In Italy, hypovirulent dsRNA-containing strains of the chestnut blight fungus, *Endothia* (*Cryphonectria*) *parasitica*, have become predominant in many areas where blight is no longer a serious problem. dsRNA-containing strains of other pathogens, with various degrees of debilitation, survive in natural populations but have not become predominant or resulted in any great reduction in disease. Examples include the Dutch elm disease fungus, *Ophiostoma* (*Ceratocystis*) *ulmi*, and the wheat take-all fungus, *Gaeumannomyces graminis* var. *tritici*. Successful biological control of such pathogens could probably be achieved, however, if methods could be developed to suppress the loss of dsRNA that occurs during the sexual and other stages of their life cycles, and to suppress the vegetative incompatibility reactions that reduce the cytoplasmic transmission of dsRNA. Systemic infection with attenuated strains of plant viruses can protect plants from later infection by virulent strains of the same or closely related viruses. Despite some notable successes, e.g. control of citrus tristeza and tomato mosaic viruses, such 'cross-protection' has not been widely applied because of the cost and difficulty of application, and caution about the widespread distribution of infectious agents in the environment. These problems could be overcome if cross-protection could be achieved by the expression of a single viral gene rather than infection with intact virus, and consideration of possible mechanisms of cross protection suggests novel ways of producing virus-resistant plants.

## 1. Introduction

There are a number of ways in which viruses might be used to control plant pathogens: (1) viruses may kill or reduce the pathogenicity of bacterial and fungal pathogens of plants; (2) viruses may kill invertebrate vectors of viruses of higher plants and thus prevent their spread; (3) mild strains causing little or no disease may protect plant hosts from later infection by more severe strains. Vidaver (1976) considered that bacteriocins were more promising and less risky than bacteriophages for control of bacterial plant pathogens, whereas the current status of insect viruses in biocontrol systems (Payne, this symposium) makes it unlikely that they will replace chemical pesticides in controlling insect vectors of plant viruses. In contrast, the recovery of blighted chestnuts in many areas of Italy associated with the spread of virus-like nucleic acids through the population of the pathogen *Endothia* (*Cryphonectria*) *parasitica* is one of the few known examples of natural biological control of a plant disease. Likewise, the protection of citrus trees in Brazil by pre-infection with mild strains of citrus tristeza virus is a spectacular example of biological control of a plant virus by the intervention of man. Reasons why these biocontrol systems have been successful, and the possibilities of applying similar

[ 185 ]

principles to other systems, will be discussed. Examples of novel ways of producing virus-resistant plants arising from consideration of the mechanisms of biological control will be presented.

## 2. Viruses of plant pathogenic fungi and their potential as biological control agents

### (a) General properties of fungal viruses

#### (i) Occurrence

Viral infections of fungi are common and have been found in all the major fungal subdivisions. Within some species a large proportion of individuals may be infected; for example, Stanway (1985) detected virus infection in 126 out of 157 field isolates of the wheat take-all fungus. *Gaeumannomyces graminis* var. *tritici*. Several morphological types of particle have been detected in different fungi, but isometric viruses with genomes of double-stranded RNA (dsRNA) are most frequent (Buck 1986a). In a few fungi, dsRNA is not enclosed in isometric particles. In *E. parasitica* the dsRNA is enclosed in lipid-rich vesicles (Hansen *et al.* 1985). The structural properties of the dsRNA (Tartaglia *et al.* 1986; Hiremath *et al.* 1986) and its association with membrane structures that contain RNA-dependent RNA polymerase activity (Hansen *et al.* 1985) suggest a viral origin, although it has also been proposed that the dsRNA may be the replicative form of a single-stranded RNA virus (Tartaglia *et al.* 1986). In *Ophiostoma (Ceratocystis) ulmi* dsRNA is associated with the mitochondria (Rogers 1987; Rogers *et al.* 1988a).

#### (ii) Transmission

Viruses of fungi differ from those of other hosts in that they generally do not lyse their host cells and are apparently transmitted only by intracellular routes (Buck 1986a). Within a fungal strain, virus particles are carried forward in the net flow of protoplasm towards the growing hyphal tip so that a fungus maintained in the mycelial state may remain infected indefinitely. Transmission into asexual spores is usually very efficient, although partial or complete loss of viral genomes has been observed at low frequency during conidiogenesis in some fungi.

Transmission between fungal strains can occur after fusion between somatic or sexual cells of the same species. Transmission by hyphal anastomosis can be limited further by vegetative incompatibility reactions when one or more vegetative compatibility (v-c) genes of the individuals are different. A fungus may have as many as seven v-c genes giving 128 possible v-c types, assuming two alleles of each gene. Transmission is usually very efficient when all v-c genes are the same, becomes increasingly less efficient with increasing number of v-c gene differences, with modulating effects caused by differing 'strengths' of individual v-c genes and different host genetic backgrounds (Anagnostakis 1983, 1984; Brasier 1984, 1986a). Sexual transmission of viruses will depend (for heterothallic organisms) on compatibility of mating-type genes. In the Basidiomycetes, transmission of viruses into sexual spores appears to be efficient, although incompatibility between dsRNA segments of different strains can lead to exclusion of some segments, e.g. in the corn smut fungus, *Ustilago maydis* (Wigderson & Koltin 1982). In a number of Ascomycetes host exclusion mechanisms result in the absence in ascospore progeny of all or most of the dsRNA segments of the parents, e.g. in *G. graminis* var.

*tritici* (McFadden *et al.* 1983), *O. ulmi* (Rogers *et al.* 1986*a*) and *Helminthosporium maydis* (Bozarth 1977). Overall, the ability of a virus to spread through a fungal population will depend on the heterogeneity of populations with respect to v-c and mating-type genes, possible host- or dsRNA-mediated exclusion reactions and the relative importance of the sexual stage in the biology of the fungus.

(iii) *Effect on fungal phenotype*

Many fungi tolerate viral infection without any apparent adverse effect. However, viral infection can alter a fungal phenotype, not as a general result of the presence of viral particles or dsRNA, but as a consequence of the expression of specific coding sequences within one or more dsRNA segments. For example, killer strains of *U. maydis* secrete protein toxins that kill sensitive strains of the same or related species. Many isolates of *U. maydis* contain multiple segments of dsRNA (Day 1981), but only those containing the specific dsRNA segments encoding protein toxins and immunity from them are killers (Koltin 1986; Shelbourn *et al.* 1987) and these are only a small proportion of natural populations (Day & Dodds 1979). Ability to produce killer toxin does not appear to alter the pathogenicity of *U. maydis* strains. However, Koltin & Day (1975) suggested that if the toxin-encoding sequences could be introduced into the genome of cereals and expressed by the plants, smut-resistant plants could be produced.

In some instances various degrees of debilitation or disease of the fungus, such as abnormal morphology, slow growth, reduced sexual and asexual sporulation, and a marked decrease in pathogenicity (often termed hypovirulence) have been shown to be associated with specific dsRNA segments. Examples include diseased or hypovirulent strains of *E. parasitica* (Van Alfen 1986), *O. ulmi* (Rogers *et al.* 1986*a*), *Helminthosporium victoriae* (Ghabrial 1986) and *Rhizoctonia solani* (Castanho & Butler 1978*a*). The role of specific dsRNA segments is inferred from observations that their transmission by hyphal anastomosis results in conversion of healthy recipients to the diseased phenotype, whereas loss of segments from diseased isolates results in recovery from the disease; proof by direct infection of healthy isolates with viral particles or dsRNA has not yet been achieved and hence the possibility that these phenotypes might be caused by defective mitochondrial DNA or DNA plasmids (Bockelmann *et al.* 1986) cannot be excluded.

(*b*) *Strategies for biological control*

Weakly pathogenic or nonpathogenic variants of a plant pathogen or related species may have the ability to protect plants from attack by the pathogen, e.g. control of *G. graminis* var. *tritici* by *Phialophora* spp. (Wong 1981). Protection may result from direct competition by prior occupation of infection sites on the host and from induction of host resistance. In weakly pathogenic organisms having multiple differences from the pathogen at the nuclear rather than the cytoplasmic level, the phenotype is not cytoplasmically transmitted. In contrast, when hypovirulence results from cytoplasmic genetic elements (H-factors), such as dsRNA, the hypovirulent strains have the potential to control a pathogen even after the latter has infected its host. Such curative properties are the result of transmission of H-factors from the weakly pathogenic (hypovirulent) to the strongly pathogenic (virulent) strains, making the latter hypovirulent.

The strategy for biological control by using isolates with cytoplasmically determined hypovirulence will depend on several variables, such as the nature of the host–pathogen interaction, the biological cycle of the pathogen, the properties of the virus-infected pathogen, the transmissibility of the virus and whether the host is annual or perennial. To illustrate how such variables may affect the strategy, two tree pathogens with different biological cycles, namely *E. parasitica* and *O. ulmi*, will be compared. Possibilities for control of annual crops with hypovirulent strains will then be assessed and ways of resolving current problems will be considered.

### (c) *Recovery of blighted chestnuts in Italy: an example of natural biological control*

The epidemic of chestnut blight in North America which started around the beginning of the twentieth century has eliminated the American chestnut, *Castanea dentata*, as an important economic tree (reviewed by Elliston (1982), Anagnostakis (1982) and Van Alfen (1982, 1986)). This devastating canker disease is caused by the fungus *E. parasitica*, which is spread by both sexual spores (ascospores), adapted for transmission by wind, and asexual spores (conidia) adapted for transmission by rain and possibly by insects, small mammals and birds. Infection is initiated at wounds in the bark, and trees are killed by mycelial fans that rapidly invade bark tissue encircling and girdling the branch or trunk, penetrate the cambium and block the vascular system. The roots of killed trees produce sprouts, but these generally only survive for up to four or five years before being killed by *E. parasitica*.

Chestnut blight was first found in Italy in 1938 and by 1950 was widely distributed in the northern and southern chestnut growing regions of the country. However, soon afterwards in a chestnut coppice near Genoa, once severely damaged by *E. parasitica*, it was noticed that although a large proportion of shoots were infected, only a few showed characteristic symptoms. On most shoots cankers were healing and the fungus was restricted to the outer layer of bark (Biraghi 1953). Isolates from the bark of such trees differed from normal *E. parasitica* in morphology and degree of pigmentation, produced fewer conidia more slowly, were nonpathogenic or only weakly pathogenic to *Castanea sativa*, and when inoculated into cankers cured existing blight (Grente 1965; Grente & Sauret 1969). A small proportion of conidia of such hypovirulent (H) strains reverted to normal virulent (V) strains, confirming their identity as *E. parasitica* and suggesting that hypovirulence is caused by a cytoplasmic genetic element (H-factor). This was proved by transmitting H-factors by hyphal anastomosis (Berthelay-Sauret 1973; Van Alfen *et al.* 1975), and correlative evidence strongly suggests that H-factors are dsRNA molecules (Day *et al.* 1977; Fulbright 1984; Elliston 1985). The spread of H strains in Italy led to a steady decline in the incidence of chestnut blight so that by 1978 it was no longer a serious problem (Mittempergher 1978; Turchetti 1978, 1979).

The current dominance of hypovirulent strains that has led to the re-establishment of the chestnut in Italy stems from a combination of several factors.

1. H strains parasitize chestnut trees but produce only superficial cankers and do not cause significant disease. There appears to be little difference in initial responses of chestnuts that are wounded and immediately inoculated with H or V strains (Hebard *et al.* 1984). In both cases, lesions or wounds are delimited initially by a zone of lignified tissue and formation of wound periderm begins at the deepest part of the wound and progresses outwards to the bark surface. Fully formed wound periderm appears to be completely resistant to mycelial fans of V or H strains. However, mycelial fans of V strains develop quickly, penetrate the lignified zone and developing wound periderm, halt wound periderm formation by killing cells in front of the

advancing hyphae and eventually colonize the vascular cambium. In contrast, mycelial fans of H strains develop more slowly and, although they can penetrate lignified zones and developing periderm, are blocked by fully formed periderm before they reach the vascular cambium. The host response therefore develops rapidly enough to control the slow-growing H strains, but not the faster-growing V strains. This explanation is consistent with the observation that even H strains can infect newly made graft wounds and kill scions of hybrid chestnuts that can only be propagated vegetatively (Turchetti 1979), presumably because they colonize exposed vascular cambium before it is protected by callus tissue.

2. Although H strains are less vigorous than V strains in that they develop more slowly on chestnut trees and produce fewer conidia, they are not too debilitated to survive in nature.

3. H strains compete successfully with compatible V strains. This is due to transmission of the cytoplasmic determinants for hypovirulence from H to V strains resulting in 'hypovirulence conversion', and not to direct competition. In fact, when H-factor transmission is blocked by vegetative incompatibility, H strains compete poorly with V strains and do not arrest canker development (Anagnostakis 1982). In Italy, conversion to hypovirulence seems to have been facilitated by strains belonging to only one or a few v-c groups in the regions where H strains have become predominant.

4. H strains do not readily revert to virulence because most conidia of H strains are hypovirulent (Van Alfen *et al.* 1978), and no European H strains are known to produce ascospores (Elliston 1982). By depressing the sexual stage of their hosts, H factors have promoted their own survival because dsRNA is normally lost during ascospore formation.

5. H strains can be transmitted from tree to tree. Their efficient spread is essential not only for survival, but also for control of V strains. Prior infection with H strains does not protect trees from infection with V strains in other locations on the tree; to be effective in control, H strains need the capacity to be transmitted to newly formed cankers caused by V strains.

In Italy all the above factors favour the establishment of equilibria not only between hypovirulent strains and the European chestnut but also between H-factors (which can be regarded as hyperparasites) and *E. parasitica*. As a result, Italian forest chestnuts are still being used as a source of timber.

Limited success in controlling blight in chestnut orchards in France and Switzerland has been obtained by treating cankers with mixtures of H strains in different v-c groups. In areas where V strains belong to one or a few v-c groups there is evidence for spread of H strains and their curative properties to other trees in the locality (Grente 1981; Bazzigher *et al.* 1981).

In North America, H strains have been obtained from naturally recovering chestnut trees in Michigan, Pennsylvania, Tennesse and Virginia (Anagnostakis 1982) with evidence for their spread in Michigan (Fulbright *et al.* 1983). Both European and American H strains are heterogeneous, varying in degree of pigmentation, morphology, sporulation and reduction of pathogenicity. This variation is probably due, at least in part, to variation of the dsRNA segments. Recent evidence suggests that a single molecule of dsRNA of about 9000 nucleotides may be sufficient to confer the hypovirulent phenotype (Hiremath *et al.* 1986; Tartaglia *et al.* 1986). A dsRNA of this size could encode five or six proteins of $M_r$ 50000, one or more of which could decrease pathogenicity to a degree varying with the dsRNA coding sequences of different H strains. Most H strains have several dsRNA segments, some being deletions of the largest dsRNA whereas others are probably satellites. Such molecules could modulate the level of hypovirulence and are a further source of variation.

Although dsRNA segments of European and North American H strains have similar terminal structures and have probably evolved from a common ancestor, they have evidently diverged considerably because no nucleotide sequence homology was detected between them by hybridization analysis (L'Hostis *et al.* 1985). However, it is likely that when the protein(s) responsible for hypovirulence is (are) identified and amino acid sequences determined, conserved functional domains will be revealed.

Attempts to use North American and European H-factors to control chestnut blight in North America have not met with widespread success. The ability of naturally occurring and introduced H-strains to spread in North America has been studied for only about 10 years whereas in Italy H-strains have been spreading for at least 36 years. It may therefore be too early to assess the situation in North America. However, possible lack of suitable vectors for spreading conidia of H-strains and the occurrence of large numbers of v-c groups in virulent isolates in North America are serious obstacles for blight control with H strains. In Connecticut, where natural spread of H-strains has not been observed, Anagnostakis (1983) classified 76 isolates in 14 forest lots of 1 acre† within Cockaponset State Forest into 35 different v-c groups. In tests of all possible combinations of 97 isolates, in pairs, all belonging to different v-c groups, transfer of the cytoplasmic determinants for curative morphology was efficient only between weakly barraging pairs that were a small proportion of the total (87 out of 4656). Possible ways in which vegetative compatibility reactions might be suppressed are considered in the next section.

### (d) Transmissible disease factors in Ophiostoma ulmi

The current epidemics of Dutch elm disease which have devastated the elm populations of Europe and North America are caused by two races of the aggressive subgroup of the ascomycete fungus *Ophiostoma (Ceratocystis) ulmi* (reviewed by Brasier (1986*b*, 1987)). The North American (NAN) race, responsible for epidemics in the U.S.A. and Canada, is believed to have been imported into the U.K. during the mid 1960s and has since spread southwards and eastwards (Brasier 1979, 1987; Houston 1985). The Eurasian (EAN) race appears to have originated from central Europe or further east and has spread westwards across Europe (Brasier 1979, 1987). In some countries, e.g. Holland and Italy, both races are now present with evidence for EAN–NAN hybrids (Brasier 1986*c*). The EAN race has not been found in North America.

The non-aggressive subgroup of *O. ulmi* is now thought to be that first recorded in northwest Europe in 1918, spreading quickly into other areas including the U.S.A. It causes relatively mild disease on European elms, competes poorly against either race of the aggressive subgroups, and may eventually become extinct (Brasier 1986*b*, 1987). The EAN and NAN races of the aggressive subgroups are sufficiently similar that they may have evolved comparatively recently from a common progenitor, perhaps through geographical isolation (Brasier & Webber 1987) although they also show important developmental differences. More extensive genetic differences are found between the non-aggressive and aggressive subgroups reinforced by reproductive isolation, precluding the possibility that the latter has arisen from the former by a simple mutation (Brasier 1982, 1987).

The biological cycle of *O. ulmi* has distinct pathogenic and saprophytic phases (see

† 1 acre = 0.405 hectare = 4046.856 m².

[ 190 ]

Webber & Brasier 1984; Brasier 1986 b). The pathogenic phase is initiated by bark beetles (Coleoptera: Scolytidae), which carry asexual spores and ascospores and feed in crotches of twigs on healthy trees in spring and summer. After spore germination and a brief mycelial phase the fungus invades xylem where it replicates as budding yeast-like cells. A host reaction, probably stimulated at least in part by various toxins produced by the fungus, such as cerato-ulmin (Richards & Takai 1984) leads to blockage of the xylem and death of the tree.

The saprophytic phase occurs in the bark, extending from late summer and autumn to spring and early summer of the following year, and originates not only from spores introduced by beetles that colonize the bark for breeding but also from fungus growing outwards from xylem into the bark. The fungus grows as a three dimensional network of interacting hyphae (Brasier 1984) in successive phases of colonization and recolonization, with distinct sequences of conidia, synnemata and perithecia (Lea & Brasier 1983; Webber & Brasier 1984). In spring, newly emerging adult beetles carry spores which initiate new disease cycles in the xylem of healthy elm trees.

Webber & Brasier (1984) have shown that *O. ulmi* has two overlapping cycles, an alternating pathogenic–saprophytic (xylem–bark) cycle and a completely saprophytic (bark–bark) cycle with direct transfer of inocula from breeding gallery to breeding gallery. It is clear that in the bark there is considerable potential for interactions between genotypes for the generation of new genotypes by sexual reproduction.

Diseased (d-infected) isolates of *O. ulmi*, characterized by slow growth, abnormal 'amoeboid' morphology, impaired ability to produce sexual spores, impaired viability of conidia and the ability to transmit the genetic determinants of the disease (d-factors) to healthy recipients by hyphal anastomosis, were described by Brasier (1983). Transmission from d-infected donor mycelia to healthy recipient mycelia is often accompanied by pigment production and by physical changes in the colony of the recipients, termed d-reactions. Studies with nuclear and cytoplasmic markers showed that the determinant was a cytoplasmic component, and indicated that it could be transmitted independently of marked mitochondria (Brasier 1983, 1986 a). Different d-factors have been designated $d^1$, $d^2$, etc., and can vary in their effects (Brasier 1986 a).

Diseased isolates have been found in the NAN and EAN races of the aggressive sub-group and in the non-aggressive subgroup (Brasier 1986 a). Multiple dsRNA segments have been found in all d-infected, and a considerable proportion of healthy, EAN and NAN isolates so far examined (Rogers *et al.* 1988 a). As in other dsRNA-determined phenotypes it appears that the diseased phenotypes are caused by specific sequences in one or more dsRNA segments. For example, $d^2$-infected isolates contain 10 dsRNA segments ranging in size from 3500 nucleotides to 340 nucleotides and numbered from 1 to 10 in order of decreasing size (Rogers *et al.* 1986 a). Transmission of the $d^2$-factor converted healthy to diseased phenotypes and conversion was accompanied by transmission of the 10 dsRNA segments. Transmission of the 10 dsRNA segments into conidia was efficient, but on the infrequent occasions when three or more dsRNA segments were lost, loss always included segments 4, 7 and 10 and the conidial isolates were healthy. Similar results were obtained after inoculating $d^2$-infected isolates into the xylem of young elm trees when the fungus multiplied in the yeast form. Recovered isolates that had lost segments 4, 7 and 10 were always healthy and it was concluded that the $d^2$-factor probably consisted of one or more of these three segments (Rogers *et al.* 1986 a). Ascospore progeny from sexual crosses between healthy and diseased isolates or between two diseased isolates were always healthy (Brasier 1983, 1986 c) and had lost all or most of the dsRNA segments of the parents (Rogers *et al.* 1986 a, 1988 a).

Although d-infected isolates survive in natural populations and are found at current epidemic fronts in Europe (Brasier 1986 a), they have not yet had a major impact on the spread or severity of Dutch elm disease. The proportion of d-infected individuals will depend on a dynamic equilibrium established by the opposing rates of acquisition and loss of d-factors by individuals and by the relative rates of propagation and death of healthy and d-infected isolates. Factors determining such gains and losses will vary with the heterogeneity of populations and their locations with respect to epidemic fronts.

Most isolates in regional collections of *O. ulmi* have been found to belong to different v-c groups. The latter would be expected to reduce the efficiency of spread of d-factors by hyphal anastomosis in the saprophytic phase in the bark because in fully vegetatively incompatible reactions d-factor spread is restricted to only *ca.* 4 % of pairings (Brasier 1984, 1986 a). However, in some locations significant proportions of isolates belong to single predominant v-c groups, (termed v-c supergroups) so that the proportion of d-infected isolates is larger than normal. For example, at the current epidemic front in Poland, 47 % of a sample of the *O. ulmi* population were in the same EAN v-c supergroup and 31 % of these were severely d-infected (Brasier 1986 c), and in more recent studies d-infection levels of 70 % have been recorded in v-c supergroup samples (C. M. Brasier, unpublished observations).

The predominance of one v-c group in populations, e.g. at the current epidemic front in Portugal where more than 90 % of the population belongs to the NAN v-c supergroup, could be due to selection for a high level of fitness (Brasier & Mitchell 1986). If so, the greater opportunity for d-factors to spread by hyphal anastomosis may be counteracted to some extent by a greater selection against d-infected members of the population.

Properties that may favour selection against d-infected individuals are reduced viability of conidia, slow hyphal growth, poor survival during flight of beetles and slower reproduction in the yeast phase (Brasier 1986 a). The decreased fitness caused by d-infection is illustrated by the observation that infection requires at least 50000 conidia of a $d^2$-infected isolate but only 1000 conidia of a healthy isolate (Webber 1988).

Sexual reproduction generally results in loss of d-factors and generates new v-c types by recombination, thus decreasing the frequency of transmission of d-factors between individuals. Sporulation is reduced by d-infection, but ascospores are still produced fairly abundantly even when both parents are d-infected (Brasier 1986 a).

Loss of d-factors can also occur during the yeast phase in the xylem (Brasier 1986 a; Rogers *et al.* 1986 a, 1988 a). Such reversion may account in part for the observation that, if sufficient spores are injected into elm trees to initiate infections, d-infected isolates are not uniformly hypovirulent (Brasier 1986 a). The frequency of loss of different d-factors during the yeast phase may vary and it is noteworthy that the d-infected isolates which are a significant proportion of isolates collected from the epidemic front in Poland (Brasier 1986 c) were obtained from the xylem.

D-infections may become latent i.e. the d-factor and specific dsRNA segments are present but the d-phenotype is not expressed. A large proportion of the viable conidia of $d^2$-infected isolates are latently d-infected (Rogers *et al.* 1986 a, b, 1988 b); reversion to overt d-infection may occur spontaneously, by hyphal anastomosis with a healthy recipient (after which either the donor or recipient may show overt d-infection), by growth on certain media, or by a second cycle of conidiogenesis (after which a small proportion of the viable conidia are overtly d-infected). Because latently d-infected isolates would not be expected to be strongly selected against, latency is probably important in maintaining the frequency of d-factors in *O. ulmi* populations.

Brasier (1986a) has suggested that d-factors might exert their greatest effects in the post-epidemic phases when *O. ulmi* populations are much smaller. Debilitation of a proportion of a small population might reduce the population size below a critical threshold level. However, the increase in the frequency of sexual, as opposed to asexual, reproduction, which occurs in the post-epidemic phase (Brasier 1986a, b; Webber *et al.* 1988) would tend to decrease the frequency and therefore the effect of d-factors.

It appears that man will have to intervene if the proportions of overt d-infections necessary to control *O. ulmi* populations are to be achieved as suggested by Brasier (1986a) by breeding and releasing bark beetles carrying inocula of d-infected isolates, probably best done by targeting the beetles on the bark in the saprophytic phase of the cycle to maximize the spread of d-factors to the resident *O. ulmi* populations. If the new generation of beetles emerging from the breeding galleries carries predominantly propagules infected with particularly deleterious d-factors, then it may be incapable of establishing infection in feeding grooves of healthy elm trees. Thus common spore loads carried by the largest vector, *Scolytus scolytus*, are 250 to 5000 spores (Webber & Brasier 1984), whereas Webber (1988) has shown that at least 50000 conidia of a $d^2$-infected isolate are required for infection of the xylem, and spore viability could be further reduced during beetle flight (see above). Hence widespread transmission of d-factors to healthy individuals in the bark could be sufficient to interrupt the saprophytic–pathogenic cycle of *O. ulmi*. It has also been suggested that the transmission of d-factors in the short mycelial phase in feeding grooves would act as a 'back-up' to attenuate any healthy propagules that had escaped transmission in the bark (Brasier 1986a; Webber 1988).

If this interesting strategy is to be successful there are several problems to overcome.

(i) Transmission of d-factors to healthy individuals must be efficient. Although substantial proportions of individuals in some locations may belong to v-c supergroups the problem of vegetative incompatibility in the rest of populations must be solved. Brasier (1986a) suggested the use of isolates in v-c 'bridging-groups', which are partly compatible with a range of isolates that are completely incompatible with each other. Alternatively, d-factors could be introduced into a range of different isolates by direct transfection of protoplasts with isolated dsRNA by adapting methods used to infect *Gaeumannomyces graminis* var. *tritici* (Stanway & Buck 1984) and *Saccharomyces cerevisiae* (Sturley *et al.* 1987) with isolated dsRNA viruses. Because of the likely large number of v-c groups in *O. ulmi* (Brasier 1984) such approaches may not be sufficient. It will probably be necessary to find a way to suppress vegetative incompatibility reactions.

Although vegetative incompatibility is widespread in fungi (Lane 1981) and is well characterized genetically, virtually nothing is known about the molecular basis. In the slime mould *Physarum polycephalum* post-fusion vegetative incompatibility can be unidirectional or bidirectional (Lane & Carlile 1979). The strength of incompatibility reactions varied with the medium on which the strains were paired, ranging from death of fused plasmodia to mild reactions in which plasmodia survived with unilateral elimination of the nuclei of one strain. Such mild incompatible reactions would be unlikely to impede transmission of a cytoplasmic genetic element. Although the 'medium' on which *O. ulmi* grows in the wild obviously cannot be altered, the *P. polycephalum* observations show that vegetative incompatibility reactions can be modified.

A possible way of completely suppressing vegetative incompatibility reactions would be by the use of anti-sense messenger RNA (mRNA) (Benedetti *et al.* 1987) to block the expression of v-c genes. General methods for transformation of fungi are now available (Yoder *et al.* 1986) and v-c genes are potentially capable of being cloned. Hence it may be possible to transform selected *O. ulmi* isolates with DNA constructs allowing production of anti-sense mRNAs to the v-c genes of these isolates to suppress their expression. A particular target could be the *w* locus which is a major locus in v-c gene expression (Brasier 1984). Then d-factors could be introduced into these isolates, before their dissemination by bark beetles bred in captivity. Alternatively, genetically manipulated d-factors carrying anti-sense v-c genes may be produced because it is now possible to construct copy DNA (cDNA) clones of RNA viruses, manipulate them at the DNA level and transcribe the cDNA back into infectious RNA (Dawson *et al.* 1986). With this approach the coat protein gene of brome mosaic virus was replaced with the gene for chloramphenicol acetyltransferase (CAT). When this construct was introduced, with the other virus genome segments, the *CAT* gene was replicated and high levels of CAT mRNA and CAT were produced (French *et al.* 1986).

An exciting possibility, if hyphal fusion between isolates of the aggressive and non-aggressive subgroups could occur without causing a vegetative incompatibility reaction, is that isolates of the non-aggressive subgroup could be used to disseminate d-factors to populations of the aggressive subgroup.

(ii) The d-infected isolate(s) selected for control purposes should be so debilitated that beetle spore inocula cannot infect xylem of healthy elm trees, but retain sufficient viability for the initial inoculum to infect bark of diseased elms. Hence careful selection of d-factors will be necessary. Fortunately, a large pool of possible d-factors, which vary greatly in their effects, exists in the aggressive (NAN and EAN) and non-aggressive subgroups (Brasier 1986a). There is also limited evidence to suggest that d-factor from one subgroup may be more deleterious when transferred to another (Brasier 1983).

Little is known about the mode of action of d-factors. One effect of the $d^2$-factor appears to be reduction in cytochrome oxidase levels (Rogers *et al.* 1988a; Rogers 1987), but whether this is its only effect and whether other d-factors cause the same effect is unknown. If more could be learned about the mode of action of d-factors it may be possible to contruct genetically manipulated d-factors designed to debilitate their hosts to specific degrees.

(iii) The selected d-factor(s) should suppress the sexual stage of the fungus, although allowing a reasonable asexual reproduction. The ability of H-factors to suppress the sexual stage in *E. parasitica* clearly is important in the current predominance of H-strains in Italy. Widespread screening will be necessary to establish whether one or more d-factors with the desired properties exists in natural populations of *O. ulmi*.

Construction of genetically manipulated d-factors able to suppress the sexual stage is possible. Little is known of the molecular genetics of sexual reproduction in the filamentous fungi, but by analogy with asexual reproduction (conidiogenesis) in *Aspergillus nidulans* (Timberlake 1980), it is likely to be very complex. However, if the gene for one essential step in the sexual stage could be identified and cloned, the anti-sense mRNA approach could be used to suppress it.

It is interesting that in some fungi there is close association between sexual compatibility and vegetative incompatibility: for example in *Neurospora crassa* the mating type locus *A/a* appears to control both (Newmeyer *et al.* 1973), and in *Podospora anserina* the *mod* genes that suppress vegetative incompatibility also cause sterility (Boucherie *et al.* 1976). Perhaps a way could be found to suppress vegetative incompatibility and the sexual stage simultaneously in *O. ulmi*, although in the latter sexual compatibility and v-c appear not to be associated (Brasier 1984).

(iv) The selected d-infected isolate(s) should not switch to latent d-infection with great frequency. Although ability to switch to latency probably helps to ensure the survival of d-factors in natural populations, it would be a disadvantage for control purposes. Investigation of the molecular nature of the switch from overt to latent d-infection, and *vice versa*, may enable genetically manipulated d-factors incapable of switching to be constructed.

In conclusion, d-factors (naturally occurring or genetically manipulated) offer exciting possibilities for the control of Dutch elm disease and the re-establishment of the elm. However, many problems remain and much further research is needed before the potential of d-factors becomes a reality.

### (e) dsRNA-associated hypovirulence in other plant pathogenic fungi

#### (i) Helminthosporium victoriae

*Helminthosporium victoriae*, which causes blight on oat cultivars with the Victoria-type of resistance to crown rust (*Puccinia coronata*), seriously decreased yields in most oat-growing areas of the U.S.A. in 1947 and 1948. Subsequently, Victoria-derived oat cultivars were abandoned in the major oat cropping areas, but continued to be grown in some of the southern states in the 1950s. Among cultures of *H. victoriae* newly isolated from oat crops in Louisiana, Lindberg (1959) encountered several stunted colonies, characterized by sectors at colony margins, collapse or lysis of aerial mycelium and almost complete inhibition of colony expansion. This 'disease' was also transmitted to healthy cultures by hyphal anastomosis and is probably caused by one of two dsRNA viruses commonly found in *H. victoriae* (Ghabrial 1986). The disease was transmitted by apparently healthy 'carrier' cultures which may be analogous to the latently d-infected isolates of *O. ulmi*. The oat crops from which diseased isolates were obtained did not suffer significant yield losses possibly because of spread of the virus in the *H. victoriae* population, because diseased isolates produced little of the toxin victorin and were much less pathogenic than normal isolates (Lindberg 1960).

#### (ii) Rhizoctonia solani

*Rhizoctonia solani* is a soil-borne pathogen of over 130 plant species (Baker 1970). Some isolates produce abnormal sectors giving cultures characterized by irregular morphology, few or no selerotia and an extremely reduced growth rate, a syndrome referred to as *Rhizoctonia* decline (Castanho & Butler 1978a). Diseased isolates of *R. solani* are weakly pathogenic and effective in reducing damping-off of sugar beet seedlings when applied to seed furrows of soil previously infected with a strongly pathogenic isolate (Castanho & Butler 1978b). Use of diseased isolates of *R. solani* is limited to short-term biological control because, unlike healthy isolates, they do not become established in either sterile or non-sterile soil, surviving for less than a month.

Control of healthy pathogenic strains by diseased strains of *R. solani* was considered to result from transmission of a cytoplasmic determinant from diseased to healthy strains. Diseased isolates contained three segments of dsRNA, whereas no dsRNA, or only traces of dsRNA segments, were detected in apparently healthy hyphal tip cultures from diseased isolates.

[ 195 ]

Transmission of the dsRNA segments by hyphal anastomosis converted healthy hyphal tip cultures to the diseased phenotype (Castanho *et al.* 1978). However, no nuclear markers were used and therefore cytoplasmic transmission has not been proved unequivocally. In addition, re-examination by Finkler *et al.* (1985) of the above hyphal tip cultures revealed the same dsRNA segments as diseased isolates. McFadden *et al.* (1983) also found that hyphal tip cultures from a dsRNA-containing strain of *G. graminis* var. *tritici* contained very small quantities of dsRNA virus particles, detectable only by very sensitive immunological or hybridization methods. However, after 18 months and a number of subcultures, the numbers of virus particles had returned to those of the parent and were easily detected by standard methods. It is likely that the hyphal tip cultures of *R. solani* (Castanho *et al.* 1978) also retained low levels of dsRNA which subsequently increased. It is now clear that dsRNA segments are present in most, if not all, pathogenic strains of *R. solani* (Zanzinger *et al.* 1984; Finkler *et al.* 1985) so that the role of dsRNA, or specific segments of dsRNA, in *Rhizoctonia* decline, remains to be clarified. It is possible that the disease is caused by small linear DNA plasmids such as those reported in some slow growing, weakly pathogenic strains of *R. solani* (Hashiba *et al.* 1984), by defects in mitochondrial DNA, which cause senescence in *Podospora anserina*, the 'poky' and 'stopper' phenotypes of *Neurospora crassa*, and the 'ragged' phenotype of *Aspergillus amstelodami* (reviewed by Bockelmann *et al.* (1986)), or even by nuclear mutations. Even if cytoplasmic transmission can be proved, the prospects for biological control may be limited by the two types of vegetative incompatibility in *R. solani*. Hyphae of isolates belonging to different anastomosis groups cannot fuse so that cytoplasmic transmission is not possible. Even within anastomosis groups, post-fusion incompatibility, as in *E. parasitica* and *O. ulmi*, is common (Anderson 1984) and it is noteworthy that Castanho *et al.* (1978) were unable to transmit the genetic determinant of the disease to four other field isolates of the same anastomosis group.

Martini *et al.* (1978) claimed that determinants for pathogenicity in *R. solani* lie on a large DNA plasmid. More recently, Finkler *et al.* (1985) obtained evidence, based on transmission by hyphal anastomosis between genetically marked strains, that a cytoplasmic factor, suggested to lie on dsRNA segments, is required for pathogenicity. Field isolates, or hyphal tip isolates from virulent dsRNA-containing strains, which lacked dsRNA were hypovirulent. Hypovirulence in these isolates resulted from specific lack of a virulence factor rather than general degeneration of the isolates, as in *Rhizoctonia* decline (Castanho & Butler 1978a), because hypovirulent isolates grew in culture as fast as virulent isolates. Hypovirulent isolates of this type are being used successfully in Israel to protect plants from infection by virulent strains of *R. solani* (Y. Koltin, personal communication). In this situation successful biological control may depend *inter alia* on failure to transmit cytoplasmic virulence factors from virulent to hypovirulent isolates because of vegetative incompatibility barriers.

Further research is needed to clarify the role of cytoplasmic factors in the biology of *R. solani*. Such research should involve direct transformation with isolated dsRNA viruses or DNA plasmids to avoid uncertainties associated with transmission by hyphal anastomosis, compounded for this fungus by the possibility that isolates may be heterokaryotic (Anderson 1984).

(iii) *Gaeumannomyces graminis var. tritici*

Pathogenicity of the wheat take-all fungus is difficult to quantify because firstly the several methods of measurement may be influenced differently by environmental factors and may not give equivalent results (Asher 1981) and secondly isolates can readily lose their pathogenicity on storage (Chambers 1970; Naiki & Cook 1983). However, isolates from natural populations do vary in pathogenicity from strongly pathogenic to hypovirulent (Asher 1980), even when obtained from lesions (Asher 1978). Such pathogenic variation shows clear evidence of being under nuclear polygenic control (Blanch *et al.* 1981) although additional effects of cytoplasmic elements in a proportion of isolates cannot be discounted.

The dsRNA virus particles are common in both strongly and weakly pathogenic isolates (reviewed by Buck (1986*b*)) and attempts to establish correlations between the presence or absence of particles have failed (Rawlinson *et al.* 1973). However, Stanway (1985) found that a greater proportion of isolates with dsRNA segments had reduced pathogenicity compared with isolates with no dsRNA, suggesting that dsRNA segments in a proportion of isolates may carry determinants for hypovirulence. One freshly isolated field isolate that was weakly pathogenic in both short-term (seedling) and long-term (full season) tests contained nine dsRNA segments. Single conidial isolates from this isolate were either hypovirulent and retaining all the dsRNA segments of the parent, or virulent and dsRNA-free. Hence there is a good correlation between the presence of the dsRNA segments and hypovirulence. Although virulent conidial isolates readily produced perithecia and ascospores (*G. graminis* is homothallic), it has not proved possible to produce these from the hypovirulent isolates, suggesting that virulence and sexual reproduction are suppressed together, as in *E. parasitica*. This would be useful in using hypovirulent strains for biological control, because virus particles and dsRNA are frequently excluded during ascospore formation in *G. graminis* (Rawlinson *et al.* 1973; McFadden *et al.* 1983).

The problem of vegetative incompatibility, which is common in field isolates (Jamil *et al.* 1984) would still need to be solved. If vegetative incompatibility could be suppressed by using methods analogous to those suggested for *O. ulmi* it may be possible to transfer the dsRNA determinants for hypovirulence to avirulent or weakly pathogenic relatives of *G. graminis* var. *tritici*. *Phialophora* spp. with lobed hyphopodia is often found on cereal roots in the U.K., whereas *P. graminicola* is common in grasslands and is found on cereal crops when these follow grass leys or are infected with grass weeds (Deacon 1981). Such *Phialophora* spp., which had been transfected with dsRNA determinants for hypovirulence, might combine their intrinsic ability for cross-protection (see above) with the ability to convert pathogenic *G. graminis* var. *tritici* to hypovirulence by transmission of the dsRNA segments. Such isolates would have considerable advantages over hypovirulent *G. graminis* var. *tritici* for widespread distribution as biological control agents because they would not become pathogenic even if they lost the dsRNA segments.

### (f) Future prospects

Cytoplasmic determinants for hypovirulence may be widespread among fungal plant pathogens. Their frequency may be low in populations of some fungi because of factors selecting directly against these determinants or against the hypovirulent isolates themselves. Searches for hypovirulence would be justified in a wide range of pathogens, but screening of several hundred isolates of a species may be necessary. Because the determinants for hypovirulence may lie on only a small fraction of the dsRNA segments or DNA plasmids found in populations of some pathogens, there is little value in attempting to establish correlations between the presence of dsRNA or DNA plasmids and hypovirulence. A more profitable approach would be to identify hypovirulent isolates, to establish cytoplasmic transmission and then identify the determinants.

Attempts to solve such problems as vegetative incompatibility, loss of determinants after sexual reproduction and latency, emphasize our ignorance of the molecular genetics, not only of plant pathogens, but of filamentous fungi in general. However, the use of recombinant DNA techniques to suppress vegetative incompatibility and the use of avirulent, close relatives of pathogens to deliver hypovirulence determinants to pathogen populations are attractive goals for the future.

## 3. Protection of plants from virulent strains of viruses by prior infection with mild strains

Infection of a plant with a virus can lead to a hypersensitive response (HR) which localizes the virus to a relatively small region of cells at the site of entry. This HR may induce rather non-specific localized or systemic resistance not only to a range of related and unrelated viruses, but also to other pathogens such as bacteria and fungi. Such resistance is caused by spread of host-induced factors to parts of the plant not carrying the virus (reviewed by Gianiazzi 1984; Ponz & Bruening 1986; Zaitlin & Hull 1987).

With many host–virus interactions the HR is not evoked and the virus infects the plant systemically. If the virus is a mild strain causing little disease, the plants become resistant specifically to pathogenic strains of the same virus. Such resistance, which is not host-induced and depends on the presence throughout the plant of the mild strain, has been called 'cross-protection'. Protection is not always complete but replication of the severe strain is usually depressed to the point where crop yields are not significantly reduced.

Potentially, any mild strain may protect against a severe strain of the same virus, but because of possible drawbacks (see later) the method has only been attempted for diseases which cause serious crop losses. Two diseases where cross-protection has succeeded are tomato mosaic and citrus tristeza.

Tomato mosaic virus, which is transmitted through seed and mechanically, is widespread. Tomatoes are grown annually from seed, and young plants can be protected by inoculation with mild virus strains by using high pressure spray guns. Protection against severe strains is usually good, yields of tomatoes are not significantly reduced by the mild virus strains and the method was used commercially for several years in Europe and Japan before being largely superseded by the use of resistant varieties (reviewed by Fulton (1986)).

Citrus tristeza virus is economically the most important citrus virus in the world (Bar-Joseph *et al.* 1981). The virus is transmitted by aphids, and spread so rapidly after its introduction from Africa into South America in the 1920s that the citrus industry in large areas of Argentina, Brazil and Uruguay was virtually wiped out in less than 20 years. A mild strain of the virus was first reported by Grant & Costa (1951) and, as a result of a U.S.A.–Brazil cooperation starting in 1961, many more have since been isolated and tested in a wide range of root stock – scion combinations for ability to protect against virulent strains of the virus. The most spectacular success has been with Pera sweet orange of which by 1980 more than eight million cross-protected trees had been planted in Brazil with very little failure of protection in successive clonal generations (Costa & Muller 1980). There are two main reasons for this success. First, the disease had caused such devastation that there was little to lose by testing

[ 198 ]

mild strains on a large scale. Secondly, many mild strains were tested to find the few with sufficiently mild symptoms combined with good cross protection.

Possible applications of cross-protection for the control of several diseases of perennial plants, such as cacao swollen shoot, papaya ringspot, avocado sun blotch and several virus diseases of stone and pome fruits, have been reviewed by Fulton (1986). However, despite the few notable successes, cross-protection has not been widely used for the following reasons.

First, it can be difficult and expensive to inoculate plants with the mild strains. This is not such a problem for perennial plants or for plants propagated vegetatively, because the virus, once introduced, persists over long periods and many clonal propagations. However, it has generally been considered impracticable for field crops of annual plants when the virus must be applied to each plant in each crop. Growers prefer to use resistant cultivars when these are available, or to use insecticidal sprays to kill insect vectors of viruses.

Secondly, there is justifiable caution about the widespread distribution in field crops of mild strains of viruses, which may give severe synergistic reactions in mixed infections with unrelated viruses, may revert to virulence or may cause severe disease if transmitted to other crops by insect vectors (Fulton 1986).

As a result of recent advances in molecular biology and recombinant DNA technology solutions to some, or all, of these problems can now be envisaged. First, construction of mild strains of viruses incapable of reverting to virulence or of vector transmission is feasible. Secondly, it might be possible to protect plants by expression of a single viral gene rather than by infection with intact virus.

Mild strains of viruses have traditionally been obtained directly from nature, by culturing infected tissue at supra-optimal temperatures for replication of the pathogenic virus strains or by nitrous acid mutagenesis (Fulton 1986). Recently, the nucleotide sequence of an attenuated strain of tomato mosaic virus has been determined and compared with that of the parent pathogenic strain (Nishiguchi *et al.* 1985). Of the ten base-substitutions found in the attenuated strain, seven occurred in the third base of codons and did not alter amino acids. The remaining three were in the common reading frame of 130 kDa and 180 kDa proteins which may be involved in viral RNA replication. Hence the mutations may reduce the capacity of the virus to replicate its RNA genome. Techniques of *in vitro* mutagenesis are now available (Smith 1985) which enable essentially any base or group of bases to be altered in a nucleic acid molecule. Hence mild virus strains could be constructed by *in vitro* mutagenesis of the genome of pathogenic strains and the effects of introducing deletions into the genome, which could not easily revert to the parental sequence, could be studied. Similarly, deletions could be made in virus genes essential for vector transmission. Non-aphid transmissible mutants of cauliflower mosaic virus with deletions in gene *II*, which encodes an aphid transmission protein, occur naturally and have also been constructed by genetic manipulation (Woolston *et al.* 1983).

The use of genetically manipulated mild strains would probably be limited to perennials and vegetatively propagated plants, because of the problems of application to annual crops outlined above. The alternative approach of expressing single virus genes in plants potentially has more general applicability. The mechanisms of cross-protection are unknown, but the following hypotheses have been put forward (reviewed by Zinnen & Fulton (1986)), some of which enable candidate genes to be identified and tested.

Coat protein of the pre-infecting strain could prevent uncoating of the challenge virus. The observation that extraneous tobacco mosaic virus (TMV) coat protein inhibited the *in vitro* co-translational disassembly of pre-swollen TMV (Wilson & Watkins 1986) is consistent with this hypothesis. Recently Abel *et al.* (1986) introduced a chimeric gene containing a cloned cDNA of the TMV coat-protein gene into the genome of tobacco cells by using a Ti plasmid vector. The resultant transgenic plants expressed the TMV coat protein as a nuclear trait. When challenged with TMV the symptoms in transgenic plants were delayed and 10–60% of the plants failed to develop symptoms, results similar to those reported for cross-protection of TMV in tomato (Cassells & Herrick 1977). Studies of virus replication indicated that symptom-less plants are not infected, showing that plants can be genetically transformed for resistance. Transgenic plants were not resistant to infection with TMV RNA (R. N. Beachy, unpublished observation quoted in Zaitlin & Hull (1987)) suggesting that blocking of virus uncoating is indeed one mechanism of resistance to virus infection.

Blocking of virus uncoating is clearly not the only mechanism of cross-protection that can be engendered by coat protein-defective or coat-less mutants of TMV (Zaitlin 1976; Sarkar & Smitamana 1981) and by viroids that are naked RNA molecules (Niblett *et al.* 1978). Palukaitis & Zaitlin (1984) suggested a more general mechanism called negative-strand capture. In the replication of positive-strand RNA viruses, which compose the majority of plant viruses, an RNA-dependent RNA polymerase catalyses the synthesis of a complementary negative strand by using the positive strand as a template; more positive strands are then synthesized by using the negative strands as templates. Palukaitis & Zaitlin (1984) proposed that positive strands of a pre-infecting mild virus strain would hybridize with the first negative strands to be produced by a related challenge virus and prevent them from acting as templates to produce more positive strands.

If cDNAs to viral RNA were linked to suitable promoters and integrated into plant genomes so that the plants produced either a whole negative strand or part of a positive strand, the replication of a challenge virus RNA could be inhibited by positive- or negative-strand capture respectively. The method could apply equally well to viroids.

Positive-strand capture is similar in principle to the use of anti-sense RNA to inhibit gene expression (Benedetti *et al.* 1987) and could suppress virus replication by preventing the synthesis of an essential viral protein. However, binding of RNA-dependent RNA polymerase to recognition sequences could also be inhibited by expression by the host plant of sequences complementary to the 3' ends of positive or negative strands. Use of positive- or negative-strand capture or anti-sense RNA is being investigated in several laboratories and information on the feasibility of this approach in producing virus-resistant plants is expected soon; mRNA-interfering complementary RNA (anti-sense RNA) is known to inhibit RNA bacteriophage replication in *Escherichia coli*, plaque formation being reduced by up to 98% (Hirashima *et al.* 1986).

Symptoms of disease development can be modified by satellite RNAs (sat-RNAs) in a virus culture. Satellite RNAs only replicate in the presence of a helper virus and are encapsidated by coat protein encoded by the helper virus; sat-RNAs have little sequence homology with the helper virus and are not required for its replication. Although some sat-RNAs increase virus symptoms, attenuation is more common (Francki 1985). It has been reported that pre-infection with a cucumber mosaic virus (CMV) strain containing a benign sat-RNA, protected against CMV and increased yield of pepper plants (Tien & Chang 1984). Also, infection of tomato plants with a CMV strain containing a benign sat-RNA protected against the effects of a CMV culture containing a virulent sat-RNA (Jacquemond 1982).

Baulcombe *et al.* (1986) introduced cDNA dimers of a benign CMV sat-RNA into the genome of tobacco plants by using an expression vector. RNA transcripts of the expected size were detected in transformed plants but there was no evidence for production or replication of unit-length sat-RNA and plants showed no symptoms. However, after infection of plants with CMV, formation and replication of sat-RNA was observed. This suggested that plants could be protected from disease symptoms caused by CMV by expressing cDNAs of sat-RNAs from the nuclear genome. However, although sat-RNAs reduce replication of their helper virus they cannot suppress it completely because of their dependence on helper virus replication. Hence they make plants tolerant of, rather than resistant to, virus infection.

In conclusion, the availability of recombinant DNA techniques to manipulate genetically both viruses and their plant hosts has led to a resurgence of interest in cross-protection. The construction of genetically engineered plants that are resistant to viral infection by the mechanisms involved in cross-protection, but without the possible hazards of the widespread dissemination of infectious agents in the environment, can now be seen as a desirable and feasible goal for the future. The use of such resistant plants may not be seen by some as biological control *sensu stricto* because it does not involve control by a third organism, but it fits nicely into the broader definition of biological control (of a plant pathogen) of Cook & Baker (1983) i.e. 'reduction in the amount of inoculum or disease-producing activity of a pathogen accomplished by or through one or more organisms other than man'. Nevertheless, it is clear that investigations of biological control have opened up several novel approaches for the control of plant virus diseases.

I am grateful to Dr Clive Brasier for many stimulating discussions regarding Dutch elm disease and d-factors and for helpful suggestions in the preparation of the manuscript.

## REFERENCES

Abel, P. P., Nelson, R. S., De, B., Hoffman, N., Rogers, S. G., Fraley, R. T. & Beachy, R. N. 1986 Delay of disease development in transgenic plants that express the tobacco mosaic virus coat protein gene. *Science, Wash.* **232**, 738–743.

Anagnostakis, S. L. 1982 Biological control of chestnut blight. *Science, Wash.* **215**, 466–471.

Anagnostakis, S. L. 1983 Conversion to curative morphology in *Endothia parasitica* and its restriction by vegetative compatibility. *Mycologia* **75**, 777–780.

Anagnostakis, S. L. 1984 The mycelial biology of *Endothia parasitica*. II. Vegetative incompatibility. In *The ecology and physiology of the fungal mycelium* (ed. D. H. Jennings & A. D. M. Rayner), pp. 499–507. Cambridge University Press.

Anderson, N. A. 1984 Variation and heterokaryosis in *Rhizoctonia solani*. In *The ecology and physiology of the fungal mycelium* (ed. D. H. Jennings & A. D. M. Rayner), pp. 367–382. Cambridge University Press.

Asher, M. J. C. 1978 Isolation of *Gaeumannomyces graminis* var. *tritici* from roots. *Trans. Br. mycol. Soc.* **71**, 322–325.

Asher, M. J. C. 1980 Variation in pathogenicity and cultural characters in *Gaeumannomyces graminis* var. *tritici*. *Trans. Br. mycol. Soc.* **75**, 213–220.

Asher, M. J. C. 1981 Pathogenic variation. In *Biology and control of take-all* (ed. M. J. C. Asher & P. J. Shipton), pp. 199–218. London: Academic Press.

Baker, K. F. 1970 Types of *Rhizoctonia* diseases and their occurrence. In *Rhizoctonia solani: biology and pathology* (ed. J. R. Parmeter), pp. 125–148. Los Angeles: University of California Press.

Bar-Joseph, M., Roistacher, C. N., Garnsey, S. M. & Gumpf, D. J. 1981 A review on tristeza, an ongoing threat to citriculture. *Proc. int. Soc. Citriculture* **1**, 419–422.

Baulcombe, D. C., Saunders, G. R., Bevan, M. W., Mayo, M. A. & Harrison, B. D. 1986 Expression of biologically active viral satellite RNA from the nuclear genome of transformed plants. *Nature, Lond.* **321**, 446–449.

Bazzigher, G., Kanzler, E. & Kubler, T. 1981 Irreversible pathogenitatsverminderung bei *Endothia parasitica* durch ubertragbare Hypovirulenz. *Eur. J. Forest Path.* **11**, 358–369.

Benedetti, A. D., Pytel, B. A. & Baglioni, C. 1987 Loss of (2′-5′) oligoadenylate synthetase activity by production of antisense RNA results in lack of protection by interferon from viral infections. *Proc. natn. Acad. Sci. U.S.A.* **84**, 658–662.

Berthelay-Sauret, S. 1973 Utilisation de mutants auxotrophes dans les recherches sur le déterminisme de 'l'hypovirulence exclusive'. *Annls Pytopath.* **5**, 318. (Abstract.)

Biraghi, A. 1953 Ulterion notizie sulla resistenze di *Castanea sativa* Mill. nei confronti de *Endothia parasitica* (Murr.) And. *Boll. Staz. Patol. veg. Roma* **11**, 149–157.

Blanche, P. A., Asher, M. J. C. & Burnett, J. H. 1981 Inheritance of pathogenicity and cultural character in *Gaeumannomyces graminis* var *tritici*. *Trans. Br. mycol Soc.* **71**, 367–373.

Bockelmann, B., Osiewacz, H. D., Schmidt, F. R. & Schulte, E. 1986 Extrachromosomal DNA in fungi-organisation and function. In *Fungal virology* (ed. K. W. Buck), pp. 237–283. Boca Raton, Florida: CRC Press.

Boucherie, H., Begueret, J. & Bernet, J. 1976 The molecular mechanisms of protoplasmic incompatibility and its relationship to the formation of protoperithecia in *Podospora anserina*. *J. gen. Microbiol.* **92**, 59–66.

Bozarth, R. F. 1977 Biophysical and biochemical characterization of virus-like particles containing a high molecular weight dsRNA from *Helminthosporium maydis*. *Virology* **80**, 149–157.

Brasier, C. M. 1979 Dual origin of recent Dutch elm disease epidemics in Europe. *Nature, Lond.* **281**, 78–79.

Brasier, C. M. 1982 Genetics of pathogenicity in *Ceratocystis ulmi* and its significance for elm breeding. In *Resistance to diseases and pests in forest trees* (ed. H. M. Heybrock, B. R. Stephan & K. von Weissenberg), pp. 224–235. Wageningen: Pudoc.

Brasier, C. M. 1983 A cytoplasmically transmitted disease of *Ceratocystis ulmi*. *Nature, Lond.* **305**, 220–223.

Brasier, C. M. 1984 Inter-mycelial recognition systems in *Ceratocystis ulmi*: their physiological properties and ecological importance. In *The ecology and physiology of the fungal mycelium* (ed. D. H. Jennings & A. D. M. Rayner), pp. 451–497. Cambridge University Press.

Brasier, C. M. 1986a The d-factor in *Ceratocystis ulmi* – its biological characteristics and implications for Dutch elm disease. In *Fungal virology* (ed. K. W. Buck), pp. 177–208. Boca Raton, Florida: CRC Press.

Brasier, C. M. 1986b The population biology of Dutch elm disease: the principal features and implications for other host-pathogen systems. *Adv. Pl. Path.* **5**, 53–118.

Brasier, C. M. 1986c Dutch elm disease – *Ophiostoma* (*Ceratocystis*) *ulmi*. The emergence of EAN and NAN hybrids in Europe. In *Report on forest research 1986*, p. 37. London: HMSO.

Brasier, C. M. 1987 Recent genetic changes in the *Ophiostoma ulmi* population: the threat to the future of the elm. In *Populations of plant pathogens: their dynamics and genetics* (ed. M. S. Wolfe & C. E. Caten), pp. 213–226. Oxford: Blackwell Scientific Publications.

Brasier, C. M. & Mitchell, A. G. 1986 Dutch elm disease – *Ophiostoma* (*Ceratocystis*) *ulmi*. Vegetative compatibility 'super-groups' in *O. ulmi*. In *Report on forest research 1986*, p. 38. London: HMSO.

Brasier, C. M. & Webber, J. F. 1987 Recent advances in Dutch elm disease research: host, pathogen and vector. In *Advances in practical arboriculture* (ed. D. Patch), pp. 166–179. (*Bull. For. Commn, Lond.* **65**.)

Buck, K. W. 1986a Fungal virology – an overview. In *Fungal virology* (ed. K. W. Buck), pp. 1–84. Boca Raton, Florida: CRC Press.

Buck, K. W. 1986b Viruses of the wheat take-all fungus, *Gaeumannomyces graminis* var. *tritici*. In *Fungal virology* (ed. K. W. Buck), pp. 221–236. Boca Raton, Florida: CRC Press.

Cassells, A. C. & Herrick, C. 1977 Cross protection between mild and severe strains of tobacco mosaic virus in doubly inoculated tomato plants. *Virology* **78**, 253–260.

Castanho, B. & Butler, E. E. 1978a *Rhizoctonia* decline: a degenerative disease of *Rhizoctonia solani*. *Phytopathology* **68**, 1505–1510.

Castanho, B. & Butler, E. E. 1978b *Rhizoctonia* decline: studies on hypovirulence and potential use in biological control. *Phytopathology* **68**, 1511–1514.

Castanho, B., Butler, E. E. & Shepherd, R. J. 1978 The association of double-stranded RNA with *Rhizoctonia* decline. *Phytopathology* **68**, 1515–1518.

Chambers, S. C. 1970 Pathogenic variation in *Ophiobolus graminis*. *Aust. J. biol. Sci.* **23**, 1099–1103.

Cook, R. J. & Baker, K. F. 1983 *The nature and practice of biological control of plant pathogens*. (539 pages.) St Paul, Minnesota: The American Phytopathological Society.

Costa, A. S. & Muller, G. W. 1980 Tristeza control by cross protection: a U.S.–Brazil cooperative success. *Pl. Dis.* **64**, 538–541.

Dawson, W. O., Beck, D. L., Knorr, D. A. & Grantham, G. L. 1986 cDNA cloning of the complete genome of tobacco mosaic virus and production of infectious transcripts. *Proc. natn. Acad. Sci. U.S.A.* **83**, 1832–1836.

Day, P. R. 1981 Fungal virus populations in corn smut from Connecticut. *Mycologia* **73**, 379–391.

Day, P. R. & Dodds, J. A. 1979 Viruses of plant pathogenic fungi. In *Viruses and plasmids of fungi* (ed. P. A. Lemke), pp. 201–238. New York: Marcel Dekker Inc.

Day, P. R., Dodds, J. A., Elliston, J. E., Jaynes, R. A. & Anagnostakis, S. L. 1977 Double-stranded RNA in *Endothia parasitica*. *Phytopathology* **67**, 1393–1396.

Deacon, J. W. 1981 Ecological relationships with other fungi: competitors and hyperparasites. In *Biology and control of take-all* (ed. M. J. C. Asher & P. J. Shipton), pp. 75–101. London: Academic Press.

Elliston, J. E. 1982 Hypovirulence. *Adv. Pl. Path.* 1, 1–33.

Elliston, J. E. 1985 Characteristics of dsRNA-free and dsRNA-containing strains of *Endothia parasitica* in relation to hypovirulence. *Phytopathology* 75, 151–158.

Finkler, A., Kolton, Y., Barash, I., Sneh, B. & Pozmak, D. 1985 Isolation of a virus from virulent strains of *Rhizoctonia solani*. *J. gen. Virol.* 66, 1221–1232.

Francki, R. I. B. 1986 Plant virus satellites. *A. Rev. Microbiol.* 39, 151–174.

French, R., Janda, M. & Ahlquist, P. 1986 Bacterial gene inserted in an engineered RNA virus: efficient expression in monocotyledonous plant cells. *Science, Wash.* 231, 1294–1297.

Fulbright, D. W. 1984 Effect of eliminating dsRNA in hypovirulent *Endothia parasitica*. *Phytopathology* 74, 722–724.

Fulbright, D. W., Weidlich, W. H., Haufler, K. Z., Thomas, C. S. & Paul, C. P. 1983 Chestnut blight and recovering American chestnut trees in Michigan. *Can. J. Bot.* 61, 3164–3171.

Fulton, R. W. 1986 Practices and precautions in the use of cross-protection for plant virus disease control. *A. Rev. Phytopath.* 24, 67–81.

Ghabrial, S. A. 1986 A transmissible disease of *Helminthosporium victoriae* – evidence for a viral etiology. In *Fungal virology* (ed. K. W. Buck), pp. 163–176. Boca Raton, Florida: CRC Press.

Gianinazzi, S. 1984 Genetic and molecular aspects of resistance induced by infections or chemicals. In *Plant–microbe interactions: molecular and genetic perspectives*, vol. 1 (ed. T. Kosuge & E. N. Nester), pp. 321–342. New York: Macmillan.

Grant, T. J. & Costa, A. S. 1951 A mild strain of the tristeza virus of citrus. *Phytopathology* 41, 114–122.

Grente, J. 1965 Les formes hypovirulentes d'*Endothia parasitica* et les espoirs de lutte contre le chancre du chataigner. *C. r. hebd. Séanc. Acad. Agri. Fr.* 51, 1033–1037.

Grente, J. 1981 Les variants hypovirulents de l'*Endothia parasitica* et la lutte biologique contra le chancre du chataigner. Ph.D. thesis, Université de Bretagne Occidentale, Brest.

Grente, J. & Sauret, S. 1969 L'hypovirulence exclusive phenomene orignal en pathologie vegetale. *C. r. hebd. Séanc. Acad. Sci., Paris* D 268, 2347–2350.

Hansen, D. R., Van Alfen, N. K., Gillies, K. & Powell, W. A. 1985 Naked dsRNA associated with hypovirulence of *Endothia parasitica* is packaged in fungal vesicles. *J. gen. Virol.* 66, 2605–2614.

Hashiba, T., Homma, Y., Hyakumachi, M. & Matsuda, I. 1984 Isolation of a DNA plasmid in the fungus *Rhizoctonia solani*. *J. gen. Microbiol.* 130, 2067–2070.

Hebard, F. V., Griffin, G. J. & Elkins, J. R. 1984 Developmental histopathology of cankers incited by hypovirulent and virulent isolates of *Endothia parasitica* on susceptible and resistant chestnut trees. *Phytopathology* 74, 140–149.

Hirashima, A., Sawaki, S., Inokuchi, Y. & Inouye, M. 1986 Engineering of the mRNA-interfering complementary RNA immune system against viral infection. *Proc. natn. Acad. Sci. U.S.A.* 83, 7726–7730.

Hiremath, S., L'Hostis, B. L., Ghabrial, S. A. & Rhoads, R. E. 1986 Terminal structure of hypovirulence-associated dsRNAs in the chestnut blight fungus *Endothia parasitica*. *Nucl. Acids Res.* 14, 9877–9896.

Houston, D. R. 1985 Spread and increase of *Ceratocystis ulmi* with cultural characteristics of the aggressive strain in north eastern North America. *Pl. Dis.* 69, 677–680.

Jacquemond, M. 1982 The phenomena of interferences between the two types of satellite RNA of cucumber mosaic virus: protection of tomato plants against lethal necrosis. *C. r. hebd. Séanc. Acad. Sci., Paris* C 294, 991–994.

Jamil, N., Buck, K. W. & Carlile, M. J. 1984 Sequence relationships between virus double-stranded RNA from isolates of *Gaeumannomyces graminis* in different vegetative compatibility groups. *J. gen. Virol.* 65, 1741–1747.

Koltin, Y. 1986 The killer systems of *Ustilago maydis*. In *Fungal virology* (ed. K. W. Buck), pp. 109–141. Boca Raton, Florida: CRC Press.

Koltin, Y. & Day, P. R. 1975 The specificity of *Ustilago maydis* killer proteins. *Appl. Microbiol.* 30, 694–696.

Lane, E. B. 1981 Somatic incompatibility in fungi and myxomycetes. In *The fungal mycelium* (ed. K. Gull & S. G. Oliver), pp. 239–258. Cambridge University Press.

Lane, E. B. & Carlile, M. J. 1979 Post-fusion somatic incompatibility in plasmodia of *Physarum polycephalum*. *J. Cell Sci.* 35, 339–354.

Lea, J. & Brasier, C. M. 1983 A fruiting succession in *Ceratocystis ulmi* and its role in Dutch elm disease. *Trans. Br. mycol. Soc.* 80, 381–387.

L'Hostis, B., Hiremath, S. T., Rhoads, R. E. & Ghabrial, S. A. 1985 Lack of sequence homology between double-stranded RNA from European and American strains of *Endothia parasitica*. *J. gen. Virol.* 66, 351–355.

Lindberg, G. D. 1959 A transmissible disease of *Helminthosporium victoriae*. *Phytopathology* 49, 29–32.

Lindberg, G. D. 1960 Reduction in pathogenicity and toxin production in diseased *Helminthosporium victoriae*. *Phytopathology* 50, 457–460.

Martini, G., Grimaldi, G. & Guardiola, I. 1978 Extrachromosomal DNA in phytopathogenic fungi. In *Genetic engineering* (ed. H. W. Boyer & S. Nicosia), pp. 197–200. Amsterdam: Elsevier/North-Holland.

McFadden, J. J. P., Buck, K. W. & Rawlinson, C. J. 1983 Infrequent transmission of double-stranded RNA virus particles but absence of DNA proviruses in single ascospore cultures of *Gaeumannomyces graminis*. *J. gen. Virol.* **64**, 927–937.

Mitemperhger, L. 1978 The present status of chestnut blight in Italy. In *Proceedings American chestnut symposium* (ed. W. L. MacDonald), pp. 34–37. Morgantown: West Virginia University Books.

Naiki, T. & Cook, R. J. 1983 Factors in loss of pathogenicity in *Gaeumannomyces graminis* var. *tritici*. *Phytopathology* **73**, 1652–1656.

Newmeyer, D., Howe, H. B. & Galeazzi, D. R. 1973 A search for complexity at the mating type locus of *Neuroscpora crassa*. *Can. J. Genet. Cytol.* **15**, 577–585.

Niblett, C. L., Dickson, E., Fernow, K. H., Horst, R. K. & Zaitlin, M. 1978 Cross protection among four viroids. *Virology* **91**, 198–203.

Nishiguchi, M., Kikuchi, S., Kiho, Y., Ohno, T., Meshi, T. & Okada, Y. 1985 Molecular basis of plant viral virulence: the complete nucleotide sequence of an attenuated strain of tobacco mosaic virus. *Nucl. Acids Res.* **13**, 5585–5590.

Palukaitis, P. & Zaitlin, M. 1984 A model to explain the 'cross-protection' phenomenon shown by plant viruses and viroids. In *Plant–microbe interactions: molecular and genetic perspectives* (ed. T. Kosuge & E. N. Nester), vol. 1, pp. 420–429. New York: Macmillan.

Ponz, F. & Bruening, G. 1986 Mechanisms of resistance to plant viruses. *An. Rev. Phytopath.* **24**, 355–381.

Rawlinson, C. J., Hornby, D., Pearson, V. & Carpenter, J. M. 1973 Virus-like particles in the take-all fungus, *Gaeumannomyces graminis*. *Ann. appl. Biol.* **74**, 197–209.

Richards, W. C. & Takai, S. 1984 Characterization of the toxicity of *Cerato-ulmi*, the toxin of Dutch elm disease. *Can. J. Pl. Path.* **6**, 291–298.

Rogers, H. J. 1987 The molecular nature of cytoplasmically inherited disease factors in *Ophiostoma ulmi*. Ph.D. thesis, University of London.

Rogers, H. J., Buck, K. W. & Brasier, C. M. 1986*a* Transmission of double-stranded RNA and a disease-factor in *Ophiostoma ulmi*. *Pl. Path.* **35**, 277–287.

Rogers, H. J., Buck, K. W. & Brasier, C. M. 1986*b* The molecular nature of the d-factor in *Ceratocystis ulmi*. In *Fungal virology* (ed. K. W. Buck), pp. 209–220. Boca Raton, Florida: CRC Press.

Rogers, H. J., Buck, K. W. & Brasier, C. M. 1988*a* Double-stranded RNA in diseased isolates of the aggressive subgroup of the Dutch elm disease fungus, *Ophiostoma ulmi*. In *Viruses of fungi and simple eukaryotes* (ed. M. J. Leibowitz & Y. Koltin). New York: Marcel Dekker Inc. (In the press.)

Rogers, H. J., Buck, K. W. & Brasier, C. M. 1988*b* The d²-factor in *Ophiostoma ulmi*: expression and latency. In *Biology and molecular biology of plant–pathogen interactions* (ed. J. A. Bailey), pp. 393–400. Berlin: Springer-Verlag. (In the press.)

Sarkar, S. & Smitamana, P. 1981 A proteinless mutant of tobacco mosaic virus: evidence against the role of a viral coat protein for interference. *Molec. gen. Genet.* **184**, 158–159.

Shelbourn, S. L., Day, P. R. & Buck, K. W. 1987 Relationships and functions of virus double-stranded RNA in a killer strain of *Ustilago maydis*. *Abstracts of the 7th International Congress on Virology, Edmonton, 9–14 August, 1987*.

Smith, M. 1985 *In vitro* mutagenesis. *A. Rev. Genet.* **19**, 423–462.

Stanway, C. A. 1985 Double-stranded RNA viruses and pathogenicity of the wheat take-all fungus *Gaeumannomyces graminis* var. *tritici*. Ph.D. thesis, University of London.

Stanway, C. A. & Buck, K. W. 1984 Infection of protoplasts of the wheat take-all fungus, *Gaeumannomyces graminis* var. *tritici*, with double-stranded RNA viruses. *J. gen. Virol.* **65**, 2061–2065.

Sturley, S. L., El-Sherbeini, M. & Bostian, K. A. 1988 The yeast killer virus as a secretion vector. In *Viruses of fungi and simple eukaryotes* (ed. Y. Koltin & M. J. Leibowitz). New York: Marcel Dekker. (In the press.)

Tartaglia, J., Paul, C. P., Fulbright, D. W. & Nuss, D. L. 1986 Structural properties of double-stranded RNAs associated with biological control of chestnut blight fungus. *Proc. natn. Acad. Sci. U.S.A.* **83**, 9109–9113.

Tien, P. & Chang, X. H. 1984 Vaccination of pepper with cucumber mosaic virus isolates attenuated with a satellite RNA. *Abstracts of the 6th International Congress on Virology, Sendai, Japan, September 1984*, p. 379.

Timberlake, W. E. 1980 Developmental gene regulation in *Aspergillus nidulans*. *Devl Biol.* **78**, 497–510.

Turchetti, T. 1978 Some observations on the 'hypovirulence' of chestnut blight in Italy. In *Proceedings of the American chestnut symposium* (ed. W. L. MacDonald), pp. 92–94. Morgantown: West Virginia University Agricultural Experiment Station.

Turchetti, T. 1979 Prospettive di lotta biologica in alcune malattie di piante forestali. *Infme fitopatol.* **29**, 7–15.

Van Alfen, N. K. 1982 Biology and potential for disease control of hypovirulence of *Endothia parasitica*. *A. Rev. Phytopath.* **20**, 349–362.

Van Alfen, N. K. 1986 Hypovirulence of *Endothia* (*Cryphonectria*) *parasitica* and *Rhizoctonia solani*. In *Fungal virology* (ed. K. W. Buck), pp. 143–162. Boca Raton, Florida: CRC Press.

Van Alfen, N. K., Jaynes, R. A., Anagnostakis, S. L. & Day, P. R. 1975 Chestnut blight: biological control by transmissible hypovirulence in *Endothia parasitica*. *Science, Wash.* **189**, 890–891.

Van Alfen, N. K., Jaynes, R. A. & Bowman, J. T.  1978  Stability of *Endothia parasitica* hypovirulence in culture. *Phytopathology* **68**, 1075–1079.

Vidaver, A. K.  1976  Prospects for control of phytopathogenic bacteria by bacteriophages and bacteriocins. *A. Rev. Phytopathol.* **14**, 451–465.

Webber, J. F.  1988  The influence of the d²-factor on survival and infection by the Dutch elm disease pathogen *Ophiostoma ulmi*. *Pl. Path.* (In the press.)

Webber, J. F. & Brasier, C. M.  1984  The transmission of Dutch elm disease: a study of the processes involved. In *Invertebrate–microbial interactions* (ed. J. M. Anderson, A. D. M. Rayner & D. W. H. Walton), pp. 271–306. Cambridge University Press.

Webber, J. F., Brasier, C. M. & Mitchell, A. G.  1988  The role of the saprophytic phase in Dutch elm disease. In *Fungal infestation of plants: establishment, progress and outcome of infection* (ed. G. F. Pegg & P. G. Ayres). Cambridge University Press. (In the press.)

Wigderson, M. & Koltin, Y.  1982  Dual toxin specificities and the exclusion relations among the *Ustilago* dsRNA viruses. *Curr. Genet.* **5**, 127–136.

Wilson, T. M. A. & Watkins, P. A. C.  1986  Influence of exogenous viral coat protein on the cotranslational disassembly of tobacco mosaic virus particles *in vitro*. *Virol.* **149**, 132–135.

Wong, P. T. W.  1981  Biological control by cross-protection. In *Biology and control of take-all* (ed. M. J. C. Asher & P. J. Shipton), pp. 417–431. London: Academic Press.

Woolston, C. J., Covey, S. N., Penswick, J. R. & Davies, J. W.  1983  Aphid transmission and a polypeptide are specified by a defined region of the cauliflower mosaic virus genome. *Gene* **23**, 15–23.

Yoder, O. C., Weltring, K., Turgeon, B. G., Garber, R. C. & Van Etten, H. D.  1986  Technology for molecular cloning of fungal virulence genes. In *Biology and molecular biology of plant–pathogen interactions* (ed. J. A. Bailey), pp. 371–384. Berlin: Springer-Verlag.

Zaitlin, M.  1976  Viral cross protection: more understanding is needed. *Phytopathology* **66**, 382–383.

Zaitlin, M. & Hull, R.  1987  Plant virus–host interactions. *A. Rev. Pl. Physiol.* **38**, 291–315.

Zanzinger, D. H., Bandy, B. P. & Tavantzis, S. M.  1984  High frequency of finding double-stranded RNA in naturally occurring isolates of *Rhizoctonia solani*. *J. gen. Virol.* **65**, 1601–1605.

Zinnen, T. M. & Fulton, R. W.  1986  Cross-protection between sunn-hemp mosaic and tobacco mosaic viruses. *J. gen. Virol.* **67**, 1679–1687.

## *Discussion*

R. J. Cook (*United States Department of Agriculture Agricultural Research Service, Washington State University, Pullman, U.S.A.*). Would Professor Buck please define the term 'hypovirulence'? Specifically, is the term to be limited to a transmissible trait or can it be used to mean 'low virulence' or 'weak virulence' that is not, by all evidence thus far, transmissible?

K. W. Buck. Hypovirulence may be defined as the reduced ability to cause disease on plant hosts that lack any specific resistance genes to the pathogen. Because it describes a phenotype, the term can be used irrespective of whether the genetic determinant is cytoplasmically transmissible or non-transmissible. In describing individual hypovirulent isolates, reference should be made to the transmissible or non-transmissible nature of the genetic determinant when this is known.

J. W. Deacon (*Department of Microbiology, Edinburgh University, U.K.*). Would Professor Buck comment on recent reports that transmissible hypovirulence in a few pathogens such as *Rhizoctonia solani* is associated with plasmid DNA? Is it possible that this has been overlooked in a wider range of pathogens because the separation procedures for extracting dsRNA have destroyed DNA?

K. W. Buck. It has not been shown unequivocally that the hypovirulence determinant in the isolates of *R. solani*, which were reported to contain linear dsDNA plasmids, is cytoplasmically transmissible. It is also noteworthy that the sizes of the linear dsDNA plasmids are the same as those of linear dsRNA molecules found in other isolates of *R. solani*. Because dsRNA survives the method used to isolate these plasmids, in my view further characterization of the plasmids, e.g. by restriction endonuclease mapping, would be desirable to prove conclusively that they are not dsRNA.

It is likely that plasmid DNA (if present) would be overlooked when extracting dsRNA by the most commonly used procedure, i.e. cellulose chromatography. If the method included DNase treatment then plasmid DNA would be destroyed along with chromosome DNA.

R. R. M. PATERSON (*C.A.B. International Mycological Institute, Kew, U.K.*). Approximately what percentage of those fungi tested have dsRNA viruses and what is the nature of the other viruses?

K. W. BUCK. About 20 %. However, only limited surveys have been done. I suspect the true figure to be higher.

Isometric single-stranded RNA and double-stranded DNA viruses have been described. Other morphological types of particle detected by electron microscopy, but not isolated, include rigid rods, filamentous rods, bacilliform particles, herpes-like particles, geminate particles and pleomorphic particles with membrane envelopes. Recently, retrovirus-like particles have been isolated from *Saccharomyces cerevisiae* and have been shown to be intermediates of DNA transposition.

C. PRIOR (*C.A.B. International Institute of Biological Control, Ascot, U.K.*). How host-specific are the viral pathogens of fungi?

K. W. BUCK. The only known method of viral transmission between different fungal strains is by hyphal anastomosis, which would be expected to contain viruses within species. However, although related viruses are generally found in the same or closely related species, there are some interesting exceptions, e.g. related viruses have been found in *Penicillium stoloniferum* and *Diplicarpon rosae*. Methods that have been developed recently for infecting fungal protoplasts with isolated viruses should allow experimental host ranges to be determined.

G. DÉFAGO (*Swiss Federal Institute of Technology, Zürich, Switzerland*). What is known about the molecular basis of hypovirulence of *Endothia parasitica*?

K. W. BUCK. Virulent strains of *E. parasitica* produce oxalic acid, which may weaken host tissue by combining with calcium, and which lower the pH, thus providing favourable conditions for the action of degrading enzymes such as polygalacturonase. Hypovirulent strains are deficient in oxalic acid production. However, there must be other factors contributing to hypovirulence. N. K. Van Alfen is currently comparing cDNA libraries of virulent and hypovirulent strains, which are isogenic in their nuclear genomes, and this work should eventually contribute to a more complete understanding of the molecular basis of hypovirulence.

C. C. PAYNE (*Institute of Horticultural Research, Littlehampton, U.K.*). Professor Buck implied that the dsDNA found in vesicles in hypovirulent *Endothia parasitica* could arise through the replication of an ssRNA virus. Is there any evidence that such a virus is related to RNA viruses of higher plants?

K. W. Buck. The comparison has been made with the animal virus poliovirus on the basis of a blocked 5′ terminus and a polyA tract at the 3′ terminus. There are several groups of plant viruses with these structural properties; in terms of size, the potyvirus (potato virus Y) group is the most similar. We must await sequence analysis of *E. parasitica* dsRNA to see if these rather superficial similarities are upheld at the level of genome organization.

*Phil. Trans. R. Soc. Lond.* B **318**, 319–333 (1988)

*Printed in Great Britain*

# Biological control of the cassava mealybug, *Phenacoccus manihoti*, by the exotic parasitoid *Epidinocarsis lopezi* in Africa

By P. Neuenschwander and H. R. Herren

*International Institute of Tropical Agriculture, Oyo Road, PMB 5320, Ibadan, Nigeria*

Since its accidental introduction into Africa, the cassava mealybug (cm) has spread to about 25 countries. The specific parasitoid *Epidinocarsis lopezi*, introduced from South America, its area of origin, into Nigeria in 1981, has since been released in more than 50 sites. By the end of 1986 it was established in 16 countries and more than 750 000 km².

In southwestern Nigeria, cm populations declined after two initial releases, and have since remained low. During the same period, populations of indigenous predators of cm, mainly coccinellids, have declined, as have indigenous hyper-parasitoids on *E. lopezi*, because of scarcer hosts. Results from laboratory bionomic studies were incorporated into a simulation model. The model, field studies on population dynamics, and experiments excluding *E. lopezi* by physical or chemical means demonstrate its efficiency, despite its low reproductive potential.

## Introduction

Some of the first introductions of biological control agents against pests were made in Africa. But only 15 insect pests have been controlled in nine countries, mostly in East Africa, a meagre record considering the opportunities and importance of biological control to African agriculture (Greathead 1986). This paper describes a large-scale biological control effort on cassava (*Manihot esculenta*), a prime source of carbohydrates (from the roots), and proteins and vitamins (from the leaves) (Sylvestre & Arraudeau 1983). The mealybug project covers most of tropical Africa from its centre in the lowland, humid tropics of West Africa and is executed and coordinated by the Africa-wide Biological Control Programme(abcp) of the International Institute of Tropical Agriculture (IITA), which collaborates with numerous institutions worldwide. The project's targets are a complete biological control programme including introduction of exotic beneficials and monitoring them after they are established, studying both their biology and their interactions with indigenous insects, particularly their host-finding capacity, then thoroughly assessing their impact on the host and on farmers' incomes.

## Accidental introduction and spread of the cassava mealybug in Africa

In 1973 an unknown species of mealybug causing serious damage to cassava in Congo (Sylvestre 1973; Matile-Ferrero 1978) and Zaire (Hahn & Williams 1973) was reported. The new pest, reproducing parthenogenetically, spread rapidly through most of the African cassava belt which extends from 15° N to 20° S (maximum distribution shown in figure 1) (Herren *et al.* 1988). Within a few years it became the major pest on cassava. Matile-Ferrero (1977) described the insect as a new species, *Phenacoccus manihoti* (Homoptera, Pseudococcidae).

In Zaire, general cm outbreaks occurred in the Bas-Zaire, Bandundu and Shaba regions; the

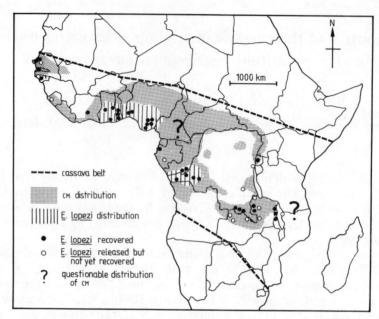

FIGURE 1. Maximum distribution of CM (shaded) and *Epidinocarsis lopezi* (stripes) in Africa showing the situation at the end of 1986.

pest gained new footholds in Senegal and Gambia in 1976, in Nigeria and Benin Republic in 1979 (Akinlosotu & Leuschner 1981), and in Sierra Leone and Malawi in 1985. From those sites, the pest spread up to 300 km per year. By the end of 1986 it had reached about 25 countries and covered about 70% of the African cassava belt. In most countries CM caused severe damage by stunting the growth points of cassava plants, sometimes totally defoliating the plants. Tuber yield losses of 84% were documented (Nwanze 1982). Weed and erosion problems, after plant growth was crippled, sometimes led to total destruction of the crops. Additionally, the poor quality of cuttings from infested plants, used as planting material, led to cassava disappearing in some regions.

Because the pest spread over large areas that are difficult to approach and mostly mixed-cropped by subsistence farmers, biological control seemed a particularly appropriate approach, needing no input by the farmers. So an effort, corresponding to the scale of the problem, was undertaken to introduce beneficial species from the original home of the CM into Africa.

## EXPLORATION FOR NATURAL ENEMIES

Since cassava, the only natural host of the CM in Africa, was introduced from South America (in the 1500s) and the genera *Manihot* and *Phenacoccus* are particularly rich in species in central and northern South America, searching for beneficial insects started there. From 1977 to 1980 the Commonwealth Institute of Biological Control (CIBC) searched in the Carribean, Venezuela, the Guyanas and northeastern Brazil; then in 1980 and 1981 IITA explored the southern U.S.A., Mexico, Central America, northern Colombia and Venezuela (figure 2). A mealybug in this region was causing the same symptoms, so it was initially thought to be identical with *P. manihoti* (Bennett & Yaseen 1980). Several parasitoid species collected failed to reproduce on CM in an insectary in the Congo (Bennett & Yaseen 1980) or on another mealybug in Trinidad (Yaseen 1988). Because of small morphological differences and the bisexual nature of the mealybug on cassava in northern Latin America, it was newly described as *P. herreni* (Cox & Williams 1981).

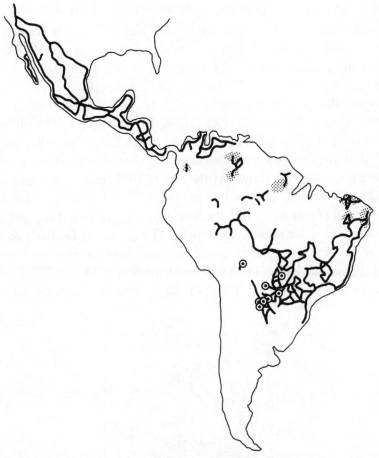

FIGURE 2. Exploration for mealybug natural enemies by the Africa-wide Biological Control Project in latin America (thick lines represent the exploration route). Recovery of *Phenacoccus manihoti* (dots) and *P. herreni* (shaded).

*P. manihoti* was finally discovered in 1981 in Paraguay by the Centro Internacional de Agricultura Tropical (CIAT). Several predators and parasitoids were collected by CIBC and sent, via quarantine at CIBC London, to IITA. The shipments were approved by the Inter-African Phytosanitary Council and passed through Nigerian Plant Quarantine.

Among the parasitoids was *Epidinocarsis* (= *Apoanagyrus*) *lopezi* (Hymenoptera, Encyrtidae), described in 1963 from northern Argentina from an unidentified mealybug. Further explorations in Paraguay, Brazil and Bolivia were sponsored by the Deutsche Gesellschaft für Technische Zusammenarbeit (GTZ) under the umbrella of IITA. Between 1983 and 1986, two entomologists covered extended regions, but discovered only eight areas where CM occurred: four in Paraguay (Löhr & Varela 1987), one in Bolivia and three in Mato Grosso do Sul, Brazil (figure 2) (Löhr 1987). In all areas CM populations were low, with peaks up to 16 CM per tip in the dry season and below 1 CM per tip during the rainy season: populations so low, that trap plants loaded with cm from a laboratory culture had to be placed into fields to attract natural enemies. That led to the collection of *E. lopezi* (and several more parasitoids and predators) from Brazil and Bolivia (Löhr 1987).

### Release, establishment, and dispersal of *E. lopezi*

*E. lopezi* (an endophagous, solitary encyrtid) was, and still is, reared at IITA on its only known host, *P. manihoti*, on potted cassava plants. First releases at IITA were made in November 1981 at the beginning of the dry season (Herren & Lema 1982) and one year later in nearby Abeokuta (figure 3) (Lema & Herren 1985). *E. lopezi* was permanently established, i.e. it was recovered after the next rainy season, which is its most difficult survival period because of low host density. By March 1983 (about 10 generations after the release) *E. lopezi* was recovered from almost all sampled fields within 100 km from where they were released, and some 170 km north of the release site in the Guinea Savannah zone. They spread more slowly south and southeast into the rain forest. At the end of 1984, three years after the first release, *E. lopezi* was found in 70 % of all fields on more than 200000 km² in southwestern Nigeria and up to the northern limit of regular cm distribution (figure 3) (Herren *et al.* 1988). This dispersal, among the fastest recorded for microhymenoptera (Tooke 1955; De Bach & Argyriou 1967; van den Bosch *et al.* 1970), occurred mostly in traditional farming environments on local cassava varieties. We do not know which mode of transport was most important: active flight, passive transport by wind, or by man transporting cassava cuttings and leaves.

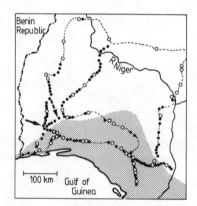

FIGURE 3. Distribution of *Epidinocarsis lopezi* in southwestern Nigeria during the survey in December 1984. The solid arrow shows the release near Abeokuta in November 1982, the broken arrow the release at IITA in November 1981; dots show where *E. lopezi* was recovered, circles show where only cm was found, and broken lines where no cm was found; shaded area represents rain forest.

On request from different governments, and in collaboration with the local agronomists and entomologists, we exported *E. lopezi* to other African countries, by the end of 1986 to more than 50 sites (confirmed distribution shown in figure 1). Although we sometimes released several thousand wasps at a site, on several occasions we used fewer than one hundred. *E. lopezi* proved to be established in almost all accessible sites the next dry season, and spread into several neighbouring countries. It is now established in 16 African countries, from north to south and west to east: Senegal, Gambia, Guinea-Bissau, Côte d'Ivoire, Ghana, Togo, Benin,

Nigeria, Cameroon, Gabon, Congo, Zaire, Angola, Rwanda, Zambia and Malawi. Recent releases in Sierra Leone and Zambia have not yet been monitored.

The area of distribution in Africa is estimated to be 750000 km$^2$. Approximately 1 % of the area (750000 ha†) is under cassava cultivation in a wide range of ecological zones (Sudan savannah, Guinea savannah, equatorial rainforest, East African highlands). The distribution already exceeds that of any other agent introduced into Africa for biological control of insect pests, and the adaptability of *E. lopezi* to different ecological conditions is without precedent in Africa (Greathead *et al.* 1971). Few other biological control agents have been spread over similarly large areas or more countries (Schuster *et al.* 1971; Bartlett 1978; Sailer *et al.* 1984).

Currently, CM is spreading farther into the East African highlands, with unconfirmed reports from Uganda, Tanzania and Mozambique. Though maximum dispersal rates of more than 100 km per dry season for *E. lopezi* were confirmed from other countries of the humid lowlands, the wasp seems to spread more slowly under the East African highland conditions of southern Shaba province in Zaire and Zambia's Luapula valley. It appears, therefore, that the strategy (ground and aerial releases) for East Africa must be changed to more numerous and closer release sites.

### RELATIONSHIP BETWEEN INDIGENOUS INSECTS AND THE INTRODUCED *E. LOPEZI*

*E. lopezi* is not the only parasitoid attacking CM. Other primary parasitoids and predators compete, and hyperparasitoids are direct antagonists. In South America, Löhr (1987) found five species of primary parasitoids on CM, but the five were attacked by six, sometimes very abundant, species of hyperparasitoids. Another 11 species of mostly polyphagous insect predators, mainly coccinellids, were attacked by five species of hymenopterous parasitoids.

Although cassava was introduced into Africa in the 16th century, it reached its current distribution in this century. Until recently it had a remarkably poor insect fauna. After CM was introduced and spread, the arthropod fauna of cassava rapidly increased in abundance and complexity. Many workers compiled lists of new insects: for Congo (Matile-Ferrero 1977; Fabres & Matile-Ferrero 1980), Nigeria (Akinlosotu & Leuschner 1981), and Gabon (Boussienguet 1986). After the introduction of *E. lopezi*, the fauna associated with CM were studied again in many countries, and more than 130 species were reported (Neuenschwander *et al.* 1987). Apparently, indigenous coccinellid predators adopted the newly arrived CM as an alternative host. A few encyrtids of the genus *Anagyrus*, parasitoids of other mealybugs like *Phenacoccus madeirensis* Green and *Ferrisia virgata* Cockerell, also adapted to the new pest, but not often. They, in turn, were followed by their own complex of parasitoids and hyperparasitoids. Simultaneously, insects of other species occupied shoot apexes that CM feeding had distorted. Polyphagous predators attracted to the enriched insect fauna added still more links to the developing food web. After *E. lopezi* was established, a complex of about 10 species of hyperparasitoids of *Anagyrus* spp. or of coccinellid parasitoids also shifted to this host.

In southwestern Nigeria, hyperparasitoids destroyed up to 50 % of all *E. lopezi* mummies the first season *E. lopezi* was established and parasitoid populations were large on the still abundant CM hosts. Similar observations were reported from Congo (Ganga 1984), Ghana

† 1 hectare = 10$^4$ m$^2$.

(Korang-Amoakoh *et al.* 1988), and Zaire (Hennessey & Muaka 1988); but the 50% fell to 20% when *E. lopezi* and CM populations in southwestern Nigeria declined in the next few years, indicating density dependence in hyperparasitism (Neuenschwander *et al.* 1988). The 20% are below the percentage reported from the same hyperparasitoids on the inefficient indigenous *Anagyrus* sp. on CM in Gabon (Boussienguet 1986), from similar species on *E. lopezi* in South America (Löhr 1987), or from many other successful biological control programmes (Bennett 1981). Finally, mathematical models predict more stability with, than without, hyper-parasitoids (Luck *et al.* 1981; Hassell & Waage 1984). So, the *E. lopezi*-hyperparasitoid system seems unlikely to change suddenly for the worse and critically affect *E. lopezi*'s performance in the future.

Establishing *E. lopezi* also influenced the abundance and composition of indigenous CM predators. On the large CM populations that existed before the exotic parasitoid was introduced, beneficial fauna consisted almost entirely of predators (98%). But within a few months after *E. lopezi* was released, it and its hyperparasitoids accounted for 61% of all specimens collected, and 84–86% of all natural enemies early in the next two dry seasons (P. Neuenschwander & W. N. O. Hammond, unpublished results). Though predators probably indiscriminately destroy active CM containing parasitoid larvae, the high percentage of *E. lopezi* indicates that it stands up well to competition.

## BIOLOGICAL STUDIES

Since the project started, the biology of *E. lopezi* had been studied for various reasons: (1) to acquire information to improve rearing, storage, and transport; (2) to understand the parasitoid's life-history and interactions with the CM host; and (3) to study the evolution of host-finding behaviour of *E. lopezi*, which seemed particularly promising for the understanding and evaluation of this and other biological control programmes. The experiments on host finding were done by the University of Leiden in collaboration with the ABCP.

### Biology of the immatures

*E. lopezi* is a solitary, internal parasitoid with four larval instars; it passes its nymphal stage inside the mummified CM often in sheltered places between leaves. Its egg and larval morphology were described (Odebiyi & Bokonon-Ganta 1986; B. Löhr, A. M. Varela & B. Santos, unpublished results). Most *E. lopezi* develop within two weeks at 27 °C, twice as fast as their host. Optimum temperature is 27 °C, and the lower thermal threshold is 13.3 °C (from Lema & Herren 1982). Male larvae grow faster than females (B. Löhr, A. M. Varela & B. Santos, unpublished results) and become smaller adults than females (Kraaijeveld & van Alphen 1986; B. Löhr, A. M. Varela & B. Santos, unpublished results). When a second instar serves as host, development is much slower. The delay affects only larval development, particularly the second instar parasitoid larvae; nymphal development remains unaffected. Thus a small proportion of *E. lopezi* emerges only after four weeks, or one parasitoid generation later, (B. Löhr, A. M. Varela & B. Santos, unpublished results), a feature that might have survival value when host populations are small. In one third of the CM with delayed development, however, the immature parasitoids die (B. Löhr, A. M. Varela & B. Santos, unpublished results). The dead parasitoid larvae are usually encapsulated within the first two weeks of development, but they reach only about 12–16% of the total (Neuenschwander &

Sullivan 1987; B. Löhr, A. M. Varela & B. Santos, unpublished results). Living parasitoid larvae that are being encapsulated can often free themselves. Most melanization, however, is restricted to wounded tissue of the host and, in the experiments that allowed the same CM to be stung several times, the supernumerary larvae have been killed (Neuenschwander & Sullivan 1988).

### Biology of the adults

After emerging, the females mate. Olfactometer experiments showed them attracted to CM-infested cassava leaves but not to CM alone. As they were also attracted to uninfested leaves from partly infested cassava plants but not to clean leaves of uninfested plants, they obviously home in on the odours (synomones) of attacked cassava to locate CM-bearing plants (Nadel & van Alphen 1986). This mechanism apparently helps the females locate very small host populations. Once they reach the plant, they are arrested by CM wax acting as contact kairomone (Langenbach & van Alphen 1986), but seem to find their hosts by chance (B. Löhr, A. M. Varela & B. Santos, unpublished results). Jerking movements of the abdomen give larger hosts a stronger defence, so attacks are concentrated more on third instar CM (Kraaijeveld & van Alphen 1986; Neuenschwander & Madojemu 1986; B. Löhr, A. M. Varela & B. Santos, unpublished results). The CM's defence is particularly strong if it has been previously attacked by a wasp, which reduces superparasitism (Iziquel 1985). Kraaijeveld & van Alphen (1986) also observed a weak rejection of already parasitized CM by a parasitoid female when testing their suitability as hosts with her antennae.

After a sting, the female parasitoid often turns and feeds on the host. Second instars are preferred, and almost as many such instars are killed as are killed by the parasitoid larva (Neuenschwander & Madojemu 1986; B. Löhr, A. M. Varela & B. Santos, unpublished results). Host-feeding is less important on older instars, and increases only slightly with increased oviposition. Eggs are rarely laid in host-fed CM (B. Santos & P. Neuenschwander, unpublished results).

The proportion of stings that leads to oviposition is highest on early fourth instars (B. Löhr & A. M. Varela, unpublished results) but varies greatly in different experiments. Younger host instars are preferred for male eggs, old ones for female eggs (Kraaijeveld & van Alphen 1986; B. Löhr & A. M. Varela, unpublished results). Mean oviposition at 25 °C was reported as high as 85 eggs per female (Iziquel 1985), but reproduction averaged 40–67 offspring per female with a maximum of 10 per day and a mean longevity of approximately 10 days. Longevity increased substantially at lower temperatures (Ganga 1984; Odebiyi & Bokonon-Ganta 1986; B. Löhr, A. M. Varela & B. Santos, unpublished results; P. Neuenschwander, unpublished results). Oviposition increased as numbers of hosts offered increased, but percentage parasitism in these experiments tended to decrease (Odebiyi & Bokonon-Ganta 1986), except at very small host populations (when it increases with an increase in host numbers) (P. Neuenschwander, unpublished results). Overall, larger females lived longer and reproduced better, which demonstrated the advantage of larger hosts for oviposition (Kraaijeveld & van Alphen 1986). The reproductive capacity of E. lopezi is limited, but mortality of the host also includes host-feeding and mutilation apart from larval parasitism. Moreover, 30 % of once stung, second instar CM, whether they contained a parasitoid egg or not, showed retarded growth and lay an average of only 37 eggs (compared with several hundred eggs by healthy CM) (B. Löhr, A. M. Varela & B. Santos, unpublished results). Collectively the other mortalities, depending on the CM instar, can far surpass mortality through mummy formation (Neuenschwander & Madojemu 1986).

[ 215 ]

IMPACT ASSESSMENT

Methods of evaluating the effectiveness of biological control agents have been reviewed (Hodek *et al.* 1972; Kiritani & Dempster 1973; van Lenteren 1980). To assess the efficiency of *E. lopezi* we chose three approaches.

*Exclusion experiments*

Physical exclusion experiments by sleeve cages were done at IITA. They demonstrated (figure 4) that, two months after artificial infestation of cassava tips, CM populations were 7.0 and 2.3 times lower on tips covered with open cages than on tips in closed cages that excluded most parasitoids. On similarly infested but uncovered tips CM populations were 24.3 and 37.5 times lower, and parasitization rates were higher (Neuenschwander *et al.* 1986). In a chemical exclusion experiment, an artificially infested field treated weekly with carbaryl had a peak CM infestation of 200 per tip because the adult parasites were killed by the insecticide. In the untreated plot, parasitism was much higher and CM populations were mostly fewer than 10 per tip (figure 5) (Neuenschwander *et al.* 1986). Those experiments were difficult, but they demonstrate the efficiency of *E. lopezi* in the field in such conditions.

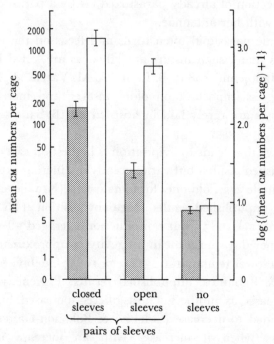

FIGURE 4. CM densities about two months after infestation in closed and open-sleeve cages, and from uncovered cassava tips without artificial infestation, in the second half of the 1983/84 dry season (shaded) and the first half of the 1984/85 dry season (white).

*Studies on CM population dynamics*

CM monitored after two early releases in southwestern Nigeria (Herren & Lema 1982; Lema *et al.* 1984) showed slight differences in the CM population dynamics in the release field and control fields (figure 6). But the so-called control fields were also invaded by *E. lopezi*, probably

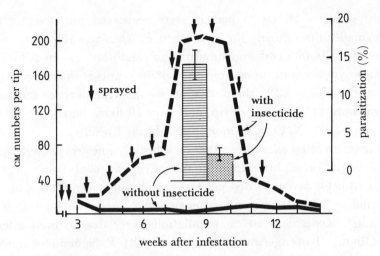

FIGURE 5. Cassava mealybug population development in insecticide treated (arrows, broken line) and untreated plots (solid line), together with mean parasitization rates for weeks 3–12 (± the standard error) by *Epidinocarsis lopezi*.

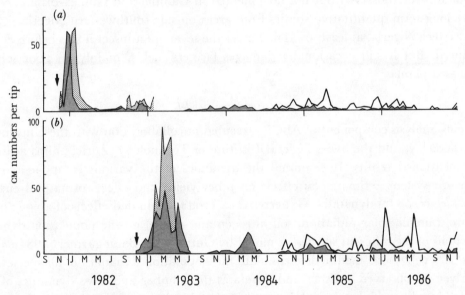

FIGURE 6. Population dynamics of CM on IITA improved (darker shade) and farmers' (white) varieties after the introduction of *Epidinocarsis lopezi* (arrows) in (a) Ibadan and (b) Abeokuta, in southwestern Nigeria. The original control field, with IITA improved variety, (lighter shade) was invaded by *E. lopezi* within 1–2 months. (Mean of 2–3 fields, 50 tips each, every 2 weeks.)

during the first month (see above under dispersal). Collapse of CM populations at the end of the dry season has also been reported where no parasitoids were established (Fabres 1982; Leuschner 1978).

Monitoring near Ibadan and Abeokuta continued on 12 fields, half planted with farmer's varieties, half with improved IITA variety TMS 30572 (figure 6) (Hammond *et al.* 1988). Every year CM populations peaked in the second half of the dry season. Peaks were generally higher near Abeokuta than in Ibadan's more humid area, averaging two to three times more on farmer's varieties than on the IITA disease-resistant variety, which grows more vigorously.

328        P. NEUENSCHWANDER AND H. R. HERREN

Occasional sharp peaks of 20–40 cm per tip were registered but, overall, cm populations remained much smaller than during the year when *E. lopezi* was released.

In surveys covering 200000 km² and hundreds of randomly chosen fields in southwestern Nigeria, cm damage symptoms declined from 88 % of the plants at the end of the first dry season after *E. lopezi* was released to 23 % the next year. By then the average cm population in 100 infested fields was only $11 \pm 1.7$ cm per tip, and only 16 fields had more than 20 cm per tip (P. Neuenschwander & W. N. O. Hammond, unpublished results).

In other countries, cm often exceeding 1000 on a heavily infested cassava tip were observed in the absence of the parasitoid but seldom quantitatively assessed. In a recent cm outbreak in Malawi, cm from 13 fields averaged 554 per tip (calculations from 50 tips per field, log of the mean density equal to $2.74 \pm 0.13$ standard error) (P. Neuenschwander & R. D. Markham, unpublished results). Reductions in cm populations were documented after *E. lopezi* was introduced in Ghana (Korang-Amoakoh *et al.* 1988; P. Neuenschwander & W. N. O. Hammond, unpublished results), in the Rift valley of Rwanda (B. Birandano, unpublished results), in Bas-Zaire (Hennessey & Muaka 1988), and in the Luapula valley of Zambia (C. Klinnert, unpublished results) despite considerable hyperparasitism. Important reductions in cm infestation were observed but not documented in Gambia and Guinea-Bissau. We still do not have long-term quantitative studies from areas outside southwestern Nigeria.

In southwestern Nigeria, at least, cm is no longer the severe pest insect it was before *E. lopezi* was introduced. But it still occasionally damages farmers' fields, mainly on poor soil and heavily diseased plants.

*Computer simulation model*

The systems-analysis component of ABCP, executed in collaboration with the University of California, Berkeley, and the Swiss Federal Institute of Technology, Zürich, aims at linking previously mentioned results. It examines the dynamics of the various components of the cassava agro-ecosystem, estimates cm effects on tuber yields and effects of natural enemies, including *E. lopezi*, on cm dynamics. Gutierrez *et al.* (1988) evaluated effects of abiotic factors (temperature, rainfall, solar radiation, soil nitrogen and water) on the population dynamics and interactions of the different species. A model by Gutierrez & Baumgärtner (1984 *a b*) and Gutierrez *et al.* (1987) was modified to simulate the population dynamics of all species. The model is driven by observed weather and simulates the number and mass dynamics of each species much like a life-table analysis. It is based on the idea that each population must acquire resources, so acquisition and demand rates determine whether the population grows or declines.

Many, but not all, of the parameters for *E. lopezi* listed in the biology section and obtained mostly in the laboratory, were superimposed on cassava and mealybug data (Nwanze *et al.* 1979; Fabres & Boussienguet 1981; Fabres & Le Rü 1986; Le Rü & Fabres 1986; Le Rü & Papierok 1986; Schulthess *et al.* 1988) and incorporated in the first simulations of the computer model (Gutierrez *et al.* 1987). Figure 7, which includes also unpublished results by A. P. Gutierrez, shows the simulated cassava yield loss due to cm during the 1983/84 season at Ibadan by introducing cm on day 50 (which gives highest loss) and reduction in yield losses due to *E. lopezi* assuming two search parameters. Though the model needs some refinement, the population curves it describes correspond well with those found (figure 6), and it predicts the impact of *E. lopezi*. Further simulations that included the effect of coccinellid predators show

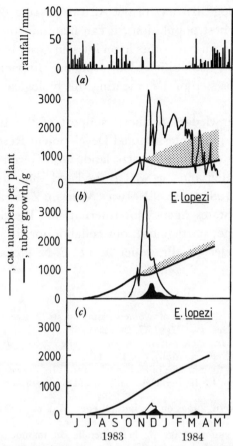

FIGURE 7. Simulated cassava tuber growth (in grams per plant) (thick line) during the 1983/84 season at Ibadan with CM populations per plant (*a*) without natural enemies (shaded area represents yield loss), (*b*) with *E. lopezi* (parasitized CM shown in black) with medium search rate assumed, and (*c*) with *E. lopezi* with a high search rate assumed.

that, contrary to the reports by Iziquel (1985) and Odebiyi & Bokonon-Ganta (1986), the introduced parasitoid is responsible for the observed small CM populations. Crop losses are now being measured directly in Ghana and Côte d'Ivoire by comparing yields in areas where the parasitoid has been established during the full or part of the growing season, or not yet. The growth characteristics of the plant, abiotic and biotic factors, farmers' opinions, and market situations are all incorporated in the simulation model.

## CONCLUSION

Results so far show that *E. lopezi*, introduced from a few localities in South America, established very successfully in several ecological zones of Africa. From the release sites it spread rapidly, at least in the lowland, humid tropics. That it displaced competing, indigenous predators attests to its efficiency. Hyperparasitism was less on the reduced parasitoid and CM populations, which reached equilibrium during the second dry season after *E. lopezi* was released. Exclusion experiments, population dynamics studies, and preliminary results of a computer-simulation model show that *E. lopezi* is an efficient biological control agent across several, but perhaps not all, ecological zones of the African cassava belt. Although *E. lopezi* cannot substantially lower large host populations, it can maintain the small CM populations that exist after the rainy season. Because it homes in on infested host plants rather than directly on CM it has a good host-finding capability. The economic impact of *E. lopezi* is being investigated now as the last major step in documenting this biological control programme.

IITA's ABCP gratefully acknowledges financial support of the International Fund for Agricultural Development, Rome; the International Development Research Centre, Canada, and governmental donor agencies of Austria, Switzerland, West Germany, and, since 1984–5, those of Denmark, Italy, The Netherlands, as well as the Food and Agriculture Organization of the United Nations, and since 1986 those of Norway. Work in Zaire and Guinea-Bissau was partly supported by the United States Agency for International Development. We thank all agencies mentioned in the text and, particularly, our collaborators in the field for their help. We also thank J. van Alphen (Leiden), L. Brandner, and L. E. N. Jackai (IITA) for reviewing the manuscript.

REFERENCES

Akinlosotu, T. A. & Leuschner, K. 1981 Outbreak of two new cassava pests (*Mononychellus tanajoa* and *Phenacoccus manihoti*) in southwestern Nigeria. *Trop. Pest Mgmt* **27**, 247–250.

Bartlett, B. R. 1978 Pseudococcidae. In *Introduced parasites and predators of arthropod pests and weeds: a world review* (ed. C. P. Clausen). (*Agric. Handb. Forest Surv.* no. **480**), pp. 137–170.

Bennett, F. D. 1981 Hyperparasitism in the practice of biological control. In *The role of hyperparasitism in biological control: a symposium* (ed. D. Rosen), pp. 43–49. Berkeley, California: Division of Agricultural Science, University of California.

Bennett, F. D. & Yaseen, M. 1980 Investigations on the natural enemies of cassava mealybug (*Phenacoccus* spp.) in the Neotropics. CIBC report. (Mimeograph.)

Boussienguet, J. 1986 Le complexe entomophage de la cochenille du manioc, *Phenacoccus manihoti* (Hom. Coccoidea Pseudococcidae) au Gabon. I. Inventaire faunistique et relations trophiques. *Annls Soc. ent. Fr.* N.S. **22**, 35–44.

Cox, J. & Williliams, D. J. 1981 An account of cassava mealybug (Hemiptera: Pseudococcidae) with a description of a new species. *Bull. ent. Res.* **71**, 247–258.

De Bach, P. & Argyriou, L. C. 1967 The colonization and success in Greece of some imported *Aphytis* spp. (Hym. Aphelinidae) parasitic on citrus scale insects (Hom. Diaspididae). *Entomophaga* **12**, 325–342.

Fabres, G. 1982 Bioécologie de la cochenille du manioc (*Phenacoccus manihoti* Hom. Pseudococcidae) en République Populaire du Congo. II. Variations d'abondance et facteurs de régulation. *Agron. Trop.* **36**, 369–377.

Fabres, G. & Boussienguet, J. 1981 Bioécologie de la cochenille du manioc (*Phenacoccus manihoti* Hom. Pseudococcidae) en République Populaire du Congo. *Agron. Trop.* **36**, 82–89.

Fabres, G. & Le Rü, B. 1986 Etude des relations plante-insecte pour la mise au point de méthodes de régulation des populations de la cochenille du manioc. In *La cochenille du manioc et sa biocoenose au Congo 1979–1984*, pp. 57–71. Brazzaville, Congo: Travaux de l'équipe Franco-Congolaise ORSTOM-DGRS.

Fabres, G. & Matile-Ferrero, D. 1980 Les entomophages inféodés à la cochenille du manioc, *Phenacoccus manihoti* (Hom. Coccoidea Pseudococcidae) en République Populaire du Congo. I. Les composantes de l'entomocoenose et leurs inter-relations. *Annls Soc. ent. Fr.* N.S. **16**, 509–515.

Ganga, T. 1984 Possibilités de régulations de la cochenille du manioc *Phenacoccus manihoti* Mat.-Ferr. (Hom. Pseudococcidae) par un entomophage exotique *Epidinocarsis lopezi* De Santis (Hym. Encyrtidae) en République Populaire du Congo. (25 pages.) Brazzaville, Congo: Office de la Recherche Scientifique et Technique Outre-Mer. (Mimeograph.)

Greathead, D. J. 1986 Opportunities for biological control of insect pests in tropical Africa. *Revue zool. afr.* **100**, 85–96.

Greathead, D. J., Lionnet, J. F. G., Lodos, N. & Whellan, J. A. 1971 A review of biological control in the Ethiopian Region. *Commonw. agric. Bur., tech. Commun.* **5**, 1–162.

Gutierrez, A. P. & Baumgärtner, J. U. 1984a Multitrophic level models of predator–prey energetics. I. Age-specific energetic models – pea aphid *Acyrtosiphon pisum* (Harris) (Homoptera: Aphididae) as an example. *Can. Ent.* **116**, 924–932.

Gutierrez, A. P. & Baumgärtner, J. U. 1984b Multitrophic level models of predator–prey energetics. II. A realistic model of plant–herbivore–parasitoid–predator interactions. *Can. Ent.* **116**, 933–949.

Gutierrez, A. P., Schulthess, F., Wilson, L. T., Villacorta, A. M., Ellis, C. K. & Baumgärtner, J. U. 1987 Energy acquisition and allocation in plants and insects: a hypothesis for the possible role of hormones in insect feeding patterns. *Can. Ent.* **119**, 109–129.

Gutierrez, A. P., Wermelinger, B., Schulthess, F., Baumgärtner, J. U., Yaninek, J. S., Herren, H. R., Neuenschwander, P., Löhr, B., Hammond, W. N. O. & Ellis, C. K. 1988 An overview of a system model of cassava and cassava pests in Africa. In *Africa-wide Biological Control Project of Cassava Pests*. (ed. P. Neuenschwander, J. S. Yaninek & H. R. Herren). (*Insect Sci. Applic.* (*spec. iss.*).) (In the press.)

Hahn, S. K. & Williams, R. J. 1973 Enquête sur le manioc en République du Zaire, 12–20 March 1973. Report to the Minister of Agriculture of the Republic of Zaire. (12 pages.) (Mimeograph.)

Hammond, W. N. O., Neuenschwander, P. & Herren, H. R. 1988 Impact of the exotic parasitoid *Epidinocarsis lopezi* on cassava mealybug (*Phenacoccus manihoti*) populations. In *Africa-wide Biological Control Project of Cassava Pests* (ed. P. Neuenschwander, J. S. Yaninek & H. R. Herren). (*Insect Sci. Applic.* (*spec. iss.*).) (In the press.)

Hassell, M. P. & Waage, J. K. 1984 Host–parasitoid population interactions. *A. Rev. Entomol.* **29**, 89–114.

Hennessey, R. D. & Muaka, T. 1988 Field biology of the cassava mealybug, *Phenacoccus manihoti*, and its natural enemies in Zaire. In *Africa-wide Biological Control Project of Cassava Pests* (ed. P. Neuenschwander, J. S. Yaninek & H. R. Herren). (*Insect Sci. Applic.* (*spec. iss.*).) (In the press.)

Herren, H. R. & Lema, K. M. 1982 CMB – first successfull releases. *Biocontrol News Inf.* **3**, 1.

Herren, H. R., Neuenschwander, P., Hennessey, R. D. & Hammond, W. N. O. 1988 Introduction and dispersal of *Epidinocarsis lopezi* (Hym., Encyrtidae), an exotic parasitoid of the cassava mealybug *Phenacoccus manihoti* (Hom., Pseudococcidae), in Africa. *Agric. Ecosystems Envir.* (In the press.)

Hodek, I. K., Hagen, K. S. & van Emden, H. F. 1972 *Methods for studying effectiveness of natural enemies*. In *Aphid technology* (ed. H. F. van Emden), p. 147–188. London: Academic Press.

Iziquel, Y. 1985 Le parasitisme de la cochenille du manioc *Phenacoccus manihoti* par l'Encyrtidae *Apoanagyrus lopezi* (= *Epidinocarsis lopezi*): induction, modalités, et conséquences agronomiques. D. E. A. d'Ecologie–Ethologie, University of Rennes.

Kiritani, K. & Dempster, J. P. 1973 Different approaches to the quantitative evaluation of natural enemies. *J. appl. Ecol.* **10**, 323–330.

Korang-Amoakoh, S., Cudjoe R. A. & Adjakloe, R. K. 1988 Biological control of cassava pests in Ghana. In *Africa-wide Biological Control Project of Cassava Pests* (ed. P. Neuenschwander, J. S. Yaninek & H. R. Herren). (*Insect Sci. Applic.* (*spec. iss.*).) (In the press.)

Kraaijeveld, A. R. & van Alphen, J. J. M. 1986 Host-stage selection and sex allocation by *Epidinocarsis lopezi* (Hymenoptera; Encyrtidae), a parasitoid of the cassava mealybug, *Phenacoccus manihoti* (Homoptera; Pseudococcidae). *Meded. Fac. Landbwet. Rijksuniv. Gent* **51**, 1067–1078.

Langenbach, G. E. J. & van Alphen, J. J. M. 1986 Searching behaviour of *Epidinocarsis lopezi* (Hymenoptera; Encyrtidae) on cassava: effect of leaf topography and a kairomone produced by its host, the cassava mealybug (*Phenacoccus manihoti*). *Meded. Fac. Landbwet. Rijksuniv. Gent* **51**, 1057–1065.

Lema, K. M. & Herren, H. R. 1982 Temperature relationships of two imported natural enemies of CM. *Int. Inst. trop. Agric. A. Rep.* **1981**, 56–57.

Lema, K. M., Herren, H. R. & Neuenschwander, P. 1984 Impact of *E. lopezi* on the CM. *Int. Inst. trop. Agric. A. Rep.* **1983**, 119–120.

Lema, K. M. & Herren, H. R. 1985 Release and establishment in Nigeria of *Epidinocarsis lopezi* a parasitoid of the cassava mealybug, *Phenacoccus manihoti*. *Entomologia exp. appl.* **38**, 171–175.

Le Rü, B. & Fabres, G. 1986 Influence de la température et de l'hyrométrie relative sur le taux d'accroissement des populations de la cochenille du manioc, *Phenacoccus manihoti* (Hom., Pseudococcidae) au Congo. In *La cochenille du manioc et sa biocoenose au Congo 1979–1984*, pp. 39–55. Brazzaville, Congo: Travaux de l'equipe Franco-Congolaise ORSTOM-DGRS.

Le Rü, B. & Papierok, B. 1986 Taux intrinsèque d'accroissement naturel de la cochenille du manioc, *Phenacoccus manihoti* Matile-Ferrero (Homoptères, Pseudococcidae). Intérêt d'une méthode simplifiée d'estimation de $r_m$. In *La cochenille du manioc et sa biocoenose au Congo 1979–1984*, pp. 14–26. Brazzaville, Congo: Travaux de l'équipe Franco-Congolaise ORSTOM-DGRS.

Leuschner, K. 1978 Preliminary observations on the mealybug (Hemiptera Pseudococcidae) in Zaire and a projected outline for subsequent work. In *Proceedings of an International Workshop on the Cassava Mealybug Phenacoccus manihoti Mat.-Ferr. (Pseudococcidae) M'vuazi, Zaire, June 26–29, 1977*. (ed. K. F. Nwanze & K. Leuschner), pp. 15–19.

Löhr, B. 1987 Report on the exploration activities for natural enemies of the cassava mealybug, *Phenacoccus manihoti*, in Paraguay, Bolivia, and Brazil. Report Deutsche Gesellschaft für Technische Zusammenarbeit, Eschborn, Federal Republic of Germany. (46 pages.) (Mimeograph.)

Löhr, B. & Varela, A. M. 1987 The cassava mealybug, *Phenacoccus manihoti* Mat.-Ferr., in Paraguay: further information on occurrence and population dynamics of the pest and its natural enemies. In *Proceedings of an International Workshop on Biological Control and Host Plant Resistance to control the Cassava Mealybug and Green Spider Mites in Africa Ibadan, Nigeria, 6–10 December 1982* (ed. H. R. Herren, R. D. Hennessey & R. Bitterli), pp. 57–69.

Luck, R. F., Messenger, P. S. & Barbieri J. F. 1981 The influence of hyperparasitism on the performance of biological control agents. In *The role of hyperparasitism in biological control: a symposium* (ed. D. Rosen), pp. 34–42. Berkeley, California: Division of Agricultural Science, University of California.

Matile-Ferrero, D. 1977 Une cochenille nouvelle nuisible au manioc en Afrique équatoriale, *Phenacoccus manihoti* n.sp. (Hom., Coccoidea Pseudococcidae). *Annls Soc. Ent. Fr.* (N.S.) **13**, 145–152.

Matile-Ferrero, D. 1978 Cassava mealybug in the People's Republic of Congo. In *Proceedings of an International Workshop on the Cassava Mealybug Phenacoccus manihoti Mat.-Ferr. (Pseudococcidae) M'vuazi, Zaire, June 26–29, 1977*. (ed. K. F. Nwanze & K. Leuschner), pp. 29–46.

Nadel, H. & van Alphen, J. J. M. 1986 The role of host- and host-plant odours in the attraction of a parasitoid, *Epidinocarsis lopezi* (Hymenoptera: Encyrtidae), to its host, the cassava mealybug, *Phenacoccus manihoti* (Homoptera: Pseudococcidae). *Meded. Fac. Landbwet. Rijkuniv. Gent* **51**, 1079–1086.

Neuenschwander, P. & Madojemu, E. 1986 Mortality of the cassava mealybug *Phenacoccus* manihoti Mat.-Ferr. (Hom., Pseudococcidae) associated with an attack by *Epidinocarsis lopezi* (Hym., Encyrtidae). *Mitt. schweiz. ent. Ges.* **59**, 57–62.

Neuenschwander, P. & Sullivan, D. 1988 Interactions between *Epidinocarsis lopezi* (De Santis) (Hym., Encyrtidae) and its host *Phenacoccus manihoti* Matile-Ferrero (Homoptera: Pseudococcidae). In *Africa-wide Biological Control Project of Cassava Pests* (ed. P. Neuenschwander, J. S. Yaninek & H. R. Herren). (*Insect Sci. Applic.* (*spec. iss.*).) (In the press.)

Neuenschwander, P., Hammond W. N. O. & Hennessey, R. D. 1988 Changes in the composition of the fauna associated with the cassava mealybug, *Phenacoccus manihoti*, following the introduction of the parasitoid *Epidinocarsis lopezi*. In *Africa-wide Biological Control Project of Cassava Pests* (ed. P. Neuenschwander, J. S. Yaninek & H. R. Herren). (*Insect Sci. Applic.* (*spec. iss.*).) (In the press.)

Neuenschwander, P., Hennessey, R. D. & Herren H. R. 1987 Food web of insects associated with the cassava mealybug, *Phenacoccus manihoti* Matile-Ferrero (Hemiptera: Pseudococcidae), and its introduced parasitoid *Epidinocarsis lopezi* (De Santis) (Hymenoptera: Encyrtidae), in Africa. *Bull. ent. Res.* **77**, 177–189.

Neuenschwander, P., Schulthess, F. & Madojemu, E. 1986 Experimental evaluation of the efficiency of *Epidinocarsis lopezi*, a parasitoid introduced into Africa against the cassava mealybug *Phenacoccus manihoti*. *Entomologia exp. appl.* **42**, 133–138.

Nwanze, K. F. 1982 Relationships between cassava root yields and infestations by the mealybug, *Phenacoccus manihoti*. *Trop. Pest Mgmt* **28**, 27–32.

Nwanze, K. F., Leuschner, K. & Ezumah, H. C. 1979 The cassava mealybug, *Phenacoccus* sp. in the Republic of Zaire. *Pest Artíc. News Summ.* **25**, 125–130.

Odebiyi, J. A. & Bokonon-Ganta, A. H. 1986 Biology of *Epidinocarsis* (= *Apoanagyrus*) *lopezi* (Hymenoptera: Encyrtidae) an exotic parasite of cassava mealybug, *Phenacoccus manihoti* (Homoptera: Pseudococcidae) in Nigeria. *Entomophaga* **31**, 251–260.

Sailer, R. I., Brown, R. E., Munir, B. & Nickerson, J. C. E. 1984 Dissemination of the citrus whitefly (Homoptera: Aleyrodidae) parasite *Encarsia lahorensis* (Howard) (Hymenoptera: Aphelinidae) and its effectiveness as a control agent in Florida. *Bull. ent. Soc. Am.* **30**, 36–39.

Schulthess, F., Baumgärtner, J. U. & Herren, H. R. 1988 Factors influencing the life table statistics of the cassava mealybug *Phenacoccus manihoti*. In *Africa-wide Biological Control Project of Cassava Pests*. (ed. P. Neuenschwander, J. S. Yaninek & H. R. Herren). (*Insect Sci. Applic.* (*spec. iss.*).) (In the press.)

Schuster, M. F., Boling, J. C. & Marony, J. J. Jr. 1971 Biological control of Rhodesgrass scale by airplane releases of an introduced parasite of limited dispersal ability. In *Biological control* (ed. C. B. Huffaker), pp. 227–250. New York: Plenum Press.

Sylvestre, P. 1973 Aspects agronomiques de la production du manioc à la ferme d'état de Mantsumba (Rep. Pop. Congo). I.R.A.T., Paris, mission report. (35 pages.) (Mimeograph.)

Sylvestre, P. & Arraudeau, M. 1983 *Le manioc*. In *Techniques agricoles et production tropicales* (ed. R. Coste), vol. 32, (262 pages.) Paris: Maisonneuve and Larose.

Tooke, F. G. C. 1955 The Eucalyptus snout beetle, *Gonipterus scutellatus* Gyll. A study of its ecology and control by biological means. *Ent. Mem. Dep. Agric. S. Afr.* **3**, 1–282.

van den Bosch, R., Frazer, B. D., Davis, C. S., Messenger, P. S. & Hom, R. 1970 *Trioxys pallidus* – an effective new walnut aphid parasite from Iran. *Calif. Agric.* **24**, 8–10.

van Lenteren, J. C. 1980 Evaluation of control capabilities of natural enemies: does art have to become science? *Neth. J. Zool.* **30**, 369–381.

Yaseen, M. 1988 Exploration for *Phenacoccus manihoti* and *Mononychellus tanajoa* natural enemies: the challenge, the achievements. In *Proceedings of an International Workshop on Biological Control and Host Plant Resistance to Control the Cassava Mealybug and Green Spider Mites in Africa Ibadan, Nigeria, 6–10 Dec. 1982* (ed. H. R. Herren, R. D. Hennessey & R. Bitterli). (In the press.)

## Discussion

I. HARPAZ (*Department of Entomology, Hebrew University of Jerusalem, Israel*). My question relates to the hyperparasites mentioned in the paper. Have these been identified, and if so, then has it been established whether these are indigenous African species that had adapted themselves to the newly introduced parasite, or that they were accidentally introduced from South America together with the primary parasite? The latter possibility seems most unlikely because the introduced material went through quarantine in London, as stated by Dr Neuenschwander.

P. NEUENSCHWANDER. Professor Harpaz is right; all hyperparasitoids of *E. lopezi* in Africa that we found are indigenous African species. The commoner ones, in fact, had already been reared previously from mummies of other mealybugs. About 10 species have been recorded up to now and identified by the British Museum (Natural History), belonging to six genera but, where identified to that level, they are different species from those in South America.

D. BADULESCU (*Faculty of Agriculture, University of Reading, U.K.*). Dr Neuenschwander said one of the goals of these kinds of programme is to leave trained teams to tackle similar problems in future; it seems to me that these programmes are very costly. Do you think that without much support from western European and American institutions such projects can be successfully repeated, such are the financial constraints in the Third World?

P. NEUENSCHWANDER. Yes, if the political will is there, but I hope the donors will continue to provide finance, because assisting in the execution of biological control programmes is a particularly good approach to achieve long-term solutions that do not make these countries even more dependent on the industrialized countries. I agree, biological control programmes are expensive to implement, because they require high quality research. Classical biological control programmes derive their benefits not from cheap initial implementation but from accruing benefits once they are successful.

A. E. AKINGBOHUNGBE (*Department of Plant Science, University of Ife, Nigeria*). Compared with the other African countries, it would appear that the mealybug outbreak in Nigeria is less severe. This I would like to think could be attributed to several factors. Firstly, the rainfall pattern within the past five years had been much better than in the late 1970s when CM was first found in the country; such rainfall removes the drought stress that helps epizootic development of CM. Secondly, within the context of a national control programme, an integrated pest management package involving date of planting, insecticide disinfestation of planting material and appropriate fertilizer application was formulated and has been implemented. Thirdly, there has been considerable shift in planting of improved, more tolerant cultivars. How do we put all of these together and account for their joint effects in assessing the efficiency of *E. lopezi* releases?

P. NEUENSCHWANDER. Without belittling other IPM components, I think we showed that *E. lopezi* was the key factor in maintaining small CM populations in southwestern Nigeria. The influence of planting time and cultivars can be tested in the simulation model as it is being developed. I would like to add that other countries, where *E. lopezi* was not established, continued to experience severe CM problems despite vastly increased rainfall compared with the early 1980s.

*Phil. Trans. R. Soc. Lond.* B **318**, 335–355 (1988)

*Printed in Great Britain*

# Biological control of bracken in Britain: constraints and opportunities

BY J. H. LAWTON

*Department of Biology, University of York, Heslington, York YO1 5DD U.K.*

Bracken (*Pteridium aquilinum*) is native to this country, but has become a major weed of marginal and hill land throughout western and northern Britain. Estimates suggest that the plant now occupies 3000–6700 km$^2$ and is spreading at 1–3 % per annum. It is a serious weed for several reasons. It causes direct loss of grazing land, is poisonous to stock, and makes shepherding very difficult. It also acts as a reservoir for sheep ticks, causing problems for farmers and managers of grouse moors (ticks transmit louping ill to grouse chicks). The plant is carcinogenic, and has been implicated in higher than average incidences of cancers in people living in bracken-infested areas. Finally, invasion by the plant leads to a loss of plant and animal communities that conservationists regard as more desirable than dense stands of bracken, for example heather moorland. Total costs to agriculture caused by bracken invasion are unknown, but probably run into several million pounds a year. The plant can be controlled by herbicides, or by cutting and rolling, but these methods are often too expensive or too labour intensive for use in many upland areas. One solution may therefore be biological control, although this has rarely been attempted against native plants anywhere in the world. This paper explains why biological control of bracken by using exotic insects from the Southern Hemisphere has a reasonable chance of success. Several potential control agents have now been found on bracken growing in temperate parts of South Africa. They include two moths: *Conservula cinisigna*, a folivorous noctuid, and one or more species of *Panotima*, pyralids that first mine the pinnae, and then bore into the rachis. Both appear to be bracken-specific. Their biologies, and those of other possible control agents are described, and constraints and problems encountered in trying to rear them under quarantine conditions are outlined. Over and above the biological and technical problems that have been encountered, and now largely overcome, are a host of political, legal, environmental and socio-economic problems that must be confronted before biological control of bracken in Britain can be attempted. The ecological and economic consequences of controlling bracken biologically need to be carefully weighed against the effects of its continuing spread, and against alternative solutions, for example, harvesting for biomass or control via markedly increased use of herbicides in upland areas.

## INTRODUCTION

Biological control has been attempted much more frequently against aliens than it has against native plants. Julien (1982), for example, documents biological control programmes against 86 naturalized weeds and 25 native species. In part, such data merely reflect the fact that many important weeds are aliens, but they are also indicative of a widely held view that native weeds are unsuitable candidates for biological control. Yet biological control of native plants can work; witness the success of *Dactylopius* released against *Opuntia* on Santa Cruz Island, California (Goeden & Ricker 1980).

This paper discusses the prospects for biological control of a British native plant, bracken fern (*Pteridium aquilinum*), by using exotic insects imported from the Southern Hemisphere. There is no tradition of biological control of either native or introduced weeds in Britain. An attempt to control the native thistle *Cirsium arvense* by using the exotic chrysomelid beetle *Haltica carduorum* failed (Baker *et al.* 1972), and did little to encourage further research on biological control of any British weeds. Yet there are good reasons for believing that well-researched programmes against specific weeds may have a reasonable chance of success, bringing with them large economic and potential environmental benefits. Bracken is a good example.

The account that follows amplifies and modifies information on constraints and opportunities that exist for the biological control of bracken in Britain, already published in Lawton (1986*a*, *b*) and Heads & Lawton (1986). The status of bracken in Britain, and reasons for regarding it as an important weed are reviewed, followed by an evaluation of biological control as a possible solution. The first thing we need to know is why native British bracken-feeding insects fail to control the plant. Consideration of this problem leads logically to the ideal characteristics of potential, exotic control agents, and then to a search for suitable species on bracken in the Southern Hemisphere, particularly South Africa. The biologies of several possible control agents are described, including two moths, *Conservula cinisigna* and *Panotima* sp., that look particularly promising. Finally, over and above the biological constraints and opportunities that exist for bracken control in Britain, there are legal, political, environmental and socio-economic factors to take into account before biological control can be attempted. These constraints are dealt with at the end of this paper.

## BRACKEN AS A WEED

Bracken is an invasive weed of marginal land, particularly hill farms in northern and western Britain. The plant's biology, ecology and status as a major weed are reviewed in Smith & Taylor (1986). According to Taylor (1986) bracken now covers approximately 6720 km² of the U.K., approximately equivalent in area to the county of Devon. Other estimates (see, for example, Lawson *et al.* 1986) put the area of infested land at about half this. What is clear is that in Britain as a whole, the plant is spreading vegetatively at about 1.3 % per year, with rates as high 3 % or more in some areas. Taylor (1986) estimates that between 1985 and 2000, at least another 1500 km² of land will be lost to bracken invasion. Put another way, for every two hectares of farming land lost each year to urban development and forestry, somewhere between half and one hectare are lost to bracken invasion. Some of the reasons for bracken encroachment are discussed by Page (1976), who summarizes the history of the plant in Britain from the Pleistocene. Originally a woodland plant, its spread can be traced to the clearance of forests by Neolithic man. More recently, a series of factors have contributed to its continuing expansion (Taylor 1986). For example, sheep rather than cattle are now the most important livestock on upland farms, but this was not always the case. Bracken is sensitive to trampling by cattle, both as dormant rhizomes (MAFF 1983) and in spring when the croziers first emerge. Sheep, with their smaller feet and lighter bodies, do much less damage. Moreover, many farmers no longer have the manpower or the money available to cut and roll bracken regularly in the spring when it is most susceptible to mechanical damage (MAFF 1983; Lowday 1986). Uncontrolled, or poorly controlled, moorland fires also encourage its spread (Brown 1986), as does improved drainage of hill land; bracken grows poorly in waterlogged soil.

*Problems caused by bracken*

Bracken is a problem for several reasons:

1. It is poisonous to domestic animals (see, for example, MAFF 1983; W. C. Evans 1986; Hannam 1986). Consumption of as little as 1 kg dry mass of bracken per day for a period of 2–4 weeks causes acute, fatal bracken poisoning in cattle; the symptoms include severe and extensive haemorrhages, ulceration of the intestinal mucosa, and leukaemia-like failure of the white blood cells. A similar condition has been described in sheep on the North York Moors, but in general sheep are more resistant than cattle to acute bracken poisoning. Instead, they tend to succumb to 'bright blindness', a progressive degeneration of the retina, and may also develop tumours, particularly in the jaw, but also in the rumen and elsewhere. In horses, eating bracken causes acute thiamine deficiency accompanied by loss of coordination and paralysis, so-called 'bracken staggers'. Invasion by the plant therefore represents not only a direct loss of grazing, but also a serious threat to livestock.

2. Dense bracken makes shepherding very difficult, because it hides both sheep and dogs, and impairs access.

3. The plant acts as a reservoir for sheep ticks (*Ixodes ricinus*) (see, for example, Hudson 1986) and hence acts as a focus of infection for two viral diseases of sheep, louping ill and tickborne fever (Hannam 1986; Johnson 1986).

4. As well as causing problems for farmers, bracken is also a serious weed on grouse moors. Red grouse (*Lagopus lagopus scoticus*) depend upon heather (*Calluna vulgaris*) as their major food, so that invasion by bracken leads directly to loss of grazing for an important upland animal. Worse, the nymphs of sheep ticks also feed on grouse chicks, to which they transmit louping ill virus disease; louping ill is implicated in the long-term decline of grouse in North Yorkshire and probably elsewhere in Britain, and its spread is linked ultimately to that of bracken (Hudson 1986; Dobson & Hudson 1986).

5. As effects on farm animals show, bracken contains one or more carcinogens (I. A. Evans 1984, 1986). There are unsubstantiated suggestions that these compounds may affect humans via milk and water supplies from bracken-infested land (Salazar 1985; Galpin & Smith 1986). Alternatively, higher than average regional incidences of human gastric and other cancers among farming communities in North Wales may be linked to inhaling or ingesting bracken spores; certainly the spores are carcinogenic in mice (I. A. Evans 1986).

6. The continuing spread of bracken poses complex and poorly studied problems for wildlife conservation. Dense stands of bracken have little to commend them in natural history or conservation terms. The plant threatens more valuable plant communities on some nature reserves (see, for example, Marrs 1985; Marrs *et al.* 1986), and on a larger scale is one of the factors contributing to the march of commercial forestry across grouse moors. The replacement of moorland by conifer plantations results in the total disappearance of grouse and other upland animals valued by conservationists (Dobson & Hudson 1986).

7. The impact of bracken on recreational use of upland areas is poorly studied and complicated (R. W. Brown 1986; I. W. Brown & Wathern 1986). In autumn, golden, bracken-covered hillsides may look nice (Heads & Lawton 1986), but walking or running through dense stands is very difficult and unpleasant; orienteers hate it (Borodino 1986)!

*Estimates of economic costs*

Together, the real and potential problems are more than enough to show that the continuing spread of bracken cannot be ignored. Yet remarkably, national figures for the economic costs directly attributable to the plant are not available. The current national average rate of spread of over 1 % per annum is the net rate after attempts at control. Economic costs include not only obvious things such as stock poisoning, lost grazing, and resources invested in existing control technology, but also less obvious 'secondary costs' such as enhanced mortality of lambs from tick-borne diseases, some of the costs of tick control by dipping, and a fall in the value of bracken-infested land. They also include things that are difficult, if not impossible, to price, such as the wildlife and conservation interests of upland areas.

Some idea of the economic costs of bracken can be obtained by reading the accounts in Smith & Taylor (1986). For example, a combination of MAFF and North York Moors National Park grants, and private investment in bracken control in the north of England in 1984 cannot have been less than £110000 (Johnson 1986). Nationally, the costs of control, lost grazing and stock poisoning must run into several million pounds a year. As Taylor (1986) points out, at current prices, the value of hill land that will be lost to bracken invasion between 1985 and 2000 amounts to some £6 million. By any criterion, bracken is an important weed.

## BIOLOGICAL CONTROL AS A POSSIBLE SOLUTION
*Biological compared with other means of control*

Bracken can be controlled by repeated cutting (MAFF 1983),or with herbicides. Asulam has been used for several years to good effect (McKelvie & Scragg 1972–73; Soper 1986), and several promising new herbicides are currently being tested (see, for example, Oswald *et al.* 1986). The problem is that hill farming and grouse shooting have precarious economies; it is difficult for individual landowners to justify investment in bracken control with average costs estimated at about £40 per ha† (Taylor 1986), and out of the question on many areas of steep and inaccessible hill land where aerial spraying is the only answer, and costs are over £100 per ha (Soper 1986). Nor do cutting and spraying provide permanent solutions. Four to ten years after spraying with Asulam, bracken has often completely regained its former dominance (Horsnail 1986; Lowday 1986; Robinson 1986; Soper 1986), although careful 'aftercare' helps to prevent reinvasion (MAFF 1983).

Against this background, biological control is attractive because it holds out the prospect of a cheap, permanent reduction in the abundance of bracken over large areas of hill land where more conventional techniques are uneconomic or impossible to apply.

*Where might suitable exotic insect control agents be found?*

Paradoxically, our capacity to adapt the techniques of classical biological weed control and use them against a native plant rests upon bracken's phenomenol success. The plant's potential Achilles heel is its world-wide distribution; it grows naturally on every continent except Antarctica (Page 1976), and may well be one of the five most abundant plants on earth (Harper 1977). In common with all other widely distributed plants (Strong *et al.* 1984), very

† 1 hectare = $10^4$ m².

different species of insects exploit bracken in different parts of its range (see, for example, Kirk 1982; Lawton 1982, 1984a, unpublished observations). This large pool of exotic insects can be regarded as a 'toolkit', from which, with time and patience, we might reasonably hope to select one or more appropriate biological control agents for use in Britain.

### Why do native, bracken-feeding insects fail to control the plant?

There is little point in searching for exotic insect control agents for bracken if they prove to be as ineffective as the plant's native British herbivores. Why do the 27 species of insects that regularly exploit the above-ground parts of the plant in Britain (Lawton 1982) cause it so little damage? Long-term studies (see, for example, Lawton 1982, 1984a, b, 1986a; Lawton & MacGarvin 1985; Lawton et al. 1986, 1987; MacGarvin et al. 1986) show that most of these herbivores are rare relative to the biomass of plant material available to them. Only very occasionally do native herbivores become common enough to cause heavy defoliation of bracken (Lawton 1976; M. F. Claridge, personal communication). However, it is possible to generate outbreaks of bracken herbivores by experimentally uncoupling them from their own enemies, broadly defined to include predators, parasitoids and diseases. Preliminary accounts of experiments on two species (the delphacid bug Ditropis pteridis and the sawfly Aneugmenus padi) are in Lawton (1984b), Lawton et al. (1986) and Lawton & MacGarvin (1985). The most dramatic results were obtained with a population of Aneugmenus padi established on an isolated, enemy-free experimental patch of bracken grown in plant pots on the University of York campus. Here, caterpillars of this species reached population densities ten times those of all the sawflies (seven species, including A. padi) at our long-term study site at Skipwith Common, near York, and bracken in the experimental patches was completely defoliated for two consecutive years. Because the bracken in the experiment was originally transplanted from Skipwith, the outbreak of Aneugmenus is unlikely to have been due to differences in the plants, something that we confirmed by taking half the bracken back to Skipwith with its sawflies. The population collapsed completely, whereas Aneugmenus on the campus continued to flourish.

Although we cannot do similar experiments with all 27 native species, a reasonable working hypothesis is that most native, bracken-feeding insects are kept rare, relative to the abundance of the host plant, by their own natural enemies. Hence, relieved of such control, exotic insects could cause extensive, permanent and ultimately debilitating damage. There is nothing particularly novel about this suggestion. A prime requisite for successful classical biological control of any insect pest or weed is to uncouple the control agent from limitation by its own predators, parasitoids and diseases (Huffaker 1974; Schroeder 1983; Goeden 1983). Hence, exotic insects released in Britain against bracken do not have to cause heavy damage to the plant in their own country; at home, they too presumably have specific enemies. What is vital is that agents are established in Britain, free from constraints imposed by higher trophic levels. Only then can we hope to damage the plant sufficiently to bring it under control.

### THE SEARCH FOR POSSIBLE CONTROL AGENTS
#### General principles

Potential insect biological control agents for use against bracken in Britain should ideally have the following characteristics.

1. They must come from a cool-temperate, seasonal climate, similar to the British Isles.

2. There are two major subspecies of bracken in the world, *aquilinum* and *caudatum*; British bracken is subspecies *aquilinum* variety *aquilinum* (Page 1976). Morphological and biochemical differences between the two subspecies could, though not inevitably, make it more difficult to establish insects from *caudatum* on *aquilinum* (see, for example, Harris 1984; Hokkanen & Pimentel 1984). In the first instance it would therefore seem wise to search for insects that normally exploit subspecies *aquilinum*.

3. The insects must be taxonomically and ecologically distinct from any of the British native bracken-feeding species. That is, they should exploit a 'vacant niche' (Lawton 1982, 1984*a*), because the more similar potential control agents are to species already resident on the plant in Britain, the more likely they are to suffer attacks from native parasitoids, predators and diseases (Goeden & Louda 1976; Jeffries & Lawton 1984; Lawton 1986*b, c*; Lawton & Brown 1986; Briese 1986), and the less likely they are to establish and control the plant.

4. The insects must be specific to bracken.

5. Finally, a search for control agents should not be confined to the above-ground parts of the plant. Little work has been done on rhizome-feeding insects on bracken in Britain (see Lawton 1982), but this should not rule out the possibility of looking for exotic rhizome feeders that also conform to characteristics 1–4. The large underground rhizome is one of the reasons why the plant is so difficult to control; a serious assault below ground could prove to be very effective.

Climatic mismatch almost certainly rules out the use of bracken feeding insects from Papua New Guinea, where the plant has a rich and varied herbivore fauna (Kirk 1982). Nothing ecologically or taxonomically distinct enough has yet been found in North America (Lawton 1982, unpublished data), and the most likely source of potential control agents therefore becomes the temperate Southern Hemisphere. South America and Australasia have the 'wrong' subspecies of bracken (*caudatum*), which leaves southern Africa. It is here that we have concentrated our search. Bracken in South Africa is not only the same subspecies, but it is also the same variety (*Pteridium aquilinum* subsp. *aquilinum* var. *aquilinum*) as British bracken (Page 1976) and grows in a similar climate, particularly in the mountains of Cape Province.

### The fauna of bracken in South Africa

The geographic range of bracken in South Africa is a broad band, from the coast inland until it becomes too dry (roughly coincident with areas that have more than 500 mm annual rainfall); that is, from the Cape, through Cape Province, and then via Ciskei and Transkei into Natal and the Transvaal, more or less parallel to the South Atlantic and Indian Ocean coasts, but extending rather further inland in the wetter Transvaal. With the exception of the Transvaal, which we have not yet searched because it is climatically very different from Britain, the rest of this area has now been reasonably thoroughly surveyed for bracken-feeding insects, commencing with preliminary work in 1983, and then detailed annual surveys in the Southern Hemisphere summers of 1984/85, 1985/86, and 1986/87 (Lawton *et al.* 1988). We have sampled bracken throughout the spring and summer in as many different habitats as possible, including various types of woodland, open sites on fynbos ('heathland'), roadside verges, burned areas, etc. At each site, the above-ground parts of a minimum of 20 fronds have been searched carefully for insects and signs of damage. In addition, in 1985–86, we collected rhizomes from four sites in the eastern Cape, and others from the southern Cape (digging up rhizomes is very hard work and time consuming, restricting the number of sites that could be

TABLE 1. SPECIES OF PHYTOPHAGOUS INSECT (AND ONE SPECIES OF PHYTOPHAGOUS MITE) FEEDING ON BRACKEN IN SOUTH AFRICA (V. K. RASHBROOK, S. G. COMPTON & J. H. LAWTON, UNPUBLISHED OBSERVATIONS OVER FOUR FIELD SEASONS)

(The stages found are indicated by +, either eggs laid on the plant, or feeding larvae and nymphs, or feeding adults.)

| species | life history stage found | | | number of sites | distribution of sites |
| | eggs | larvae/ nymphs | adults | | |
|---|---|---|---|---|---|
| Thysanoptera | | | | | |
| *Mycterothrips* sp. | – | + | + | 12 | Cape Province Natal |
| Hemiptera | | | | | |
| Cicadellidae | | | | | |
| *Eupteryx maigudoi* | – | + | + | 33 | Cape Province Natal |
| Cicadellid sp. 1 | – | + | + | 1 | Natal |
| Cicadellid sp. 2 | – | + | + | 3 | Natal |
| Psyllidae | | | | | |
| Psyllid sp. 1 | – | + | – | 7 | Natal |
| Pseudococcidae | | | | | |
| Mealybug sp./spp. | – | + | + | † | Cape Province |
| Aphididae | | | | | |
| Miscellaneous aphids | – | + | + | ‡ | Cape Province Natal |
| Homopteran sp. 1 | – | + | + | 2 | Cape Province |
| Pentatomidae | | | | | |
| *Erachtheus spinosus* | + | + | + | 8 | Natal |
| Anthocoridae | | | | | |
| *Orius* sp. | – | + | + | 17 § | Cape Province Natal |
| Coleoptera | | | | | |
| Curculionidae | | | | | |
| *Holcolaccus* sp. | – | – | + | 1 | Natal |
| Lepidoptera | | | | | |
| Pyralidae | | | | | |
| *Panotima* sp./spp. | + | + | – | 45 | Cape Province Natal |
| Noctuidae | | | | | |
| *Conservula cinisigna* | + | + | – | 53 | Cape Province Natal |
| *Conservula minor* | + | + | – | 7 | Cape Province Natal |
| Hadeninae sp. 1 | – | + | – | 2 | Cape Province |
| Arctiidae | | | | | |
| *Dionychopus amasis* | – | + | – | 3 | Cape Province |
| *Diacrisia eugraphica* | – | + | – | 1 | Cape Province |
| Geometridae | | | | | |
| *Nopia saxaria* | – | + | – | 1 | Cape Province |
| *Epigynopterix maeviaria* | – | + | – | 3 | Cape Province |
| Acari | | | | | |
| Eriophyidae sp. 1 | + | + | + | 46 | Cape Province Natal |

All the taxa dealt with in the following notes have been omitted from the list of 13 species, found more than once, definitely feeding on the above-ground parts of the plant in South Africa (see text).

† Mealybugs occur regularly on potted bracken in cultivation, and we have occasionally found single mealybugs on wild bracken, although it is unclear whether the same species is involved, or whether the 'wild' specimens are feeding and established on the plant.

‡ At least three species of aphids have been found, but we have no evidence that any species forms permanent colonies on the plant.

§ Although *Orius* sp. are common on bracken in some localities, this genus is not normally regarded as phytophagous. The relationship of this species with bracken remains to be determined.

examined). As expected after more than 3 years of field work, we are now finding new species at a very slow rate, and feel reasonably confident that we know all the important herbivores (table 1).

Thirteen species have been found more than once, feeding on the above-ground parts of the plant. (There are 12 insects and 1 mite; in the analyses that follow, the phytophagous mite has been included with the insects). No rhizome-feeders were discovered in the limited below-ground samples. There may be more than one species in the genus *Panotima* (see below); if so, this will raise the number of definite species of herbivores accordingly. At least seven other species (or more correctly, taxa) probably or possibly feed on the plant in South Africa.

Widespread plants are fed on by more species of phytophagous insects than are rare plants. Examples of these species–area relations are now many, both for different species of plants within any one region, and for the same species of plant in different regions (Strong *et al.* 1984). Bracken is no exception, with richer insect faunas in parts of the world where it is more common and widespread (Lawton 1982, 1984*a*). Figure 1 shows the geographic species–area relation

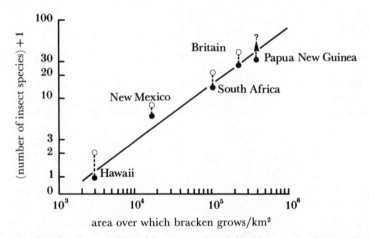

FIGURE 1. Species–area relation for the number of insect species definitely (●) feeding on bracken in different parts of the world, from previously published data in Lawton (1984*a*), with the addition of new information from South Africa (see text for a description of the areas surveyed in South Africa, and table 1 for a list of insects found). Also shown (○) are numbers of species including doubtful or very infrequent associates of bracken. Species + 1 has been used on the ordinate to allow the inclusion of a zero count in Hawaii. Bracken in South Africa has been recorded from 156 grid squares (average area 660 km²) (W. B. G. Jacobsen, personal communication to V. K. Rashbrook, plus additional records from V. K. Rashbrook and S. G. Compton), giving a total area within which bracken grows of *ca.* 103000 km². Similar methods were used to calculate the areas within which bracken grows elsewhere in the world. The area for South Africa is certainly an underestimate, because records of the plant's distribution are incomplete. However, the insect list may also be incomplete, because the Transvaal has not been surveyed in detail for insects, and *Panotima* may contain more than one species (see text). Hence the close relation between area and number of species apparent in earlier plots (Lawton 1984*a*), and now reinforced by the South African data may be weakened by further work. It is extremely unlikely, however, that further work in South Africa, either on the distribution of bracken, or on its insect herbivores, will alter the relation enough to make it no longer statistically significant. The fitted regression line on the definite records is:

$$\log_{10}(\text{species}+1) = 0.696 \log_{10}\text{area} - 2.33, \quad r = 0.987; f = 112.1; 0.005 > p > 0.001.$$

for bracken and its herbivores, incorporating the new South African data. It suggests that our surveys are now reasonably complete and that further searches are unlikely to be a good investment in time or money (see Lawton & Schroeder 1978).

Among the species that have been discovered in South Africa, two stand out as potential biological control agents for bracken in Britain: *Conservula cinisigna* and *Panotima* sp. (spp.?). Some of the other species may also be suitable, particularly the unidentified mite. I now consider what is known about each.

## STUDIES ON POTENTIAL CONTROL AGENTS
### *Conservula cinisigna*

Adult *Conservula cinisigna* are typical, brown noctuids with a wing span of about 2.5 cm. Identification of our material was made by the Commonwealth Institute of Entomology Identification Service, and by V. M. Swain at the National Collection of Insects, South Africa. Taxonomic details are in Lawton *et al.* (1988).

Eggs are laid singly or in groups, tucked and glued tightly into crevices on the tips of new bracken fronds; they are further protected by a light covering of small hairs, presumably from the female's abdomen. The newly hatched caterpillars are green; later instars are dramatically polymorphic in colour, either vivid green, olive brown, or almost black, with white, longitudinal stripes. The significance of this larval polymorphism is unknown. Final instars are large (up to 4 cm long), with voracious appetites. All instars are typical, free-living, chewing folivores, exploiting the pinnae ('leaves') of bracken. Eggs are laid very early in the spring on newly emerging fronds, and caterpillars become abundant soon after. However, there appears to be at least a partial second generation later in the year; some eggs and caterpillars can be found throughout the growing season, and fresh adults emerged in the laboratory only 19–36 ($n = 15$) days after larvae from the spring generation had pupated. The mechanisms controlling voltinism are not yet known. *Conservula* is abundant and widespread on bracken throughout South Africa (table 1), and tolerates a wide range of climates, including high-altitude sites with frost and snow in winter.

Although there are several free-living Lepidoptera among the 27 'core species' feeding on bracken in Britain, and several others that do so very occasionally (see, for example, Lawton 1982), and although several of these species are noctuids, there are reasons for believing that *Conservula cinisigna* may make a good biological control agent. First, its main feeding period is much earlier in the year than any native British species, with the exception of the much smaller geometrid *Petrophora chlorosata*. It could therefore occupy a 'temporally vacant niche', and hence avoid enemies, particularly parasitoids, known to attack such species as *Ceramica pisi*, *Laconobia oleracea*, *Euplexia lucipara* and *Phlogophora meticulosa*, all noctuids found on British bracken later in the season. A spring-feeding control agent also attacks the plant when it is most vulnerable to damage (see above). Secondly, and much more important, unlike these British noctuids, all of which are polyphagous on a wide range of plants, *Conservula* appears to be virtually monophagous on bracken in the laboratory and totally so in the field (table 2). The only fern other than bracken on which newly hatched *Conservula* larvae grew and developed in the laboratory was *Pellaea viridis*, but we have never found *Conservula* eggs or caterpillars on this, or any other ferns in the field in South Africa (table 2). A reasonable conclusion from these field surveys is that adult female moths will not oviposit on anything other than their normal host plant, bracken.

The final reason for thinking that *Conservula* may sufficiently damage the plant to make a good biological control agent in Britain is the heavy frond damage sometimes observed in South Africa. Large populations of caterpillars are not uncommon despite attacks by

TABLE 2. LABORATORY AND FIELD OBSERVATIONS ON USE OF SOUTH AFRICAN FERNS BY *PANOTIMA* AND *CONSERVULA*

(Fern species after Jacobsen (1983). No eggs, larvae or feeding damage of either *Panotima* or *Conservula* were found on any ferns examined in the field, except bracken.)

| fern species and families | laboratory trials† Panotima no. of larvae tested | Panotima feeding damage | Panotima no. of larvae surviving beyond first instar | Conservula cinsigna no. of larvae tested | Conservula feeding damage | Conservula no. of larvae surviving beyond first instar | no. of fronds examined in field for both species | notes |
|---|---|---|---|---|---|---|---|---|
| **Schizaeaceae** | | | | | | | | |
| *Mohria caffrorum* | 22 | trace | 0 | 30 | trace | 0 | 75 | — |
| **Gleicheniaceae** | | | | | | | | |
| *Gleichenia polypodioides* | — | — | — | — | — | — | 31 | — |
| **Cyatheaceae** | | | | | | | | |
| *Alsophila dregei* | — | — | — | — | — | — | 10 | — |
| **Dennstaeditiaceae** | | | | | | | | |
| *Pteridium aquilinum* | 45 | heavy | 41 | 62 | heavy | 58 | not applicable | — |
| *Hypolepis sparsisora* | 30 | 1–5 % | 0 | 30 | trace | 0 | 40 | — |
| **Adiantaceae** | | | | | | | | |
| *Adiantum poirettii* | 27 | trace | 0 | 25 | 0 | 0 | 0 | British genus |
| *Pteris dentata* | 30 | trace | 0 | 30 | trace | 0 | 5 | — |
| *Cheilanthes hirta* | — | — | — | 20 | trace | 0 | 3 | — |
| *Pellaea calomelanos* | — | — | — | — | — | — | 8 | — |
| *P. viridis = Cheilanthes viridis* | 23 | 1–5 % | 0 | 35 | extensive | 7 | 238 | — |
| *P. quadripinnata = C. quadripinnata* | — | — | — | — | — | — | 30 | — |
| **Davalliaceae** | | | | | | | | |
| *Nephrolepis cordifolia* | 27 | 1–5 % | 0 | 30 | trace | 0 | 0 | — |
| **Aspleniaceae** | | | | | | | | |
| *Asplenium aethiopicum* | 24 | trace | 0 | 30 | 0 | 0 | 0 | British genus |
| **Thelypteridaceae** | | | | | | | | |
| *Amouropelta bergiana = Thelypteris bergiana* | 24 | 1–5 % | 0 | 30 | 1–5 % | 0 | 10 | British genus |
| **Athyriaceae** | | | | | | | | |
| *Cystopteris fragilis* | — | — | — | 25 | 1–5 % | 0 | 0 | British species |
| **Aspidiaceae** | | | | | | | | |
| *Dryopteris inaequalis* | 20 | trace | 0 | 30 | trace | 0 | 76 | British genus |
| *Polystichum lucidum* | 26 | trace | 0 | 30 | 1–5 % | 0 | 37 | British genus |
| *Rumohra adiantiformis* | 24 | trace | 0 | 30 | 0 | 0 | 378 | — |
| **Blechnaceae** | | | | | | | | |
| *Blechnum punctulatum* | — | — | — | — | — | — | } 67 | British genus |
| *B. australe* | — | — | — | — | — | — | | British genus |

† Laboratory feeding trials were done by dissecting eggs from bracken and placing them on test fronds. Only healthy eggs that hatched are included in the analyses. Dissected eggs were placed singly on excised, fresh pinnae, maintained on damp filter paper in a petri dish. Experiments were inspected at least once a day, and fresh pinnae provided as required. 'Trace' signifies that the newly hatched larvae attempted to feed; '1–5 %' is the area consumed, given ca. 3 cm² of frond material; 'extensive' is less feeding damage than 'heavy'.

parasitoids (table 3), and what is from our point of a view a very unwelcome enemy in the form of an unidentified, but quite devastating infectious disease (Heads & Lawton 1986). We have repeatedly lost laboratory stocks of *Conservula* to this disease, and in consequence, with only one main generation a year to work with, have not been able to import enough material into quarantine in Britain to establish experimental cultures. Accordingly, it has not yet been possible to repeat the encouraging screening results in table 2 by using British ferns. However, many of the species tested in South Africa are in the same genus as, or in genera very close to, British ferns. The host-specificity tests in table 2 are therefore very encouraging.

TABLE 3. PARASITOIDS REARED FROM *CONSERVULA CINISIGNA* AND *PANOTIMA* IN SOUTH AFRICA
(DATA OF S. G. COMPTON, PERSONAL COMMUNICATION)

| stage attacked | parasitoid life history | parasitoid taxonomy | status |
|---|---|---|---|
| *Conservula* | | | |
| eggs | solitary | Trichogrammatidae, genus indeterminable | rare |
| larvae | solitary | Ichneumonidae, ?*Ophion* sp. | rare |
| larvae | gregarious | Eulophidae, *Euplectrus* sp. | common |
| larvae | solitary | Braconidae, genus indet. | widespread |
| larvae | solitary | Braconidae, genus indet. | uncommon |
| larvae | solitary | Ichneumonidae, genus indet. | rare |
| *Panotima* | | | |
| eggs | solitary | Trichogrammatidae, genus indet. | locally common |
| small lv. | solitary | Eulophidae, genus indet. | uncommon |
| larvae | solitary | Ichneumonidae, genus indet. | rare |
| larvae | solitary | Braconidae, genus indet. | uncommon |
| larvae | gregarious | Braconidae, genus indet. | locally common |

*Panotima sp./spp.?*

*Panotima* is referred to as *Parthenodes angularis*, or a species very close to it, in earlier publications (Lawton 1986a, b; Heads & Lawton 1986). Unfortunately, the taxonomic situation is now confused. L. Vári (personal communication) has informed us that a photograph of an adult reared during our work 'is a perfect match' with a series of *Parthenodes angularis* in the Transvaal museum (actual specimens have not yet been compared). However, the genus is poorly known taxonomically, and the Commonwealth Institute of Entomology recently transferred our material to *Panotima* and suggested that more than one species may be involved. Difficulties in rearing adults in the laboratory mean that material for taxonomic work is very limited, and the specific identity of the moth and the number of species feeding on bracken in South Africa have yet to be resolved. Because of these difficulties we have kept separate material from bracken in different localities, and ensured that all our experiments have been conducted on animals of known origin. If more than one species is involved, we have so far found nothing to indicate that their biology differs sufficiently to influence their use as biological control agents. The discussion that follows therefore treats all our material as one species. However, these taxonomic problems will have to be resolved before there can be any question of employing *Panotima* as a biological control agent in Britain.

Adult *Panotima* are golden-brown moths, with silver marks on the fore-wings and a wing-span of about 2 cm. No pyralids feed on bracken in Britain, and its life history is totally different from anything found on the plant in this country. Eggs are laid early in the season, singly on the underside of expanding fronds, and the newly hatched caterpillars tunnel and feed in surface mines protected by folds at the edge of the pinnae, with a mixture of silk and frass spun over the back of the frond. They spend the first two or three instars there, often causing very heavy damage to the undersides of the pinnae before migrating to the rachis ('stem') of the plant, into which they tunnel to complete their development. The rachis is usually mined between ground level and the first pair of pinnae. Each larva occupies a single mine, but there can be several mines per stem (the maximum we have found is nine; some typical figures are in table 4). Frass is expelled through an exit hole, and the larvae eventually leave the mine to pupate. Mines cut through vascular bundles in the rachis, and if several larvae occupy one frond, damage is severe; growth of the plant is restricted, and all but the basal pair of pinnae usually die.

TABLE 4. REPRESENTATIVE SAMPLES OF *PANOTIMA* MINES IN BRACKEN FRONDS FROM SITES IN SOUTHEASTERN CAPE PROVINCE, SOUTH AFRICA

(Hogsback and Katberg are mountain sites. Samples taken in the autumn and winter (March–July) represent cumulative attacks on fronds over the previous Southern Hemisphere spring and summer.)

| locality | date | fronds examined | no. of *Panotima* mines occupied | no. of *Panotima* mines unoccupied | mines per frond |
|---|---|---|---|---|---|
| Featherstone Kloof, Grahamstown | 25.III.83 | 20 | 0 | 28 | 1.40 |
| | 26.III.83 | 15 | 0 | 25 | 1.67 |
| | 17.XII.84–4.II.85 | 80 | 5 | — | 0.06† |
| Mountain Drive, Grahamstown | 1.IV–9.VII.85 | 67 | 0 | 4 | 0.06 |
| Hogsback | 28.XII.84 | 20 | 11 | 7 | 0.90 |
| | 30.III.85 | 126 | 2 | 13 | 0.12 |
| Katberg | 11.XII.84–3.II.85 | 180 | 23 | 11 | 0.19 |
| | 31.III–5.IV.85 | 344 | 356 | 53 | 1.19 |

Distribution of attacks in representative samples (unpublished data of J. H. Lawton, S. G. Compton & V. K. Rashbrook)

| | | mines per frond | | | | | | | |
|---|---|---|---|---|---|---|---|---|---|
| | | 0 | 1 | 2 | 3 | 4 | 5 | 6 | 7 |
| Featherstone Kloof, Grahamstown | 25.III.83 | 11 | 2 | 0 | 3 | 3 | 1 | 0 | 0 |
| Grahamstown | 26.III.83 | 8 | 1 | 2 | 0 | 1 | 2 | 1 | 0 |
| Katberg | 31.III.85 | 6 | 11 | 11 | 2 | 1 | 0 | 0 | 1 |
| Katberg | 11.XII.84–3.II.85 | 153 | 22 | 3 | 2 | 0 | 0 | 0 | 0 |
| Hogsback | 28.XII.84 | 9 | 5 | 5 | 1 | 0 | 0 | 0 | 0 |

† Unoccupied mines not counted.

Because *Panotima* is so different biologically and taxonomically, it is unlikely to be heavily attacked by any specific natural enemies of British bracken-feeding insects. The only vaguely similar species is a gelechiid, *Paltodora cytisella*, whose larvae attack bracken early in the spring by mining into the costa ('main stems' of the pinnae) and rachis, where they often induce gall-like swellings. *Panotima* larvae enter the rachis later in the season, feed much lower down, and do not induce swollen galls. There are also at least two species of rachis-mining fly larvae in Britain (Lawton 1982; McGavin & Brown 1986), but these are unlikely to share enemies with *Panotima*.

*Panotima* is widespread in South Africa (table 1), and common over a wide range of climatic conditions. (If more than one species is involved, it may be that each does best under different climatic regimes, something that will require further investigation.) The main generation is in spring, but in the laboratory a small number of adults emerged 14–19 days ($n = 3$) after larvae from the spring generation had pupated, and in the field small numbers of larvae occur in stem-mines in late summer (e.g. table 4), suggesting that there is a small, second generation. The control of voltinism is not understood.

*Panotima* seems a very promising control agent. It attacks the plant most heavily in spring and early summer when damage has the greatest impact, but unlike *Conservula*, it causes two kinds of damage (first it defoliates, then it attacks the rachis). It also appears to be bracken-specific. We have been unable to rear it on anything else in the laboratory (table 2) and have never found either eggs, larvae, or its highly characteristic feeding damage to fronds or stems, on any other ferns in the field (table 2). Populations occasionally reach high levels (e.g. table 4), despite some parasitoids that attack it in its own environment (table 3). Without such enemies in Britain, the effects of *Panotima* could be dramatic.

*Panotima*'s peculiar life-history has made it very difficult to rear in the laboratory. Small larvae are easy to culture on cut pinnae, but the rachis-mining larger instars are very difficult to keep. Cut sections of rachis do not stay fresh long enough for caterpillars to complete development; they either dry out, or go mouldy when in water, and because the rachis is hard and tough, it is extremely difficult to remove larvae for transfer to fresh material without damaging them. A few pupae reared on cut stems were small and often mishapen. Most failed to emerge. Caterpillars can be reared on pot-grown bracken, but this needs much space, and they tend to kill the plants! With only one main generation a year, progress in the laboratory has been slow and we have not been able to rear sufficient material either to solve the taxonomic problems or to establish cultures in quarantine in Britain. However, we now appear to have solved the rearing problems by the simple device of making artificial bracken 'stems' from tightly rolling and clipping sections of pinnae to make crude, green 'cigars'. The larger instars readily burrow into these, and the rolls stay fresh much longer than stems. Moreover, when they eventually dry up or go mouldy, they are easily undone, and the larvae rehoused in fresh rolls. This technique has now produced nearly 100 large, healthy-looking pupae, and when applied on a larger scale, should make possible the establishment of good, quarantine stocks of *Panotima* in Britain.

### Eriophyid mites

Bracken at many sites in South Africa (table 1) is attacked by a gall-forming mite (Acari, Prostigmata; Eriophyidae). The pinnae, costae and rachis of galled plants are badly swollen and distorted, and photosynthetic tissue is greatly reduced on heavily attacked plants. The species is undescribed (S. Neser, personal communication), but it appears to be bracken specific; nothing resembling its highly distinctive and conspicuous galls has been found on other ferns in South Africa (e.g. table 2, and during many more casual inspections of ferns throughout the southern and eastern Cape). Most eriophyids are extremely host-specific (S. Neser, personal communication), so failure to find it on other ferns is not surprising. We know little else about the biology of this herbivore, nor have we done laboratory specificity tests. However, we know that some bracken patches in South Africa are heavily attacked (e.g. 39 from 67 fronds in a sample near Grahamstown in 1985) and severely damaged, whereas others are apparently mite-free. Dispersal may be a problem, and this, combined with the potential difficulties of working with animals as small as eriophyids, may make them less than ideal as a biological control agent. However, the damage caused may well compensate for these disadvantages.

An eriophyid gall-mite has been reported on bracken in Britain (*Phytopus pteridis*) (Lawton 1976), but I have not seen it during more than 15 years of field work on the plant. (C. Rigby reported few galls that she identified as this species on the North York Moors (Rigby & Lawton 1981). I did not see the specimens then, nor since. Perhaps Rigby's specimens were abnormal *Dasineura* galls.) Descriptions of the damage caused by *Phytoptus* vary (see Lawton 1976), but none resemble the large swollen galls formed by the South African species. On present evidence, therefore, the latter would appear to be another possible biological control agent for use in Britain.

*Other South African species*

With one exception, either too little is known about the other taxa in table 1 to evaluate them as possible biological control agents or they are ecologically too similar to species already on the plant in this country. The exception is the homopteran *Eupteryx maigudoi*. This feeds only on bracken in South Africa (J. G. Theron, personal communication) and in the Katbergs may cause heavy damage, giving the fronds a silvery appearance presumably by removing most of the cell-contents from the epidermis. Moreover, some Homoptera are important vectors of plant disease, so *Eupteryx* may possibly be exploited in this way. (The control of bracken by diseases has been explored by Burge *et al.* (1986), so far without success.) Against these positive characteristics of *Eupteryx* must be set the presence of native British species in the genus, including *E. filicum* on several ferns, but not bracken (Ottosson & Anderson 1983). That introduced *E. maigudoi* might recruit parasitoids or other enemies from native congeners could greatly reduce its efficiency.

*Potential control agents from South Africa: a review*

Biological and technical problems have constrained the work in South Africa. Failure to find a rhizome-feeder is disappointing, although few sites have been searched below ground. Above ground, bracken in South Africa has yielded some potentially promising control agents, but disease and other rearing difficulties have made detailed studies frustratingly slow, as has the predominantly univoltine life cycle of the two most interesting species (*Panotima* and *Conservula*). These difficulties now seem to have been overcome, and should make it possible to establish quarantine populations of both species in Britain. We now need to repeat the encouraging host-specificity trials (table 2) with British ferns, although it seems very doubtful that the results will differ substantially or significantly from those obtained with closely related South African ferns. On biological grounds, therefore, the opportunities for controlling bracken in Britain by using one or more exotic insects from South Africa look hopeful.

POSSIBLE BIOLOGICAL CONTROL AGENTS FROM ELSEWHERE IN THE
SOUTHERN HEMISPHERE

A search for possible biological control agents on subspecies *caudatum* has been made on my behalf by J. A. Thomson and colleagues in southeastern Australia. The insect fauna is rather disappointing, and, despite herculean efforts, no rhizome feeders have been found. However, they discovered a new species of moth in Tasmania, the larvae of which mine the pinnules of mature fronds, destroying the entire mesophyll and palisade layers. Several caterpillars occupy one frond, and damage is severe. There is nothing similar on bracken in Britain, making this new microlepidopteran another potentially useful control agent. It is not known whether it will feed on subspecies *aquilinum*.

## THE LIKELIHOOD OF SUCCESSFUL CONTROL

Looking ahead, and assuming that one or more safe (i.e. bracken-specific) species will soon be available for use in Britain, what are the chances of successful control? The history of biological control is littered with the corpses of very promising agents that failed to live up to expectations. Worse, we often have no idea why some agents fail and others succeed (Schroeder 1983). A potential cause of failure on bracken could be climatic mismatch (see Hokkanen (1986) for a recent review). Cape Province is at the same latitude south as North Africa or southern Spain, and although winters in the mountains bring snow and frost, summers are sunnier and drier than in Britain. Unfortunately, detailed climatic records are not available for Hogsback or Katberg, the two main mountain study sites near Grahamstown (e.g. table 4), but even if they were imperfectly matched with British sites, little further could be done. Africa stops at Cape Aghulas. So we have to make do with the available study areas (Schroeder 1983).

It is equally difficult to predict the impact of resident natural enemies on introduced control agents. Natural enemies have been implicated in the failure of classical weed control programmes (Goeden & Louda 1976), and as pointed out on p. 340, they might be a particular threat to exotic insects introduced to control a native plant. However, the proposed agents are all ecologically and taxonomically distinct from the resident herbivores of the British bracken community. Probably the only way to see if they are distinct enough is to introduce them.

These considerations aside, bracken is such a vigorous plant that it seems unduly optimistic to expect control by a single species of insect. Several agents are often needed in biological weed control (Hokkanen 1986, and references therein). Harris (1986) discusses the idea of a critical damage threshold, arguing that plants must sustain a certain amount of damage before they can be brought under biological control. More than one agent may be neccesary to do this. Whether *Conservula*, *Panotima* and other agents would together impose sufficient stress on bracken to slow down, halt, or even reverse its rate of spread, is impossible to say with certainty. But the signs are hopeful. *Panotima* alone scores well on Goeden's (1983) system for evaluating potential control agents (Lawton 1986a), and would appear to have a good chance of contributing to effective control. Both *Conservula* and *Panotima* cause greatest damage in spring and early summer when bracken is at its most vulnerable, another very desirable property for control (Schroeder 1983; Harris 1986). Finally, experience of previous biological control successes suggests that species that 'destroy the vascular support tissue' and that 'damage the plant in several different ways' may, though not always, make the best control agents (Hokkanen 1986, and references therein). Both criteria apply to *Panotima*.

THE BROADER IMPLICATIONS OF BIOLOGICAL CONTROL OF BRACKEN

In many ways, the constraints and problems encountered during the search for bracken biological control agents are insignificant compared with legal, political, environmental and socio-economic questions that confront us (Heads & Lawton 1986). The opportunity to control bracken biologically looks technically feasible; but do we actually want to do it, and who should decide? The great advantage of biological control is that it could provide a permanent, cheap solution to the bracken problem. But the permanence worries many people, as does the uncontrolled nature of the experiment; a successful agent will spread widely and can potentially reduce or eliminate bracken wherever it occurs. Not everybody will regard this as self evidently good, however appealing it may seem to hill farmers. Conflicts of interest are a feature of biological control programmes anywhere in the world (Schroeder 1983), but may be particularly strong when the target is a native plant.

### The legal position and the problem of consultation

Under the Wildlife and Countryside Act 1981, permission to release alien insects into Britain for biological control purposes rests ultimately with the Secretary of State for the Environment, but how is information for and against such a release to be obtained? There are no precedents for the release of exotic biological control agents against a native weed in Britain. For example, there is no obligation under the Act for consultation with the Nature Conservancy Council (Stubbs 1987), although its opinions are obviously important. So are the opinions of other individuals and organizations, from the Ministry of Agriculture, Fisheries and Food, and voluntary conservation bodies, to land owners and other individuals. The Central Directorate for Environmental Protection (CDEP) in the Department of the Environment ultimately has responsibility for coordinating information for and against a release (Stubbs 1987), but how CDEP might get its information is unclear.

One potential legal problem centres on commoners rights of 'estovers', the right to cut bracken for winter bedding (Hughes & Aitchison 1986). Although the practice is not now so prevalent, reflecting the decline in cattle on upland farms, it is still regarded as a valuable right on many Welsh commons (Hughes & Aitchison 1986), and doubtless elsewhere. Would commoners have any redress against a very successful biological control programme that deprived them of their crop? Indeed, would any individual landowner who did not wish their bracken controlled have any legal redress?

### Other problems

It is easier to pose other problems and questions that need to be resolved than to answer them. The main problems and questions seem to be as follows.

1. What scale of economic benefits might be expected to follow successful biological control of bracken? These are not difficult to work out for individual farms and estates, assuming various levels of control and no change in the *status quo* of other components, for example, patterns of taxation and government subsidies for hill farms. Likely effects on the economic infrastructure of upland areas, subsidies, taxes, land values and so on are much more difficult to take into account.

2. What effects will successful biological control have on ecological communities? One way to examine this problem is to assume that success will do no more than restore the open, more

bracken-free uplands, forests and heaths of a hundred or so years ago. Yet bracken is not without some benefits, because it provides an important habitat for some British native animals. But it can be argued that its spread excludes many more plants and animals of greater conservation importance. My view, based on evidence that no biological control agent has ever eliminated its host plant and that extermination of bracken in Britain is inconceivable, is that biological control poses much less of a threat to native flora and fauna than the continuing spread of bracken, or massive aerial spraying of herbicide, or blanket afforestation of uplands. None of these alternatives looks very attractive for conservation, but a proper assessment has not been done. What is needed is an 'environmental balance sheet' setting out the ecological pros and cons of biological control of bracken. It would also help to know NCC's Policy and Position Guidelines on introductions into Britain; these have never been made public, but are known to be extremely conservative (Stubbs 1987). The Nature Conservatory Council do, however, maintain an open mind about the use of exotic insects to control the spread of bracken in Britain (Key 1987).

3. Will biological control be safe? Above all, we must be sure that any introduced biological control agent feeds exclusively on bracken. Existing data for several of the potential control agents are very encouraging, but more host-plant specificity tests are needed. If control agents pass these standard tests (e.g. CIBC 1978; Schroeder 1983), there are no grounds for believing that they pose a threat to any other native plants. Whenever the standard protocol has been followed, biological weed control has an excellent and enviable safety record; there have been no adverse or unpredictable effects from introductions made against more than 86 species of weeds, in some twenty countries over the past 75 years (Julien 1982; Batra 1982; Schroeder 1983; Kelleher & Hulme 1984; Lawton 1986 b).

4. Can anything useful be done with bracken-infested land that does not involve biological control, herbicide control, or commercial afforestation? The answer is a guarded 'yes'. One interesting suggestion is that bracken could be cut for biomass, dried or treated in some other way, and burned as a renewable energy source (Lawson et al. 1986, and references therein). On a local scale, the idea looks economically feasible. The problem is that harvesting bracken for biomass on many steep, rocky or remote hillsides is impossible. Here bracken will continue to spread and cause problems. Again, there are no clear answers to questions of alternative land-use strategies, national priorities, and economics.

5. What are the other real or perceived problems? This is not a frivolous question. Release of a biological control agent is essentially irreversible, and therefore to be taken very seriously. How do we consult people in general, and how are their views to be heard? Should we even bother if the experts' considered opinion of is that, on balance, biological control is a good idea? The solution for analogous problems of regional or national concern is a public enquiry. Perhaps, in the end, something similar will be needed before attempting the biological control of bracken in this country. These are deep and uncomfortable waters for a biologist!

CONCLUDING REMARKS

Constraints on the biological control of bracken in Britain are many and varied, the most difficult being human, not biological. It may seem odd that legal, political, environmental and socio-economic problems were not resolved before spending time and money looking for suitable control agents. But in the absence of promising agents, it made no sense to spend even more time and money exploring a thorny and multi-disciplinary problem embracing everything from the legal rights of estovers, to the economics of hill farming, and the ecology of upland Britain. The problem now is to try and develop both the biological control work and the complementary, but essentially much larger and more complex studies side by side, until either an insurmountable technical difficulty rules out biological control; or it is deemed too risky and the idea has to be abandoned, or permission to go ahead is finally granted. The bracken problem will not be resolved on its own. Continuing with present policies, or lack of them, has a price in economic, social and environmental terms. So does a massive increase in the use of herbicides to halt or reverse the relentless spread of the plant, and so do alternative land use strategies. The prospects for biological control deserve a fair hearing within this much larger context.

Work on South African insects is supported by an AFRC Grant to the University of York, and is a joint venture with C.A.B. International Institute of Biological Control, Imperial College, London, and the Department of Zoology and Entomology at Rhodes University. Ms Vanessa Rashbrook, Dr Steve Compton and Professor Cliff Moran have all made work in South Africa possible; I am extremely grateful to all of them. Cliff Moran first helped me to find *Panotima* and has continued to provide help and support throughout the study. Vanessa Rashbrook has done the main burden of field work and laboratory screening, and without her efforts, and the interest and support of Steve Compton the project would have been impossible. Dr Matthew Cock at CIBC has been stoic and helpful throughout, not least when surrounded by dead caterpillars. Dr Brad Hawkins made valuable comments on the manuscript. *Conservula* and *Panotima* are imported under a MAFF licence to CIBC

## REFERENCES

Baker, C. R. B., Blackman, R. L. & Claridge, M. F. 1972 Studies on *Haltica carduorum* Geurin (Colepotera: Chrysomelidae) an alien beetle released in Britain as a contribution to the biological control of creeping thistle, *Cirsium arvense* (L.) Scop. *J. appl. Ecol.* **9**, 819–830.

Batra, S. W. T. 1982 Biological control in agroecosystems. *Science, Wash.* **215**, 134–139.

Borodino 1986 *Pteridium aquilinum* – the orienteer's scourge. *Compass sport: the orienteer* **7** (7), October/November, p. 14.

Briese, D. T. 1986 Factors affecting the establishment and survival of *Anaitis efformata* (Lepidoptera: Geometridae) introduced into Australia for biological control of St. John's wort, *Hypericum perforatum*. II. Field trials. *J. appl. Ecol.* **23**, 821–839.

Brown, I. W. & Wathern, P. 1986 Bracken control and land management in the Moel Famau Country Park, Clwyd, North Wales. In *Bracken, Ecology, land use and control technology* (ed. R. T. Smith & J. A. Taylor), pp. 369–377. Carnforth: Parthenon Publishing.

Brown, R. W. 1986 Bracken in the North York Moors: its ecological and amenity implications in national parks. In *Bracken, Ecology, land use and control technology* (ed. R. T. Smith & J. A. Taylor), pp. 77–86. Carnforth: Parthenon Publishing.

Burge, M. N., Irvine, J. A. & McElwee, M. 1986 The potential for biological control of bracken with the causal agents of curl-tip disease. In *Bracken, Ecology, land use and control technology* (ed. R. T. Smith & J. A. Taylor), pp. 453–458. Carnforth: Parthenon Publishing.

CIBC 1978 *Screening organisms for biological control*. Farnham Royal: Commonwealth Agricultural Bureaux.

Dobson, A. P. & Hudson, P. J. 1986 Parasites, disease and the structure of ecological communities. *Trends Ecol. Evol.* **1**, 11–14.

Evans, I. A. 1984 Bracken carcenogenicity. In *Chemical carcinogens* (ed. C. E.Searle), pp. 1171–1204. (American Chemical Society Monograph 182.) Washington, D.C.: American Chemical Society.

Evans, I. A. 1986 The carcinogenic, mutagenic and teratogenic toxicity of bracken. In *Bracken, Ecology, land use and control technology* (ed. R. T. Smith & J. A. Taylor), pp. 139–146. Carnforth: Parthenon Publishing.

Evans, W. C. 1986 The acute diseases caused by bracken in animals. In *Bracken, Ecology, land use and control technology* (ed. R. T. Smith & J. A. Taylor), pp. 121–132. Carnforth: Parthenon Publishing.

Galpin, O. P. & Smith, R. M. M. 1986 Bracken, stomach cancer and water supplies: is there a link? In *Bracken, Ecology, land use and control technology* (ed. R. T. Smith & J. A. Taylor), pp. 147–159. Carnforth: Parthenon Publishing.

Goeden, R. D. 1983 Critique and revision of Harris' scoring system for selection of insect agents in biological control of weeds. *Protection Ecol.* **5**, 287–301.

Goeden, R. D. & Louda, S. M. 1976 Biotic interference with insects imported for weed control. *A. Rev. Ent.* **21**, 325–342.

Goeden, R. D. & Ricker, D. W. 1980 Santa Cruz island – revisited. Sequential photography records the causation, rates of progress, and lasting benefits of successful biological weed control. In *Proceedings of the Vth International Symposium on the Biological Control of Weeds, July 1980, Brisbane, Australia* (ed. E. S. Delfosse), pp. 355–365. Melbourne: CSIRO.

Hannam, D. A. R. 1986 Bracken poisoning in farm animals with special reference to the North York Moors. In *Bracken, Ecology, land use and control technology* (ed. R. T. Smith & J. A. Taylor), pp. 133–138. Carnforth: Parthenon Publishing.

Harper, J. L. 1977 *Population biology of plants*. London: Academic Press.

Harris, P. 1984 *Euphorbia escula–virgata* complex, leafy spurge and *E. cyparissias* L., Cypress spurge (Euphorbiaceae). In *Biological control programmes against insects and weeds in Canada 1969–1980* (ed. J. S. Kelleher & M. A. Hulme), pp. 159–169. Farnham Royal: Commonwealth Agricultural Bureaux.

Harris, P. 1986 Biological control of weeds. *Fortsch. Zool.* **32**, 123–138.

Heads, P. & Lawton, J. 1986 Beat back bracken biologically. *New Scient.* **111** (1525), 40–43.

Hokkanen, H. M. T. 1986 , Success in classical biological control. *CRC Crit. Rev. Plant Sci.* **3**, 35–72.

Hokkanen, H. & Pimentel, D. 1984 New approach for selecting biological control agents. *Can. Ent.* **116**, 1109–1121.

Horsnail, G. B. 1986 A comparison of methods of control of bracken regrowth following aerial application of asulam in northern Britain. In *Bracken, Ecology, land use and control technology* (ed. R. T. Smith & J. A. Taylor), pp. 425–430. Carnforth: Parthenon Publishing.

Hudson, P. J. 1986 Bracken and ticks on grouse moors in the north of England. In *Bracken, Ecology, land use and control technology* (ed. R. T. Smith & J. A. Taylor), pp. 161–170. Carnforth: Parthenon Publishing.

Huffaker, C. B. (ed.) 1974 *Biological control*. New York: Plenum/Rosetta.

Hughes, E. J. & Aitchison, J. W. 1986 Bracken and the common lands of Wales. In *Bracken, Ecology, land use and control technology* (ed. R. T. Smith & J. A. Taylor), pp. 93–99. Carnforth: Parthenon Publishing.

Jacobsen, W. B. G. 1983 *The ferns and fern allies of southern Africa*. Durban and Pretoria: Butterworths.

Jeffries, M. J. & Lawton, J. H. 1984 Enemy free space and the structure of ecological communities. *Biol. J. Linn. Soc.* **23**, 269–286.

Johnson, J. 1986 Current policies on the reclamation of bracken land with particular reference to northern England. In *Bracken, Ecology, land use and control technology* (ed. R. T. Smith & J. A. Taylor), pp. 325–330. Carnforth: Parthenon Publishing.

Julien, M. H. (ed.) 1982 *Biological control of weeds. A world catalogue of agents and their target weeds*. Farnham Royal: Commonwealth Agricultural Bureaux.

Kelleher, J. S. & Hulme, M. A. (eds) 1984 *Biological control programmes against insects and weeds in Canada 1969–1980*. Farnham Royal: Commonwealth Agricultural Bureaux.

Key, R. S. 1987 Bracken control – an open mind. *Farmers Weekly* 6 November 1987, pp. 9–10.

Kirk, A. A. 1982 Insects associated with bracken fern *Pteridium aquilinum* (Polypodiaceae) in Papua New Guinea and their possible use in biological control. *Acta Oecol./Oecol. Appl.* **3**, 343–359.

Lawson, G. J., Callaghan, T. V. & Scott, R. 1986 Bracken as an energy resource. In *Bracken, Ecology, land use and control technology* (ed. R. T. Smith & J. A. Taylor), pp. 239–247. Carnforth: Parthenon Publishing.

Lawton, J. H. 1976 The structure of the arthropod community on bracken. *Bot. J. Linn. Soc.* **73**, 187–216.

Lawton, J. H. 1982 Vacant niches and unsaturated communities: a comparison of bracken herbivores at sites on two continents. *J. Anim. Ecol.* **51**, 573–595.

Lawton, J. H. 1984a Non-competitive populations, non-convergent communities, and vacant niches: the herbivores of bracken. In *Ecological communities: conceptual issues and the evidence.* (ed. D. R. Strong, Jr, D. Simberloff, L. G. Abele & A. B. Thistle), pp. 67–101. Princeton University Press.

Lawton, J. H. 1984b Herbivore community organisation: general models and specific tests with phytophagous insects. In *A new ecology: novel approaches to interactive systems* (ed. P. W. Price, C. N. Slobodchikoff & W. S. Gaud), pp. 329–352. New York: Thomas Wiley.

Lawton, J. H. 1986a Biological control of bracken: plans and possibilities. In *Bracken, Ecology, land use and control technology* (ed. R. T. Smith & J. A. Taylor), pp. 445–452. Carnforth: Parthenon Publishing.

Lawton, J. H. 1986b Ecological theory and choice of biological control agents. In *Proceedings of the VIth International Symposium on the Biological Control of Weeds, August 1984, Vancouver, Canada* (ed. E. S. Delfosse), pp. 13–26. Ottawa: Agriculture Canada.

Lawton, J. H. 1986c The effect of parasitoids on phytophagous insect communities. In *Insect parasitoids* (ed. J. Wagge & D. Greathead), pp. 265–287. London: Academic Press.

Lawton, J. H. & Brown, K. C. 1986 The population and community ecology of invading insects. *Phil. Trans. R. Soc. Lond.* B **314**, 607–617.

Lawton, J. H. & MacGarvin, M. 1985 Interactions between bracken and its insect herbivores. *Proc. R. Soc. Edinb.* B **86**, 125–131.

Lawton, J. H., MacGarvin, M. & Heads, P. A. 1986 The ecology of bracken-feeding insects: background for a biological control programme. In *Bracken, Ecology, land use and control technology* (ed. R. T. Smith & J. A. Taylor), pp. 285–292. Carnforth: Parthenon Publishing.

Lawton, J. H., MacGarvin, M. & Heads, P. A. 1987 The effects of altitude on the abundance and species richness of insect herbivores on bracken. *J. Anim. Ecol.* **56**, 147–160.

Lawton, J. H., Rashbrook, V. K. & Compton, S. G. 1988 Biocontrol of British bracken: the potential of two moths from Southern Africa. *Ann appl. Biol.* (In the press.)

Lawton, J. H. & Schroeder, D. 1978 Some observations on the structure of phytophagous insect communities: the implications for biological control. In *Proceedings of the IVth International Symposium on the Biological Control of Weeds, August 1976, Gainesville, Florida* (ed. T. E. Freeman), pp. 57–73. Gainesville: University of Florida.

Lowday, J. E. 1986 A comparison of the effects of cutting with those of the herbicide asulam on the control of bracken. In *Bracken, Ecology, land use and control technology* (ed. R. T. Smith & J. A. Taylor), pp. 359–367. Carnforth: Parthenon Publishing.

MacGarvin, M., Lawton, J. H. & Heads, P. A. 1986 The herbivorous insect communities of open and woodland bracken: observations, experiments and habitat manipulations. *Oikos* **47**, 135–148.

MAFF 1983 *Bracken and its control.* Northumberland: Ministry of Agriculture, Fisheries and Food (Publications). (Leaflet 190.)

Marrs, R. H. 1985 The effects of potential bracken and scrub control herbicides on lowland *Calluna* and grass heath communities in East Anglia, UK. *Biol. Cons.* **32**, 13–32.

Marrs, R. H., Hicks, M. J. & Fuller, R. M. 1986 Losses of lowland heath through succession at four sites in Breckland, East Anglia, England. *Biol. Cons.* **36**, 19–38.

MacGavin, G. C. & Brown, V. K. 1986 Variation in populations of mine- and gall-forming Diptera and the growth form of their host plant, bracken (*Pteridium aquilinum* (L.) Khun). *J. nat. Hist.* **20**, 799–816.

McKelvie, A. D. & Scragg, E. B. 1972–3 The control of bracken by Asulam. *Scott. Agric.* **51**, 474–480.

Oswald, A. K., Richardson, W. G. & West, T. M. 1986 The potential control of bracken by sulphonyl-urea herbicides. In *Bracken, Ecology, land use and control technology* (ed. R. T. Smith & J. A. Taylor), pp. 431–439. Carnforth: Parthenon Publishing.

Ottosson, J. G. & Anderson, J. M. 1983 Number, seasonality and feeding habits of insects attacking ferns in Britain: an ecological consideration. *J. Anim. Ecol.* **52**, 385–406.

Page, C. N. 1976 The taxonomy and phytogeography of bracken – a review. *Bot. J. Linn. Soc.* **73**, 1–34.

Rigby, C. & Lawton, J. H. 1981 Species–area relationships of arthropods on host plants: herbivores on bracken. *J. Biogeog.* **8**, 125–133.

Robinson, R. C. 1986 Practical herbicide use for bracken control. In *Bracken, Ecology, land use and control technology* (ed. R. T. Smith & J. A. Taylor), pp. 331–339. Carnforth: Parthenon Publishing.

Salazar, J. V. 1985 Carcinogenicidad del *Pteridium aquilinum* y alta incidencia del cancer gastrico en Costa Rica. *Rev. Cost. Cienc. Méd.* **6**, 131–139.

Schroeder, D. 1983 Biological control of weeds. In *Recent advances in weed research* (ed. W. W. Fletcher), pp. 41–78. Farnham Royal: Commonwealth Agricultural Bureaux.

Smith, R. T. & Taylor, J. A. (eds) 1986 *Bracken, Ecology, land use and control technology.* Carnforth: Parthenon Publishing.

Soper, D. 1986 Lessons from fifteen years of bracken control with asulam. In *Bracken, Ecology, land use and control technology* (ed. R. T. Smith & J. A. Taylor), pp. 351–357. Carnforth: Parthenon Publishing.

Strong, D. R., Lawton, J. H. & Southwood, T. R. E. 1984 *Insects on plants: community patterns and mechanisms.* Oxford: Blackwell Scientific.

Stubbs, D. 1988 *A report on introductions and reintroductions of living organisms into the wild in Great Britain.* Wildlife Link (In the press.)

Taylor, J. A. 1986 The bracken problem: alocal hazard and global issue. In *Bracken, Ecology, land use and control technology* (ed. R. T. Smith & J. A. Taylor), pp. 21–42. Carnforth: Parthenon Publishing.

*Discussion*

M. J. WAY (*Imperial College at Silwood Park, Ascot, U.K.*). In the face of the problems you mention could you indicate the way ahead? How will you deal with the potential environmental issues without evidence from some form of experiment in an ecologically isolated site?

J. H. LAWTON. If and when we get to the point of wanting to release one or more agents, the safest and wisest course of action would be to do the introductions on one of the many small, bracken-infested, isolated offshore islands that lie along the west coast of Britain. Several offers from owners or tenants, of such islands have already been received to use their islands as release sites. There is great interest in the project and I do not think finding suitable sites will be difficult.

J. S. NOYES (*Department of Entomology, British Museum (Natural History), U.K.*). In light of the fact that Professor Lawton is introducing an exotic phytophage to control a native plant pest does he not think it is possible or even likely that a native parasite or parasites will switch from native insects on bracken to the introduced phytophage and stop it before it can effectively control the bracken?

J. H. LAWTON. As I have explained in the paper, the insects we have chosen as the most suitable potential control agents have been chosen to avoid this possibility as far as possible; i.e. they are ecologically and taxonomically as different as possible to native, bracken-feeding insects. But we cannot rule out attack from native enemies as a possible cause of failure.

*Phil. Trans. R. Soc. Lond.* B **318**, 357–373 (1988)

*Printed in Great Britain*

# Commercial application of biological control: status and prospects

By A. R. Jutsum

*I.C.I. Plant Protection Division, Jealott's Hill Research Station, Bracknell,
Berkshire RG12 6EY, U.K.*

The global market value of control agents used in crop protection and public health is approaching $16000 million annually, but less than 1 % of this market is penetrated by biological control agents (BCAs). This paper examines the suitability of different types of BCA to research and commercialization, bearing in mind the sharply targeted approach employed by much of the industry. Advantages and disadvantages are discussed along with examples of failures and successes with BCAs. Commercialized products described range from specific chemical control agents which have no adverse effects on beneficial organisms to true BCAs such as pheromones, mass-produced bacteria, and predatory mites.

From a commercial viewpoint, greatest potential resides with the utilization of bacteria and fungi, particularly for insect control, but registerability (particularly for genetically engineered agents) patentability, reliability and cost-effectiveness must be achieved. Industry believes that biotechnology will increase the usefulness of BCAs and is therefore encouraging cooperation with academic researchers and performing in-house research to advance the technology. Even so, BCAs will not replace chemicals in the foreseeable future, but will complement them and allow the development of improved integrated control measures.

## 1. Introduction

The agrochemical industry has defined and quantified targets for pest, disease and weed control, and sets itself the goal of obtaining safer and more effective agents for use in the market place. Historically, the use of agrochemicals has been the most common approach, but the agrochemical industry is an effects business and the compounds used, for example in insect control, cover many modes of action from rapid kill to disruption of growth and the use of chemosterilants. For instance, plants can be protected from nematode attack without killing nematodes, whereas insect sex pheromones are employed to disrupt mating which reduces or eliminates the production of damaging progeny.

The stance of the agrochemical industry on using bacteria, viruses, fungi, nematodes and insects, and even plants for pest, disease and weed control has changed over the past decade. Technology has advanced and many examples of acceptable control can be cited. This paper concentrates on the benefits and drawbacks of biological control agents, bearing in mind factors such as reliability, patentability and registerability, and indeed cost-efficacy compared with conventional control techniques. It sets out to examine the common and erroneous thesis that all chemicals are bad and all biological control agents are good. Industry's views on the development of the different types of biological control agent are presented within this context, along with prospects for successful commercialization. Generally I shall try to encapsulate the stances of both large and small companies, but obviously the content reflects my personal views, although many, if not most, of the views expressed will be shared by my colleagues in my own company and in other agrochemical companies.

## 2. Definition of biological control

Biological control, by definition, can cover a broad spectrum of approaches ranging from the use of obligate parasites and pathogens, to facultative parasites and pathogens, to competitors, to toxin-producing pathogens, to toxins produced by pathogens, and finally non-toxic behaviour-modifying chemicals. This spectrum is outlined in figure 1, with some examples.

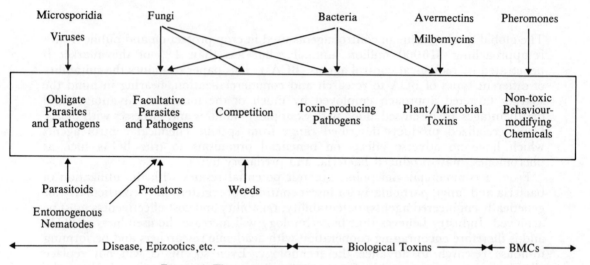

FIGURE 1. The spectrum of biological control agents.
(In this figure BMCs stands for behaviour-modifying chemicals.)

The group of biological control agents encompassed by this definition, which includes parasites, parasitoids, predators, pathogens and pheromones, will be referred to as BCAs (biological control agents) through the paper.

In addition to examining this range of BCAs, the use of selective agrochemicals, that is highly specific compounds such as insect growth regulators, will also be described.

Examples of the use of BCAs for reducing or controlling problem weeds and diseases will be cited, but the paper will concentrate primarily on pest examples, and particularly on entomological ones, as this is the area in which most commercial interest has been shown to date.

## 3. Pest, pathogen and weed markets

To examine the present and future impact of BCAs on the global pesticide, fungicide and herbicide markets, it is necessary to give a breakdown of the major commercial opportunities in the world.

An analysis of the global market for insecticides, fungicides and herbicides in 1985 (figure 2) shows that 44 % of world sales are accounted for by herbicides, 31 % by insecticides (including acaricides) and 18 % by fungicides (Wood Mackenzie 1986). In total, sales in 1985 were estimated at $15 900 million.

These figures represent a 4.6 % increase over 1984 (Wood Mackenzie 1986). However, the increase to the year 2000 is expected to be 2–3 % per year throughout the period.

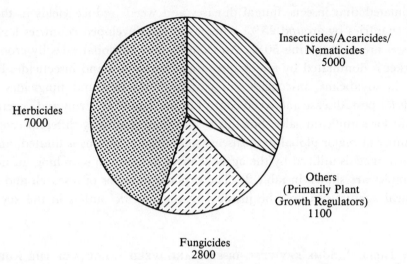

FIGURE 2. Global pesticide, fungicide and herbicide sales (end-user value given in millions of U.S. dollars at 1985 value).


TABLE 1. GLOBAL SALES OF PESTICIDES, FUNGICIDES AND HERBICIDES ON THE WORLD'S MAJOR CROPS (END-USER VALUE GIVEN IN MILLIONS OF U.S. DOLLARS AT 1985 VALUE)

| herbicides | millions of U.S. dollars | percentage of sector |
|---|---|---|
| maize | 1575 | 22 |
| soya | 1475 | 21 |
| wheat | 920 | 13 |
| rice | 650 | 9 |
| fruit and vegetables† | 610 | 9 |
| sugar beet | 350 | 5 |
| cotton | 340 | 5 |
| | | total 84 |
| insecticides | | |
| cotton | 1335 | 27 |
| fruit and vegetables† | 1260 | 25 |
| rice | 825 | 17 |
| maize | 470 | 9 |
| soya | 155 | 3 |
| sugar beet | 145 | 3 |
| wheat | 95 | 2 |
| | | total 86 |
| fungicides | | |
| fruit and vegetables† | 1290 | 46 |
| rice | 430 | 15 |
| wheat | 380 | 14 |
| soya | 55 | 2 |
| maize | 40 | 1 |
| sugar beet | 40 | 1 |
| cotton | 40 | 1 |
| | | total 80 |

† Includes vines.

It is estimated that insects, fungal diseases and weeds reduce yields in the agriculturally developed countries by around 25%, whereas in less developed countries losses run at 40%. In rice, losses are a staggering 50%. An examination of global sales by crop shows that the world market is dominated by five major crops: herbicides and insecticides in maize (corn), herbicides in soyabeans, insecticides in cotton, herbicides and fungicides in wheat, and compounds for pest, disease and weed control in rice (table 1). Fruit and vegetables as a group also account for significant sales, but this is split between many different crops.

The number of major global pest, disease and weed problems is limited, and a selection of these major targets is utilized by the agrochemical industry in searching for novel toxophores (some examples are shown in table 2). The expense in terms of research and development of new chemical agents, can only be justified in the specific outlets in the key market sectors listed.

TABLE 2. SOME KEY PEST, DISEASE AND WEED TARGETS OF THE WORLD

| target | species | common name |
|---|---|---|
| insects | *Heliothis* spp. | cotton bollworm, etc. |
| | *Spodoptera* spp. | cotton leafworm, etc. |
| | *Diabrotica* spp. | corn rootworms |
| | *Myzus persicae* | peach potato aphid |
| | *Nilaparvata lugens* | brown planthopper |
| | *Nephotettix* spp. | green leaf hoppers |
| diseases | *Pyricularia oryzae* | rice blast |
| | *Erysiphe graminis* | wheat powdery mildew |
| | *Botrytis cinerea* | grey mould |
| | *Plasmopara viticola* | vine downy mildew |
| | *Venturia inaequalis* | apple scab |
| weeds | *Avena fatua* | wild oats |
| | *Sorghum halepense* | Johnsongrass |
| | *Agropyron repens* | couch grass/quack grass |
| | *Cyperus* spp. | sedge |
| | *Ipomoea* spp. | morning glory, etc. |
| | *Galium* spp. | cleavers |
| | *Xanthium* spp. | cocklebur |

## 4. UTILITY OF BCAS

### Niches for commercial exploitation

BCAs may ultimately be exploited in virtually any market provided that they are as good as (or better than) existing control agents in terms of cost, efficacy and reliability, or have a significant toxicological or environmental advantage. At present, however, there are only four specific market niches that can be commercially exploited.

1. Outlets where conventional chemical agents give insufficient levels of control, such as in certain diseases caused by soil-borne pathogens, or where there is insecticide resistance.

2. Outlets where conventional chemical agents are too expensive, for example the potential control of the bracken-fern (*Pteridium aquilinum*) with lepidopterous natural enemies (Heads & Lawton 1986).

3. Outlets where governments restrict the application of conventional chemical agents, as practised in Canadian forestry.

4. Outlets where the environment is contained and controlled, for instance in glasshouses where the fungus *Verticillium lecanii* is used to control aphids and whitefly.

### *Commercial and non-commercial successes and failures of BCAs*

*Successes*

1. Use of the moth *Cactoblastis cactorum* to control prickly pear, *Opuntia* spp., in Australia.

2. Introduction of the predatory *Vedalia* ladybeetle, *Rodolia cardinalis*, for controlling cottony cushion scales on citrus in California in 1888–1889.

3. Introduction of the ectoparasite *Aphytis holoxanthus*, for controlling Florida red scale on citrus in Israel in 1956–1957.

4. Use of the parasitic chalcid wasp *Encarsia formosa*, for controlling whitefly under glass or plastic.

5. Use of the predatory mite *Phytoseiulus persimilis*, for controlling mites under glass or plastic.

6. Use of the bacterial pathogen *Bacillus thuringiensis*, for controlling lepidopterous and dipterous pests.

7. Use of the fungal mycoherbicide *Colletotrichum gloeosporioides*, for controlling Northern jointvetch.

8. Use of *Peniophora gigantea* to control *Heterobasidion annosum*, in forestry.

*Failures*

1. Extensive work to control Bermuda cedar scales failed despite the introduction of over fifty species of natural enemies, mainly coccinellid predators to cedar forests in Bermuda between 1946 and 1951.

2. Introduction of cane toads in sugar in Australia failed to control cane beetles and the toads became pests.

3. Release of sterile fruit flies in California was unsuccessful when non-sterile flies were released by mistake.

4. Commercialization of the nematode *Romanomermis culicivorax* for use against mosquito larvae failed due to difficulties in handling, storage and shipping, environmental limitations, host specificity, expense and user acceptance.

5. *Heliothis* spp. nuclear polyhedrosis virus (NPV) although technically successful, failed commercially because of poor forecasting of market needs and trends.

Overall, only 34% of predators and parasites released for insect control become established, and of these only 16% give satisfactory control. This means that only 5% of all deliberate releases actually achieved their aim.

Further examination of such examples yields technical and commercial insights of value in appraising the potential of BCAs and the level of commitment of industry to different types of BCA (see §5).

### *Penetration of the global market*

Sales of BCAs and selective chemicals account for 1% of the world market of crop protection products, but the majority of sales are in the insecticide sector where they account for 2.5% of sales. This is attributed to sales of selective chemicals and *Bacillus thuringiensis*, with little contribution from other BCAs (table 3), although sales figures for predators and parasites may be underestimated.

Some analysts predict that BCAs will have a 50% market share by the year 2000, but industry in general believes this is highly unlikely despite political pressure such as that seen in Canadian forestry, and the potential for genetic manipulation.

TABLE 3. PENETRATION OF THE GLOBAL INSECTICIDE MARKET BY BIOLOGICAL CONTROL AGENTS (END-USER VALUE GIVEN IN MILLIONS OF U.S. DOLLARS AT 1985 VALUE)

1. sales of selective chemicals/pheromones

| | | |
|---|---|---|
| selective chemicals | | 90 |
| pheromones | | 2 |
| | total | 92 |

2. sales of predators/parasites and pathogens

| | | |
|---|---|---|
| Bacillus thuringiensis (products for forestry, agriculture and public health) | | 30 |
| viral insecticides | ca. | 1 |
| predators/parasites/other pathogens | ca. | 3? |
| | total | 34 |

5. INDUSTRY VIEW OF BCAS
*General objectives*

Many of the objectives implicit in developing BCAs are being achieved with chemicals by the agrochemical industry. These include reduced application rates, better application techniques, improved selectivity, and reduced toxicological and environmental hazards. However, as an effects business, the industry considers the value of BCAs very seriously, even though selective BCAs, by their very nature, are likely to command a small fraction of the global market. This has historically led industry to develop broad spectrum compounds, for sound commercial reasons (Braunholtz & Tietz 1980). The use of BCAs requires re-education of farmers, growers and pest-control operatives, especially if the apparent speed of effect is slow, because the user is generally looking for control as good as, or better than, that obtained with the product he now uses at the same, or a lower, price.

None the less, many large multinationals are now pursuing BCAs as control agents, where markets of sufficient size exist. The research programmes include genetic manipulation of pathogens, expression of genes from pathogens in plants, and plant or microbial toxins as starting points for developing other control agents. Generally, large companies are interested in selling selective agents if they complement their existing portfolio of products or if a series of small outlets can be identified which add up to make a robust business case. However, it is usually the small companies that provide supplies of predators, parasites and some naturally occurring pathogens, as they are usually specialized and have a limited product range, whereas large companies will run a large number of projects simultaneously, which must compete for the same resource.

In recent years, the agrochemical industry has tried to incorporate its products into integrated programmes. This has been prompted by practical and commercial reality, by a more responsible attitude within industry, and by the availability of certain control agents. In the sections following, selective chemicals and different types of BCA are discussed, with entomological examples.

*Selective chemicals*

Industry supports the use of selective chemicals such as insect growth regulators, antifeedants and repellents, provided they form an attractive financial proposition. The structures of three such specific insecticides are shown in figure 3: pirimicarb (I.C.I.) is a specific aphicide, chlorfluazuron (Ishihara Sangyo Kaisha) is an insect growth regulator for lepidopterous, coleopterous and dipterous pests, and buprofezin (Nihon Nohyaku) is an insect growth regulator for homopterous pests.

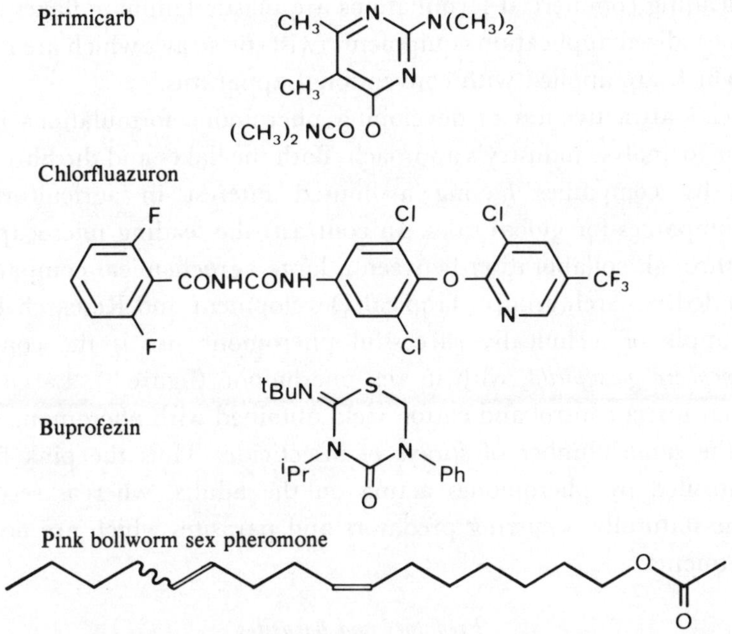

FIGURE 3. Examples of selective chemicals and a pheromone which are commercially available for use in pest control.

Pirimicarb is a fast-acting, selective carbamate aphicide which is active through contact, fumigant, translaminar and root-systemic routes, but at the rates necessary for good aphid control has no significant activity against other insects, including the beneficial pollinating and predatory insects, such as bees, ladybirds and lacewings. In addition, the compound is non-phytotoxic and causes no accumulation problems in the environment. The compound was discovered and developed by industry and is probably the best selective aphicide available. However, it does not dominate the market as it is one of a number of aphicides that are available, and most are broader-spectrum compounds and some are cheaper.

Similarly, many insect growth regulators have not enjoyed the success that might be derived from fairly specific control agents, probably because of the drawback of limited sales potential. Major changes in farmer perception are needed before compounds such as chlorfluazuron and buprofezin become a dominant force, even though they preserve essential beneficial organisms, are active on resistant strains, and can be used selectively as a management tool.

## Pheromones

Insect pheromones have been commercialized by a few companies and can be used in four ways: for monitoring purposes, for mass trapping, as mating disruptants, and in mixtures with conventional insecticides. Exploitation of pheromones for monitoring purposes is pursued by some small specialist companies, whereas some multinationals have developed controlled release formulations to allow sex pheromones to be used as mating disruptants, or with conventional insecticides in mixtures that function by attracting and then killing specific pests.

The present leading commercial formulations are plastic laminate flakes and hollow fibres which require specialized application equipment, twist–tie straws which are hand-applied, and microcapsules which are applied with conventional apparatus.

The commercial attractiveness of developing pheromone formulations is small and it is therefore of value to analyse industry's approach. Both the flakes and the fibres were researched and developed by companies having a limited interest in agriculture, who licensed multinational companies for global sales. In contrast, the leading microcapsule formulation was developed through collaboration between a large agrochemical company (I.C.I.) and a Government funded research group (Tropical Development and Research Institute).

The best example of technically successful pheromone use is the control of the pink bollworm, *Pectinophora gossypiella*, with its sex pheromone (figure 3). Large-scale trials have demonstrated that insect control and cotton yield obtained with pheromone is as good as that obtained with the same number of sprays of insecticide. Thus the pink bollworm can be successfully controlled by pheromones acting on the adults, whereas secondary pests are controlled by the naturally occurring predators and parasites which are not affected by the pheromone treatments.

## Predators and parasites

The utilization of mass-released entomophagous insects and mites has been reviewed recently by van Lenteren (1986). At present, few natural enemies are mass produced and applied for pest control, and marketing is restricted to small specialist companies such as Koppert BV in The Netherlands. The large agrochemical companies do not find the market, as presently perceived, to be of sufficient size to warrant production bearing in mind overheads and internal competition for development resource. None the less, such agents can be cost-effectively employed in a repeated fashion, for instance, on glasshouse crops. Some examples of predators and parasites presently used are shown in table 4.

Similarly, 'one-off' attempts to eradicate specific pests with predators and parasites are not the domain of industry, as others are much better suited to exploiting this niche.

The use of predators and parasites will not supplant chemical means in the foreseeable future, but can be a valuable approach in integrated pest management, and some researchers are already working on the development of pesticide resistance in natural enemies. However, it is worth noting that as with agrochemicals, pests are capable of developing resistance to entomophagous control agents, by developing thicker cuticles, encapsulating parasite eggs, or changing behaviour, for instance by developing cryptic habits.

| | |
|---|---|
| predators | *Phytoseiulus persimilis* |
| | *Amblyseius mckenziei* |
| | *A. cucumeris* |
| parasites: | *Encarsia formosa* |
| | *Opius pallipes* |
| | *Trichogramma evanescens* |
| pathogens: | |
| viruses | *Neodiprion sertifer* NPV |
| | *Autographa californica* NPV |
| bacteria | *Bacillus thuringiensis* var. *kurstaki* |
| | *B. thuringiensis* var. *israelensis* |
| fungi | *Hirsutella thompsonii* |
| | *Verticillium lecanii* |
| microsporidia | *Nosema locustae* |

## *Pathogens*

The utilization of pathogens, such as viruses, bacteria and fungi has been reviewed recently (Payne, this symposium), and fits closely with the skills and channels of trade of the agrochemical industry, particularly as such agents have considerable potential for use as pesticides. However, genetic engineering will be necessary before many potential applications are developed. Many species of virus, bacteria, fungi and microsporidia have been identified as biological control agents, but few have been commercialized, and only some of these can be regarded as successful. Some examples of pathogens which are commercially available are shown in table 4.

The agents with greatest usage at the present time are bacteria and fungi, then viruses. Generally, the user expects the agrochemical industry to provide new products which are as cost-effective as chemicals now used. However, there are a number of limitations that must be overcome. These include breadth of spectrum, speed of action, field persistence, shelf-life and cost of production. Some small companies and a few large ones are producing and selling pathogens, especially *Bacillus thuringiensis* for insect pest control. This approach is sound in the short term so long as targets, such as forestry, are selected in which the characteristics of existing BCAs are advantageous or, at least, not deleterious. However, in the medium-term, BCAs will have to be improved considerably if they are to penetrate the market in a big way, probably through rigorous strain selection, and in the long-term by introducing, for example, genes from *Bacillus thuringiensis* into plants to confer resistance to attack by insect pests.

## *Conclusions on industry's stance opposite BCAs*

The level of interest shown by the agrochemical industry to the different types of BCA available is summarized in table 5, and it is evident that, at present, only bacteria stimulate as much interest as selective chemicals.

Industry, however, is committed to integrating BCAs into control programmes. A range of selective compounds is available which can be used in an integrated manner (see, for example, Collins *et al.* (1984)) and pheromones have been incorporated into spray programmes quite successfully (Critchley *et al.* 1984). Selective agents that spare beneficial organisms which can

TABLE 5. TYPES OF BIOLOGICAL CONTROL AGENT AND LEVEL OF INTEREST FROM INDUSTRY

| biological control agent | interest from industry |
|---|---|
| selective chemicals | * * * * |
| pheromones: | |
| monitoring | * |
| mass trapping | * |
| mating disruption | * * * |
| use in mixtures | * * * |
| predators/parasites | * |
| pathogens, etc. | |
| microsporidia | * |
| viruses | * |
| bacteria | * * * * |
| fungi | * * |
| nematodes | * |
| insects | * |

Key to interest from industry: *, Least interest; ****, greatest interest.

exert further control are used early in the season. Later in the season, broad-spectrum compounds are used when pest pressure increases and natural control fails. As additional BCAs become available commercially, further strategies can be formulated.

## 6. COMMERCIALIZATION OF BCAS
### Characteristics essential for commercialization

Commercialization of BCAs involves selling such products in a competitive market with the expectation of recovering research and development costs and making a reasonable margin of profit. A number of factors are critical to achieving success, and four of these are described below.

### Reliability

Once produced, a BCA has to be formulated and packed to maintain biological activity during storage and distribution, and to retain effectiveness when applied or released on to a target or substrate. Selective chemicals and pheromones, usually perform reliably provided that recommendations for use are adhered to, but pathogens, predators and parasites, on the other hand, are not always reliable.

Efficacy can be strongly affected by environmental conditions such as moisture, temperature, sunlight and pH. Timing of application can be critical, and persistence of effect may be disappointing.

Failings in terms of reliability of pathogens will be overcome through improvements, for instance in formulation and application. These include improving the stability of the product by using better stabilizers and gelling agents, obtaining better adhesion and spread on targets or substrates or both, and by improving persistence by incorporating ultraviolet stabilizers and the like. The sensitivity of microbial BCAs to ultraviolet light and humidity could be overcome by selecting targets where these environmental factors can be minimized or avoided, such as soil and rice paddy; by the production of more resistant mutants through strain selection; or by genetic engineering of the toxin coding genes either into the plant genome or into, for example, a bacterial epiphyte.

*Patentability*

Protection of a discovery by industry usually involves the filing of patents or keeping secret the nature of the discovery. Novel selective chemicals newly identified can be patented *per se* whereas industrial property for known published pheromones can be obtained through patenting new controlled release systems for delivering pheromones. Little protection can be obtained in producing predators and parasites, and reliance on intellectual property protection for naturally occurring pathogens is problematical. Production methods and formulations can be patented, but there is nothing to prevent competitors from developing other products based on the same agent.

There are, however, significant opportunities for patenting in this area when improved BCAs are obtained through the modern techniques of genetic manipulation, which can also provide improvements in biological effect. This approach can also be policed by the owner who has proprietary rights.

*Registerability*

The registration requirements for a so called 'biorational' pesticide, such as a pheromone or a naturally occurring pathogen, are less stringent than for a selective chemical, and hence can be obtained more quickly and at less cost. This process is being questioned, however, especially where non-indigenous organisms, pathogenic organisms or genetically engineered organisms are concerned. Commercially available BCAs have proved to be uncompetitive with the natural macro- and micro-fauna under field conditions and are thus often unreliable, but pose a limited environmental threat. The risk is that by producing reliable BCAs, undesirable pathogenicity may become a real problem, as has been demonstrated by myxomatosis and certain plant diseases. This may, however, be overcome by building into the BCA, sensitivity to factors such as ultraviolet light, oxygen, or high or low temperature. The stance of registration authorities is still developing, as is evidenced by responses to industrial requests to field test engineered organisms. None the less, in the U.S.A. the Environmental Protection Agency has stated its intention not to restrict progress in this area of biotechnology by over-regulation, otherwise BCAs will only be developed in the largest markets.

The importance of speed of registration cannot be over-emphasized. A company with proprietary property can only guarantee profitable sales for the life of the patent and if registration procedures are protracted then the sales life of the product may be reduced. If registration requirements were more harmonized between countries, the introduction of BCAs may become more likely as markets would be accessible at lower cost, and hence industry would be more likely to proceed with their development.

*Cost-effectiveness*

In a limited number of outlets, BCAs may be sold at a premium, but in the majority of markets globally, users will expect at least the same effect at the same price as can be obtained with conventional chemicals.

*Bacillus thuringiensis* is sold successfully in Canadian forestry at nearly twice the price of an acceptable chemical, fenitrothion. However, this is probably going to be the exception rather than the rule, in the future.

If production costs for microbial BCAs can be reduced by improving fermentation systems, reducing media costs, increasing yield, modifying culture systems, or even by inserting genes coding for toxins into 'easy to grow' organisms such as *Pseudomonas* spp., and efficacy can be improved, such agents should be able to compete effectively with conventional chemicals.

## Collaboration between the public and private sectors

Most of the presently commercialized BCAs were known to be of limited potential, but were seen to be of value in overcoming significant local problems and were exploited through collaborative research between the public and private sectors.

Interaction continues to increase at all levels between government institutes, independent institutes and universities on the one hand, and biotechnology companies and agrochemical producers on the other. Successes include microencapsulated pheromones and *Verticillium lecanii*. This positive approach to understanding and exploiting 'the basic science' is laudable, but to market the product successfully, involvement of large multinational companies will be imperative.

## BCAs as sources of novel control agents

Some toxins produced by pathogens have been isolated and identified, and examples include the β-exotoxin and δ-endotoxin from *Bacillus thuringiensis* and the avermectins from *Streptomyces avermitilis*.

Chemicals identified from pathogens showing promise as biological control agents can be exploited in three possible ways.
1. As commercially viable products in their own right.
2. As starting structures for the chemical synthesis of analogues.
3. As building blocks for further chemical/microbial modification.

Some success has already been achieved with these approaches in developing insecticides, acaricides, and nematicides, and some experts (Poole & Chrystal 1985) believe that this will be the only successful approach for exploiting microbial phytotoxins as herbicides.

## BCAs: options for pest control

An examination of the BCA options available for insect, disease and weed control is an enormous task, but it is valuable to focus on a few such options. The best examples are the microbial BCAs and microbial toxins that have potential for controlling insect pests. Fungi have the widest spectrum of activity and have potential for controlling foliar chewing and sucking pests, soil pests, and insects of public health importance. Bacteria and viruses have the greatest potential for controlling foliar Lepidoptera, whereas bacteria show most promise for use in public health.

The microsporidia and avermectins, on the other hand, appear to have the least potential as insecticides, but it should be noted that avermectins, for example, also possess acaricidal and nematicidal properties.

If the characteristics of the three microbial BCAs – viruses, bacteria and fungi – which show greatest potential as insecticides are examined, then technical shortcomings which need to be reduced or overcome to ensure successful commercialization can be listed (table 6). The major failings of viruses are those of spectrum of activity and difficulty of production on a large scale.

Research is progressing in the mapping and identification of genes in some baculoviruses, and genes of particular interest are those that control specificity, host range and virulence.

TABLE 6. TECHNICAL SHORTCOMINGS OF VIRUSES, BACTERIA AND FUNGI FOR COMMERCIALIZATION AS BIOLOGICAL CONTROL AGENTS

| characteristic | viruses for soil application | viruses for foliar application | bacteria for soil application | bacteria for foliar application | fungi for soil application | fungi for foliar application |
|---|---|---|---|---|---|---|
| lack of contact activity | * * * | * | * * * | * | — | — |
| speed of action | * | * * * | * | * * | * | * * * |
| ultraviolet sensitivity | — | * * * | — | * * ? | — | * |
| moisture tolerance | — | — | — | * | * | * * * |
| mobility | * * | * | * * | * | — | — |
| spectrum | * * * | * * * | * * | * * | * | * |
| ease of production | * * * | * * * | — | — | * * | * * |
| formulation stability | * | * | * | * | * * * | * * * |

Key to symbols used: *, minor shortcomings; ***, major shortcomings.

Virus production at present involves *in vivo* methods, as insect larvae are efficient producers of baculoviruses, and it is possible that one easily cultured insect host could be employed to produce several different viruses. None the less, industry would probably favour *in vitro* production if this proved cost attractive, but opinions on the feasibility of developing such a process at present are diverse. Other shortcomings include sensitivity to ultraviolet light and speed of action when used as foliar applications, and lack of contact activity against the pest species in soil use. Problems with ultraviolet light can be overcome through formulation optimization, but the other problems remain to be tackled.

The technical shortcomings of bacteria are perceived as less acute than for viruses but much work must still be done to improve the spectrum of activity, to make the control agent more mobile and faster acting, to improve dispersion in the soil, and to enhance effectiveness under ultraviolet light. Some improvements here are already promised as genetic manipulation can be used to broaden the spectrum of activity and optimize the speed of action, while formulation research will yield a more persistent agent under field conditions.

The third group of pathogens with greatest potential for commercialization is the fungi. Ease of production is a problem, but the major technical problems are associated with formulation stability, moisture tolerance and speed of action when used on foliage. These shortcomings will have to be overcome before fungi can be exploited to any extent outside 'protected environments'. Again, genetic manipulation and formulation technology should allow fungi to be exploited as BCAs on a reasonable scale.

## 7. CONCLUSIONS AND PROSPECTS FOR THE FUTURE

Braunholtz & Tietz (1980) were 'uncertain that the present agrochemical industry would in the short to medium term become involved in any major way in the provision and practice of biological control measures'. However, they did believe that industry could aid progress though the development of new formulations, new target oriented chemicals and new application methods. Seven years later, science and technology have made great strides forward, and industry is interested in, and committed to, developing selected BCAs and selective chemicals.

BCAs for insect control are commercially available, but agents for controlling weeds and diseases are generally less developed. However, mycoherbicides, insects and competitive plants hold promise for weed control, and antagonists have potential for controlling disease. Of the agents at present available, predators and parasites provided by government agencies and a few small specialized companies, will continue to be used to decrease damage caused by pests, whereas selective chemicals and pheromones produced by the agrochemical industry will increase in importance if compatible with integrated practices (see papers by van Emden and Pickett, this symposium).

The most radical changes occurring in industry are in response to the perceived potential value of exploiting pathogens. The options available range from selling naturally occurring pathogens, which could even be produced by cottage-type industries in less developed countries, to the low technology approach of undirected mutagenesis, to the high technology options of genetically manipulating pathogens to improve the efficiency of production or widen the spectrum of activity, and getting genes from BCAs expressed in plants. The choice of option to pursue will be critical for a company which will have to weigh up the risks of factors such as increased research and development costs, uncertain registerability, unproven markets, and the impact of plant biotechnology. In fact, some small companies which market microbial pest control agents have already gone out of business.

Industry, and the large multinationals in particular, will be instrumental in commercializing BCAs for pest, disease and weed control, as the foundation is laid for the introduction of very exciting control techniques in the 1990s and the next century. However, even though the future looks bright for BCAs, the agrochemical industry does not expect them to replace chemicals, but to complement them and allow the development of better integrated control programmes.

I thank Dr M. D. Collins for the many valued discussions we have had on biological control, and Dr C. N. E. Ruscoe, Dr K. A. Powell, Dr N. J. Poole, Dr R. A. Brown, Mr C. A. Manley, Mr R. E. Griggs and Mr N. D. Bishop for their valuable comments about the manuscript.

## REFERENCES

Braunholtz, J. T. & Teitz, H. 1980 The future of integrated pest control – commercialisation constraints. In *Conference of Future Trends of Integrated Pest Management, Bellagio.*

Collins, M. D., Perrin, R. M., Jutsum, A. R. & Jackson, G. J. 1984 Insecticides for the future: a package of selective compounds for the control of major crop pests. In *Proceedings of the 1984 British Crop Protection Conference – Pests and Diseases, Brighton, U.K.*, pp. 299–304. BCPC Publications.

Critchley, B. R., Campion, D. G., McVeigh, E. M., McVeigh, L. J., Jutsum, A. R., Gordon, R. F. S., Marrs, G. J., Nasr, El Sayed A. & Hosny, M. M. 1984 Microencapsulated pheromones in cotton pest management. In *Proceedings of the 1984 British Crop Protection Conference – Pests and Diseases, Brighton, U.K.*, pp. 241–245. BCPC Publications.

Heads, P. & Lawton, J. H. 1986 Beat back bracken biologically. *New Scient.* **111** (1525), 41–43.

Lenteren, J. C. van 1986 Evaluation, mass production, quality control and release of entomophagous insects. In *Biological plant and health protection* (ed. J. M. Franz) (*Fortschr. Zool.* **32**, 31–56).

Poole, N. J. & Chrystal, E. J. T. 1985 Miocrobial phytotoxins. In *Proceedings of the 1985 British Crop Protection Conference – Weeds, Brighton, U.K.*, pp. 591–600. BCPC Publications.

Wood Mackenzie 1986 *Agrochemical Service*, March 1986.

*Discussion*

J. M. FRANZ (*Gundolfstrasse* 14, 6100 *Darmstadt, F.R.G.*). During the past forty years I have heard many forecasts as to the future application of biological control issued by representatives of the pesticide industry. They were all wrong, and I am afraid that the present outlook is not correct either. Some examples may suffice to indicate the fundamental differences: first the difficulty of using the U.S. dollar as a basis for evaluation, considering its instability. Secondly, the dependence of public acceptance of BCAs for quite different (partly political) reasons. Thirdly, the increasing tendency to make the producer responsible for environmental problems (including resistance of pests to pesticides) caused by his products. The future will show who is right.

A. R. JUTSUM. I would like to comment on the three specific points raised by Professor Franz. First, the U.S. dollar is the accepted currency for making comparisons in the agrochemical business, and the figures presented were given in dollars at 1985 values throughout. Secondly, I agree that there will be increased use of BCAs in some countries in response to political pressures, but this may be followed by counter pressure when people start to consider genetically engineered BCAs as hazardous. Thirdly, industry does take a responsibility for the environmental acceptability of its products, hence GIFAP's (International Group of National Associations of Manufacturers of Agrochemical Products) support for the International Code of Conduct on the Distribution and Use of Pesticides developed by the FAO (Food and Agriculture Organization of the United Nations, Rome). It is also worth emphasizing that the belief that 'pesticides are harmful to the environment' is a meaningless generalization and just not true.

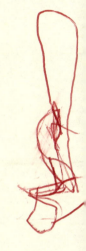

J. W. DEACON (*Department of Microbiology, Edinburgh University, U.K.*). I suggest that the agrochemical industry will wish to exploit biocontrol in conjunction with any newly developed, basipetally translocated fungicides. If these have similar properties to those of currently available systemic fungicides then they are likely to have single-site modes of action, and resistance to them could develop quite rapidly. Effective biocontrol agents could be integrated with their usage to prevent or delay the build-up of resistance in target pathogens.

A. R. JUTSUM. Preventative resistance management is a major target for the Fungicide Resistance Action Committee (FRAC), and is being tackled quite effectively with fungicide mixtures. Integration of chemical fungicides with BCAs will help preserve product life, but will only be acceptable, in the absence of legislation, if the BCA works at cost-effective rates and hence gains grower support.

C. C. PAYNE (*Glasshouse Crops Research Institute, Littlehampton, U.K.*). Would Dr Jutsum please comment on the rate at which new, active chemical ingredients are likely to be developed by the agrochemical industry? My understanding is that their rate of development is likely to be slowed and that the economics may shift in favour of diversification and greater exploitation of biological control agents.

A. R. JUTSUM. Chemical invention rates are declining across the agrochemical industry, but this may be counterbalanced by biotechnology directed at improved inventiveness. Thus we may get a renaissance period. Development is another matter, and obviously rests on the outcome of cost and benefit analysis. As the agrochemical market matures, it becomes more difficult to justify development, particularly as registration costs increase. This makes effective BCAs relatively attractive but will require changes in acceptance at grower level before significant market penetration is achieved. On the subject of diversification, I agree in principle with Dr Payne if he is referring to niche specialization (for example for control of rice water weevil in a mature Japanese market) but if specialized means small yet expensive to register, then industry will not be able to afford to exploit such niches.

T. Lewis (*Rothamsted Experimental Station, Harpenden, U.K.*). How could the prospects for biological control change, and how would the agrochemical companies respond, if, for environmental reasons, governments decided to tax pesticides?

A. R. Jutsum. I am appalled by the concept of introducing an environmental tax which seems impossible to implement fairly: it would be preferable to register only environmentally acceptable pesticides and get away from the 'pesticides are nasty' syndrome. However, if a tax were levied, the agrochemical industry would either stop developing new products for particular markets if returns became unattractive, or develop broader spectrum products to add value to the development case, which may be less attractive to the advocates of integrated pest management but not to the growers.

It would be much better to encourage industry by providing incentives to develop selective chemicals and BCAs which are compatible with integrated pest management. In this way, environmental acceptability can be attained whilst retaining a viable agricultural economy.

R. R. M. Paterson (*C.A.B. International Mycological Institute, Kew, U.K.*). Would a purified pesticidal metabolite from a microbe be defined as a BCA or a conventional chemical?

A. R. Jutsum. I believe that purified pesticidal metabolites from microbes will be classified as chemicals. Both avermectin, a secondary metabolite from *Streptomyces avermitilis*, and thuringiensin, the purified β-exotoxin from *Bacillus thuringiensis* (*Bt*) have not achieved bio-rational registration. However, *Bt* endotoxin would, I suspect, be classified as a BCA in terms of bio-rational registration. Yet, *Bt* is in effect the crystal toxin enclosed in a bacterium which can even be dead.

Thus, microbial metabolites should be generally regarded as chemicals, but *Bt* remains effectively an anomaly.

J. K. Waage (*C.A.B. International Institute of Biological Control, Ascot, U.K.*). In the context of industrial development, what is the future of small biological control industries? Are they transient or stable? If stable, what makes them able (or willing) to develop BCAs which major industry is currently not doing?

A. R. Jutsum. Within the biological control industry, companies such as Koppert BV who work primarily with predators and parasites are relatively stable, but specialist microbial pesticide companies are inherently unstable, particularly when they have relied upon venture capital and have been unable to provide monetary returns in a short time period. Those biotechnology groups working in the area currently under venture capital or industrial sponsorship or both will probably get taken over by industry if they are good, or cease trading if they are not. As far as your final point is concerned, the successful small biological control industries concentrate on specialized, limited markets which are financially unattractive to companies with large overheads, and this allows them to operate in a different competitive environment.

H. F. van Emden (*Departments of Horticulture, and Pure & Applied Zoology, University of Reading, U.K.*). Could Dr Jutsum forecast future trends in the tonnage of pesticide chemicals used on those crop areas currently receiving some pesticide?

A. R. Jutsum. Wood Mackenzie's (1986) view is that there will be slow, sustained growth of the agrochemical business world-wide at a rate of 2.5 % per year. However, as more efficacious chemicals are developed (but usually at a higher price per unit of active ingredient), the actual tonnage of chemicals used will decrease as rates of active ingredient applied are reduced. Use of BCAs will increase, but will not significantly erode the conventional business before the year 2000.

*Phil. Trans. R. Soc. Lond.* B **318**, 375–376 (1988)

*Printed in Great Britain*

# General discussion

A. K. Minks (*Research Institute for Plant Protection, Wageningen, The Netherlands*). The organizers should be given much credit for arranging this meeting on biological control where attention has been given not only to entomological but also to the other disciplines of plant protection. It is my belief that a multidisciplinary approach is the only way to develop biological control methods and to implement them successfully. In our Institute we became aware of this and recently we decided to leave the classical organizational division in entomology, mycology, plant virology, etc. sections and to change to sections named: detection, ecology, genetics and resistance breeding, and control, in which entomologists, mycologists, etc. have a much better possibility to work together. Another example of this in the Netherlands is the operation (since 1980) of the experimental farm 'Development of Farming Systems', recently followed by a second farm with a similar set-up where systems can be studied at the farm level.

R. M. May, F.R.S. (*Department of Biology, Princeton University, New Jersey, U.S.A.*). Many speakers have emphasized the need to think about the population- or even community-level consequences of releasing viral, bacterial or other pathogenic microorganisms into the environment. In particular, such questions arise for the release of genetically engineered microorganisms. Although it is obviously difficult to plan systematic studies of the unanticipated, I think that two approaches may deserve more attention than they have received here.

First, as seen in several of the papers dealing with insect pests, mathematical models can serve as strategic tools for exploring possibilities, for formulating testable ideas and for guiding the design of focused experiments and data gathering. I do not believe that mathematical models are intrisically either more or less useful in illuminating the population dynamics of host–pathogen associations than they provenly are for insect pests and enemies; as shown in my paper with Hassell, there are many useful parallels between the dynamical behaviour of insect and of pathogen systems.

Second, I think there is need for studies of the ecology of microorganisms in controlled laboratory settings (as well as in the field), as part of the safety programmes that must accompany the release of the pathogens, particularly genetically modified ones, as control agents. Such studies of 'microcosms' may require expenditures on a scale more customary for chemists and physicists than ecologists!

C. C. Payne (*Institute of Horticultural Research, Littlehampton, U.K.*). I would like to endorse these comments. Biological control has had its few successes with trial and error on 'enlightened empiricism' approaches. There is urgent need to consider now a more analytical and quantitative approach.

K. Jones (*Tropical Development and Research Institute, Porton Down, U.K.*). Emphasizing the need to consider all aspects when using biological control in the field, we need to be aware of relationships of pest with crop, pathogen and crop, and so on.

Taking *Spodoptera littorolis ruru* as an example, the slow speed of action of the virus on this crop is not a disadvantage. The cotton leaf can stand a large amount of damage before there is a loss in yield. Looking further, the target is found on the lower leaf surface; here we find protection against the effects of ultraviolet light due to shading and hence ultraviolet light is not such a problem as it would seem. Here also we need to bring in spray application specialists to get the virus to the area we need.

D. BADULSESCU (*Faculty of Agriculture, University of Reading, U.K.*). I think that one of the reasons for the lack of widespread practical application and success of biological control measures is the fact that the projects are directed and run in most cases very far away from the farmer. How can a scientist sitting in central London understand and visualize the real needs of a farmer in Peru or China? I believe that it is important to understand that needs may vary between farmers even if they grow the same crop and have to fight against the same pest. A multidisciplinary approach and a better understanding of farmers' needs are essential.

A. R. JUTSUM (*I.C.I. Plant Protection Division, Jealott's Hill, U.K.*). In response to the request [not printed] for comments on approaches to developing control agents aimed at outlets which are small on a global basis, I would like to describe the process pursued in developing controlled-release pheromone formulations which can be applied by using conventional application equipment. Development of the microcapsule formulation involved collaboration between industry (I.C.I.) and the Tropical Products Institute (T.P.I., now T.D.R.I.) which culminated in the filing of a joint patent. Field trials using the sex pheromone of the adult pink ballworm, *Pectinophora gossypiella* in this formulation were performed by I.C.I. with T.P.I. and the Centre for Overseas Pest Research (now also T.D.R.I.) in conjunction with the Egyptian Government. Highly successful trials were done over a number of seasons which finally led to commercialization of the product 'Pectone'. Thus a market of significant local value, but of limited value globally, was entered through effective collaboration. The formulation is now also being progressed in countries such as Pakistan and Peru.

C. C. PAYNE (*Institute of Horticultural Research, Littlehampton, U.K.*). Factors important in the implementation of practical biological control include:

(*a*) economic necessity: this way is the driving force for the uptake of biological control under glass. Growers have few if any chemical alternatives;

(*b*) political will: creation of a national or international atmosphere for the preferential deployment of biological control, e.g. *Oryctes* virus, and biological control of cassava pests.

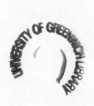